THE DEFINITIVE GUIDE TO THE **OSCE**

The Objective Structured Clinical Examination as a performance assessment

Ronald M. Harden OBE MD FRCP (Glas) FRCPC FRSCEd

Professor Emeritus Medical Education, University of Dundee, UK;
General Secretary, Association for Medical Education in Europe (AMEE)

Pat Lilley BA (Hons)

Operations Director, Association for Medical Education in Europe (AMEE)

Madalena Patrício PhD

Professor of Education, Faculty of Medicine, University of Lisbon, Portugal

Foreword by

Geoff Norman PhD

Professor Emeritus, Department of Clinical Epidemiology and Biostatistics,
McMaster University, Hamilton, Ontario, Canada

ELSEVIER

Edinburgh   London   New York   Oxford   Philadelphia   St Louis   Sydney   Toronto
2016

ELSEVIER

ISBN 978-0-7020-5550-8

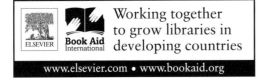

Contents

SECTION A

SECTION B

CONTENTS

Foreword

When Ron Harden approached me to write the foreword, I viewed it as a distinct honour. It was also a bit of a watershed. There was a time, now two decades ago, when I would have been the last person Ron would have asked (and, yes, it's Ron to me, not Professor Harden – entirely as a result of the incident I am about to relate). And if he had asked me to write the foreword, to paraphrase Lyndon Johnson, "If asked, I would not write". But something happened twenty years ago that has a bearing on both the book itself and my authoring of the foreword.

Prior to 1995, Ron and I were at opposite poles. With my PhD in physics, I was a purist ivory-tower researcher whose goal was to advance the science of education. Consequences of my actions were of no consequence. Ron's goals were almost diametrically opposed. He genuinely wanted to improve the education of medical students and physicians, and the more people he could influence, the more impact he could have. I was the elitist; Ron the populist. To me, no standards could be rigorous enough; to Ron, engagement was the issue, and so he would bring in the novices and nurture them to higher standards.

Then, in 1995, we met at a small conference in Islamabad, and ended up in my hotel room – just me, Ronald and a third participant named Johnnie Walker. And we have become good friends and confidants ever since. In hindsight, I began to understand better where he was coming from, and moreover, I began to realize that the inclusiveness of meetings like AMEE and the Ottawa Conference, both of which had a large Harden *imprimatur* (along with Ian Hart, rest in peace, one of the loveliest men ever to grace this planet), served an ulterior motive. By making a conference presentation accessible to almost all, he created a venue where even novices could come and fall under the influence of some of the masters. Moreover, the large number of participants enabled the conference to "buy" top class people as plenary speakers. So my arrogance was misplaced and arguably Ron, with his inclusiveness, has done more to improve the quality of medical education than all of us academics.

At another level, perhaps we were both right. Both of us went on to be awarded the Karolinska Prize, the highest award in medical education research. We have both been widely recognized for our contributions – far more than I (and my wife) could ever have dreamed possible. And despite the fact that our world views remain distinct, each has come to appreciate the contribution of the other.

Back to Ron, and the underlying rationale for this book. Nowhere is his genuine concern more evident than in the development and success of the OSCE. Ron describes the concerns he had about assessment in Chapter 2. Recognizing the failings of the traditional clinical examination, which bore more resemblance to the Spanish Inquisition than anything in education, he devised the OSCE strategy to provide a more equitable test of clinical skills.

However, left unstated in his narrative is just why the OSCE became so popular. (And it is popular. I do a workshop on assessment around the world. I used to ask people if they know what an OSCE is. I don't anymore. Everyone, in every land, knows what OSCE is.) To understand its popularity requires an expanded history lesson.

Back in the early 1970s when I was first hired into medical education, we were all preoccupied with "skills" – problem-solving skills, critical thinking skills, communication skills, physical examination skills, evidence-based medicine skills, etc. I was hired (Why me, Lord? Goodness knows.) to investigate clinical problem-solving skills. We put doctors and students into rooms with simulated patients, videoed them, reviewed their tapes, and pored over the transcripts seeking the mysterious elixir of problem-solving skill. We never found it. Instead what we found, looming large, was "content specificity", as identified by the group at Michigan State (Elstein et al. 1978). In brief, successful problem-solving was dictated as much by the specific knowledge required to solve the problem as by any general intellectual skill. And when we looked at other measures of "problem-solving" we found the same issue. Patient Management Problems or PMPs (McGuire and Babbott 1967) were a written objective case-based test, requiring about 45 minutes per case. For them as well, the correlation of performance measures across problems was 0.1 to 0.3. Since each PMP took about 45 minutes, it was not long before PMPs were dropped from licensing and specialty examinations.

The solution to the psychometric problem was simply one of sampling. To get good measurement required multiple samples rated by multiple observers (and, incidentally, sampling across cases was more important than sampling across raters). The larger issue, as noted by Ron in Chapter 2, was that removing the PMP meant that most examinations were now multiple choice only. While that may be acceptable for a specialty examination where the goal is just precise and valid measurement, it is not acceptable for educational programs because of the potential steering effect (Newble and Jaeger 1983). What was required was something that, on the one hand, efficiently sampled over cases and raters, and on the other, measured actual performance. Enter OSCE! And as they say, the rest is history.

Not surprisingly, though, as an innovation gets disseminated, it also gets diluted and mutated. Strategies like problem-based learning, small group learning, multiple-choice tests – just about everything we do in education – eventually get reborn in so many variations as to be almost unrecognizable. It's not like a drug – there is no equivalent of 300 mg t.i.d. As a result, it is critical to develop standards of best practice, based on evidence. To some degree this is achieved by approaches like Best Evidence Medical Education (another Harden innovation), although the constraints of systematic review methodology limit the usefulness of these reviews as guidelines for educational practice. And that is where this book is an invaluable addition. It pulls together in one place pretty well everything that is known about the OSCE; what works and what doesn't. It is a welcome addition to the bookshelf of any educational leader. Please enjoy!

Geoff Norman
Professor Emeritus, Department of Clinical Epidemiology and
Biostatistics, McMaster University, Hamilton, Ontario, Canada

References

Elstein, A.S., Shulman, L.S., Sprafka, S.A., 1978. Medical Problem Solving: An Analysis of Clinical Reasoning. Harvard University Press, Cambridge MA.

McGuire, C.H., Babbott, D., 1967. Simulation technique in the measurement of clinical problem-solving skills. J. Educ. Meas. 4, 1–10.

Newble, D.I., Jaeger, K., 1983. The effect of assessments and examinations on the learning of medical students. Med. Educ. 17, 165–171.

Preface

The assessment of the competence of a student, trainee or healthcare professional, it can be argued, is the most challenging task facing the teacher or educator today. There are many reasons why it is an important task. The public needs to be reassured that the doctor certified by the medical school as competent to practise has the necessary knowledge, skills and attitudes. In the undergraduate curriculum, the student has to show that he/she has achieved the competencies necessary to move on to the next stage of the curriculum. The junior doctor or trainee has to demonstrate that he/she is qualified to work as a specialist in medicine, surgery, general practice or some other field. Assessment of the learner is a key element in the move to outcome-based or competency-based education, with an answer to the question – has the learner achieved the necessary learning outcomes?

There are other reasons why assessment is important. What we choose to assess is perceived by the learner as an indication of what we value in a training programme, and this impacts directly on the learner's behaviour and study pattern. There is also a new understanding of the relationship between learning and assessment that embraces more than 'assessment *of* learning'. In 'assessment *for* learning', or 'assessment *as* learning', assessment is an integral part of the overall educational programme. So, although this book is about assessment and, indeed, one approach to assessment, it is relevant to everyone who is engaged with curriculum planning, teaching and learning, instructional design, quality assurance and student selection.

Over the years there has been an increasing interest in both the theoretical principles underpinning assessment and the tools used to implement assessment in practice (McGaghie 2013). Whilst much has changed, much has remained the same. Reliability (consistency), validity (measuring what we need to measure) and feasibility or practicality remain key criteria on which an assessment tool can be judged, with the acceptability and impact that the assessment method has on the learner also attracting attention. In the past, much emphasis had been placed on reliability as an assessment matrix and on the assessment of knowledge acquisition. The importance of the validity of an assessment and the need to assess clinical skills and competencies rather than simply knowledge acquisition, however, is now recognised. It was with this in mind that the OSCE was developed as a reliable and valid tool to assess the clinical skills of the learner (Harden et al. 1975). The OSCE has come to dominate performance assessment (Norman 2002) and is recognised as the best method of formally assessing clinical skills (Reznick et al. 1997). The OSCE has proved to be a useful tool for both summative assessment with judgements as to the examinee's competence to practise or move on to the next step of training and for formative assessment with feedback to the examinee. The OSCE has also been used extensively in the evaluation of curricula, courses or teaching methods and is now used also as a tool to select students for admission to medical studies.

A key factor in the acceptance and increasing use made of the OSCE has been its flexibility, with the process being readily adapted to meet local needs, simple or complex, and to assess a range of learning outcomes in different phases of the curriculum. Outcomes assessed include traditional competencies relating to communication and physical examination skills and also competencies attracting attention more recently, including patient safety, professionalism and teamwork. There has been increasing interest, too, in the selection of students for admission to medical studies, and a version of the OSCE – the multiple mini-interview (MMI) approach – has been used for this purpose. For all of these reasons the OSCE and this book have a place in the assessor's toolkit.

When administered well, the OSCE is a powerful and valuable tool to assess a learner's competence in the area tested. Examples can be found where the OSCE is administered in an inappropriate manner and one that does not reflect best practice (Gupta et al. 2010; Huang et al. 2010; Sturpe 2010). This can be a serious problem, particularly when the OSCE is used as a summative assessment to certify that a graduating doctor has the skills necessary to practise or that a trainee is competent to practise as a specialist. The adoption of the approaches presented in the book should ensure that problems are avoided in the implementation of an OSCE and only high-quality OSCEs are used in the assessment of students and trainees.

We have written the book to provide the reader with an easily accessible account of the basic concepts underpinning the OSCE and how an OSCE can be implemented in practice. We thought that the reader might also be interested in the story of how the OSCE was initially developed and introduced as an assessment tool in medicine. The practical guidelines and tips provided are based on the extensive experience that we and others have gained over the past 40 years. You will find in the text, as well as in the case studies, information and ideas about how the OSCE can be used in a wide range of settings and in different professions to assess the expected learning outcomes. In the boxes, you will find personal accounts and anecdotes that illustrate the points made in the text.

We look at the OSCE from the perspectives of the examiner, the student and the patient and address issues, including advance planning, possible venues, the design of stations, alternative approaches to scoring the examinee's performance, the provision of feedback and the evaluation of the OSCE. We also look at how the OSCE can be implemented when the available resources are constrained. The OSCE has not been without its critics, and in Section C of the book we address limitations on the use of the OSCE and common misconceptions. Finally, we look at the continuing development of the OSCE and the changes we might see in the years ahead.

The book will be of interest to teachers or trainers in the healthcare professions working in undergraduate, postgraduate or continuing education. Many teachers, trainers or clinical supervisors will be engaged with an OSCE as an OSCE station developer, an examiner, a curriculum or programme planner, a student/trainee advisor or counsellor or an education researcher. The book should also have a wider appeal outside the healthcare professions and be of value in any context where there is an interest in performance assessment. As demonstrated by the police force in England and Wales, the approach can be readily adapted for use in different situations.

More than 1,800 papers have been published on the OSCE. This book is based on our own personal experience with OSCEs and informed by the work of others from around the world. The case studies included in Section D and referred to throughout the book provide valuable examples of how the OSCE can be implemented in practice in different situations.

It is not our intention to provide a complete systematic review of the published literature on the OSCE. We have studied the publications on the OSCE, however, and have referred to papers where we feel they add to an understanding of the OSCE as it is presented in this book. We refer throughout the text to key papers in the area and to examples that illustrate the different ways in which an OSCE can be employed in practice, highlighting the use of the OSCE in different subjects and professions. There are many more examples of its use that we could have included but have had to omit them because of space constraints.

You may choose to read systematically through the book and address the themes as we have presented them or to dip into the chapters and topics most relevant to your needs. Whatever approach you adopt, we hope that you find the book an interesting read and that it includes ideas that you can employ with advantage in your own setting.

Ronald Harden
Pat Lilley
Madalena Patrício

About the Authors

Ronald M. Harden

Professor Ronald Harden graduated from medical school in Glasgow, Scotland, UK. He completed training and practised as an endocrinologist before moving full time to medical education. He is Professor of Medical Education (Emeritus), University of Dundee, Editor of *Medical Teacher* and General Secretary and Treasurer of the Association for Medical Education in Europe (AMEE).

Professor Harden has pioneered ideas in medical education, including the Objective Structured Clinical Examination (OSCE), which he first described in 1975; has published more than 400 papers in leading journals; is co-editor of *A Practical Guide for Medical Teachers*; and is co-author of *Essential Skills for a Medical Teacher: An introduction to learning and teaching in education*. His contributions to excellence in medical education have attracted numerous international awards, including the Hubbard Award by the National Board of Medical Examiners, USA; an OBE by Her Majesty the Queen for services to medical education, UK; the Karolinska Institute Prize for Research in Medical Education, which recognises high-quality research in medical education; and a Cura Personalis Honour, the highest award given by Georgetown University, Washington, DC, USA.

Pat Lilley

Pat Lilley joined the University of Dundee in 1995 and worked on a range of projects in the Centre for Medical Education. In 1998 she joined the Association for Medical Education in Europe (AMEE) and has been part of its development into a leading healthcare educational association with members in over 90 countries. Now AMEE Operations Director, Pat is closely involved in all of AMEE's projects and initiatives. Since 2006 she has assisted in the development and execution of the AMEE Essential Skills in Medical Education (ESME) face-to-face courses for teachers and is a course tutor for the online ESME Course. Pat is also Managing Editor of AMEE's journal *Medical Teacher*.

Madalena Patrício

Madalena Folque Patrício is Past President of AMEE and an ex officio member of its Executive Committee. She is Chair Elect of the Best Evidence Medical Education (BEME) Collaboration, a member of the Editorial Board of the journal *Medical*

Teacher and external adviser to the World Federation for Medical Education. She is Professor at the Institute of Introduction to Medicine at the Faculty of Medicine of the University of Lisbon and Head of the Lisbon BEME Group at the Center for Evidence Based Medicine (CEMBE), where she coordinates a systematic review on the reliability, validity and feasibility of the Objective Structured Clinical Examination (OSCE). Her special interests are evidence-based teaching, humanization of medicine, community-based teaching, social accountability of medical schools and the Objective Structured Clinical Examination (OSCE). She was awarded the 2013 AMEE Lifetime Achievement Award.

Contributors to Case Studies

Case Study 1: Dundee Medical School – Year 2 OSCE

Rob Jarvis, MA MB ChB MPH FHEA
Academic Mentor (Educational Guidance and Support Tutor), Medical School, University of Dundee, UK

Case Study 2: King Saud bin Abdulaziz University for Health Sciences Cardiovascular System Block Phase 2 OSCE

Tarig Awad Mohamed, BSc (Hons) MSc MHPE
Lecturer, Department of Medical Education, College of Medicine, King Saud bin Abdulaziz University for Health Sciences, Ministry of National Guard Health Affairs, Riyadh, Kingdom of Saudi Arabia

Bashir Hamad, MB BS MD DTPH DCMT DET FRSTM FFSMSB
Professor of Medical Education, College of Medicine, King Saud bin Abdulaziz University for Health Sciences, Ministry of National Guard Health Affairs, Riyadh, Kingdom of Saudi Arabia

Ali I AlHaqwi, MD MRCGP(UK) ABFM MHPE PhD (Med Edu)
Associate Professor, Chairman, Department of Medical Education, College of Medicine, King Saud bin Abdulaziz University for Health Sciences, Ministry of National Guard Health Affairs, Riyadh, Kingdom of Saudi Arabia

Mohi M.A. Magzoub, MBBS MSC PhD MFPHM
Professor of Medical Education, College of Medicine, King Saud bin Abdulaziz University for Health Sciences, Ministry of National Guard Health Affairs, Riyadh, Kingdom of Saudi Arabia

Case Study 3: Manchester Medical School MBChB – Phase 2 Formative OSCE

Alison Quinn, MBBS FRCA FCARCSI PgC Med Edu
Honorary Lecturer, Medical School, University of Manchester, UK

Clare McGovern, FRCA
Consultant Anaesthetist, Medical School, University of Manchester, UK

Emyr Wyn Benbow, BSc MB ChB FRCPath
Senior Lecturer in Pathology, Medical School, University of Manchester, UK

Kamran Khan, MBBS FRCA MMedEd FAcadMed
Consultant Anaesthesiologist, James Paton Memorial Hospital, Gander, NL, Canada

Case Study 4: Monash University Malaysia Formative OSCE

Wee Ming Lau, MD MMed AM Grad Dip FP Derm PG Dip Occ Health GCHE
Senior Lecturer, Jeffrey Cheah School of Medicine and Health Sciences, Monash University Malaysia, Malaysia

Case Study 5: UCL Medical School Final Examinations – Short Station OSCE

Kazuya Iwata, BSc(Hons) MBBS MRCPsych MSc FHEA
Honorary Clinical Lecturer in Medical Education, University College London Medical School, UK

Daniel S. Furmedge, MBBS MRCP(UK) DRCOG MAcadMEd FHEA AKC
Honorary Clinical Lecturer in Medical Education, University College London Medical School, UK

Alison Sturrock, BSc(Hons) MRCP PGCMedEd FHEA
Clinical Senior Lecturer in Medical Education, University College London Medical School, UK

Deborah Gill, MBBS MRCGP MMEd FHEA EdD
Interim Director of University College London Medical School, University College London Medical School, UK

Case Study 6: Culture OSCE for Pediatric Residents

Elizabeth K. Kachur, PhD
Medical Education Consultant – Maimonides Medical Center/Director, Medical Education Development, National & International Consulting, NY, USA

Lisa Altshuler, PhD
Associate Director of Evaluation and Assessment, Program for Medical Education Innovations and Research (PrMeir), New York University School of Medicine, NY, USA

Ingrid Walker-Descartes, MD MPH
Program Director, Pediatrics Residency Training Program, Maimonides Medical Center, NY, USA

Lita Aeder, MD
Director, Board Review Course, Brookdale University Hospital and Medical Center, NY, USA

Members of the Maimonides Pediatrics OSCE Committee

Case Study 7: Medical Council of Canada's Qualifying Examination Part II

Sydney Smee, PhD
Assessment Advisor, Medical Council of Canada (MCC), ON, Canada

Members and Consultants of MCC OSCE Test Committee who are Faculty members of Canadian Medical Schools

Case Study 8: OSCE for Postgraduate Year-1 Resident Physicians – Madigan Army Medical Center

Matthew W. Short, MD FAAFP
Madigan Army Medical Center, WA, USA

Patricia A. Short, MD FACP
Madigan Army Medical Center, WA, USA

Case Study 9: Dundee Undergraduate BSc in Nursing Programme – First-Year OSCE

Arlene Brown, MPhil BSc Nursing PGCert(THE) RGN
Lecturer in Nursing, School of Nursing and Midwifery, University of Dundee, UK

Iain Burns, MSc Nursing BA Business Organisation DipEd DipNurs RGN
Senior Lecturer in Nursing, School of Nursing and Midwifery, University of Dundee, UK

Case Study 10: OSCE in Undergraduate Dentistry

Anthony Damien Walmsley, BDS MSc PhD FDSRCPS
Professor of Restorative Dentistry, School of Dentistry, University of Birmingham, UK

Case Study 11: Diploma in Veterinary Nursing

Martin Barrow, BVM&S
Chair of Governors, Central Qualifications (CQ), Examination Board and Awarding Organisation, UK

Denise Burke
Quality Assurance Manager, Central Qualifications (CQ), Examination Board and Awarding Organisation, UK

Case Study 12: Summative OSCE for a Clinical Pharmacy Course, Malaysia

Ahmed Awaisu, PhD MPharm BPharm
Assistant Professor of Clinical Pharmacy and Practice, College of Pharmacy, Qatar University, Doha, Qatar

Siti Halimah Bux Rahman Bux, BPharm
Senior Academic Fellow and Deputy Dean (Student Affairs), Faculty of Pharmacy, International Islamic University Malaysia, Kuantan, Malaysia

Mohamad Haniki Nik Mohamed, PharmD BPharm
Associate Professor and Deputy Dean (Academic Affairs), Faculty of Pharmacy, International Islamic University Malaysia, Kuantan, Malaysia

Case Study 13: Postgraduate Year 1 – Patient Safety OSCE

Dianne P. Wagner, MD
Professor of Medicine, Associate Dean for College-wide Assessment, College of Human Medicine, Michigan State University, East Lansing, MI, USA

Ruth B. Hoppe, MD
Professor of Medicine, Senior Associate Dean for Academic Affairs Emeritus, College of Human Medicine, Michigan State University, East Lansing, MI, USA

Carol J. Parker, MPH
Executive Director of Academic Affairs, College of Human Medicine, Michigan State University, East Lansing, MI, USA

Case Study 14: Basic Abdominal Ultrasound Course

Matthias Hofer, PD Dr med MPH MME
Arzt für Diagnostische Radiologie, Leiter der AG Medizindidaktik, Studiendekanat, Heinrich-Heine-Universitat Düsseldorf, Germany

Case Study 15: Dundee Medical School Multiple Mini-Interview (MMI)

Adrian Husbands, MSc
Lecturer in Medical Education, School of Medicine, University of Dundee, UK

Jon Dowell, MRCGP MD FHEA
Chair of UK Medical Schools Electives Council, and Admissions Convener, School of Medicine, University of Dundee, UK

Acknowledgements

Over the past 40 years we have benefitted from working with many colleagues in different settings and have gained from them a wealth of experience on the OSCE. We are indebted to those who made possible the early efforts to introduce the OSCE into the medical school assessment programme in Dundee. In particular we would like to thank Sir Alfred Cuschieri, Paul Preece, Robert Wood and James Crooks, who played a leading role in the initial implementation of the OSCE in Dundee. As a senior member of staff in the Dundee Centre for Medical Education, Fergus Gleeson worked on the development of the OSCE and its implementation and co-authored one of the two initial key publications on the topic. We would also like to acknowledge the other members of staff of the Centre for Medical Education who have supported the ongoing work on the OSCE.

Special thanks should go to two medical educators who are, sadly, no longer with us. Ian Hart spent several sabbaticals in Dundee working on the OSCE, amongst other things. As described in the text, Ian made a significant contribution to the dissemination of the OSCE internationally through the Ottawa Conferences, the first of which was held in 1985. Miriam Friedman Ben-David also spent a sabbatical in Dundee, and her contributions to the OSCE and to assessment more widely deserve special mention. We remember both Ian and Miriam with great fondness, and the discipline of medical education is all the richer for their contributions.

On our last count, more than 1,800 papers had been published on the OSCE. We are grateful to everyone who took the time and effort to record their experiences on paper, and we have learned a lot from these reports. In the same way, the OSCE has featured prominently in medical education conferences, and this, too, has provided a powerful learning opportunity for us. We are also grateful for the many invitations we have received to visit other schools to see the OSCE in action in different locations throughout the world.

We are grateful to the students who have given us constructive feedback on the OSCE over the years and hope that all examinees, whatever their stage of training, believe the OSCE contributed to their development as learners, rather than remembering it as a traumatic method of assessment.

The case studies described in Section D, we believe, represent an important part of the book, and we would like specially to thank the contributors who have openly shared their experiences with us.

Finally, we would like to thank everyone who supported us in the preparation of this book, including Cary Dick from AMEE for help with typing and preparation of graphics; Alex Haig and Valerie Harden, who undertook an initial review of the papers published on the OSCE; Jim Glen, who drew the cartoons, which we hope will entertain the reader; Geoff Norman who has written the Foreword; and Laurence Hunter, Carole McMurray and Anne Collett from Elsevier.

Ronald Harden
Pat Lilley
Madalena Patrício

What is an OSCE? 1

An introduction to the OSCE for readers unfamiliar with the concept and, for those already familiar with the OSCE, a more in-depth insight into the characteristics that define the OSCE as an assessment tool.

A definition

This book is about the *Objective Structured Clinical Examination,* or the 'OSCE', the acronym by which the approach has become widely known. The concept is well established in health professions education and the approach is familiar to many teachers. We start, however, by defining an OSCE and outlining the features that set it aside from other assessment tools. It is as Hodges (2003) suggested, *'An examination like no other.'* In short, the OSCE is a performance-based examination in which examinees are observed and scored as they rotate around a series of stations according to a set plan (Figure 1.1). Each station focuses on an element of clinical competence, and the learner's performance with a real patient, a simulated patient (SP), a manikin or patient investigations is assessed by an examiner. An example of a 20-station OSCE is given in Table 1.1.

To understand better what an OSCE is and the features that characterise the approach, it is helpful to look more closely at the elements in the name (Table 1.2).

Objective

The OSCE was introduced, as described in Chapter 2, to replace the traditional clinical examination, which had been demonstrated to be an unreliable form of assessment. Problems with the traditional clinical examination included the small sample of skills assessed and the subjectivity or bias associated with the examiner's rating of the candidate. The OSCE was designed to avoid these problems. It has attracted attention as the 'gold standard' in performance assessment at least in part because of its perceived objectivity. The notion of objectivity is, however, a relative one. Even multiple-choice questions and other so-called objective tests are not as truly objective as their designers may claim. The issues of objectivity and reliability in an OSCE are discussed in more depth in Chapter 3.

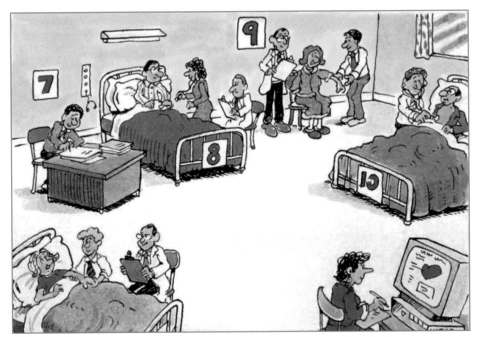

Figure 1.1 In an OSCE students rotate around a series of stations. At each station an element of competence is assessed.

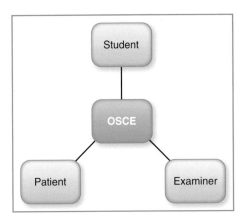

Figure 1.2 In any clinical examination there are three variables: the patient, the examiner and the candidate.

In any clinical examination there are three variables: the patient, the examiner and the candidate (Figure 1.2). In the OSCE, any bias as a result of the patients seen and the examiners is reduced so that the result is a truer assessment of the examinee's clinical competence.

A number of stations

The first key feature of the OSCE is that examinees are assessed over a **number of stations**. The OSCE has sometimes been referred to as a multistation clinical examination. This is very different from the traditional clinical examination with a single long case. In a typical OSCE, there may be 20 or more such stations. The number

Table 1.1 Example of a 20-station OSCE

Station	Description	Patient	Examiner
1	History from a patient with pain in the hip	SP	Yes
2	Questions relating to Station 1	–	–
3	Auscultation of chest in a patient with a murmur	Harvey manikin	Yes
4	Explain insulin administration to a diabetic patient	SP	Yes
5	Examination of neck in a patient with goitre	Real patient	Yes
6	Questions relating to Station 5	–	–
7	Examination of hands in a patient with rheumatoid arthritis	Real patient	Yes
8	Preparation of case notes relating to Station 7	–	–
9	History from a patient with dysuria	SP	Yes
10	Referral letter to hospital for a patient in Station 9	–	–
11	Catheterisation of a patient	Cystoscopy manikin	Yes
12	Interpretation of chest X-ray	X-rays	–
13	Interview with a psychiatric patient	Video recording	–
14	Discuss interview with examiner	–	Yes
15	Questions relating to ward prescription chart	Patient's drug chart	–
16	Questions relating to drug advertisement	Drug advertisement	–
17	Examination of leg for a patient with hemiplegia	Real patient	Yes
18	Questions relating to Station 17	–	–
19	Measurement of blood pressure in a patient with hypertension	Real patient	Yes
20	Questions relating to Station 19	–	–

SP, simulated patient.

Table 1.2 The OSCE

Objective	A number of stations Examinees assessed on the same stations Clear specification of what is assessed A number of examiners Specification of standards required
Structured	OSCE blueprint
Clinical	Students watched performing a clinical task on real and standardised patients

of stations may vary, as described in Chapter 6; this may be as low as 6 or as high as 40. What is known, however, is that the reliability of the examination increases as the number of stations increases. Each domain to be assessed, such as communication skills or physical examination skills, is usually tested at several stations.

To allow a smooth rotation of examinees around the OSCE stations, the time allocated to each station is uniform. In some examinations this may be 5 minutes and in other examinations it may be 15 to 20 minutes. Each examinee starts at a different station and on a given signal at the end of the set time period they move forward to the next station. The exception to this is a *double station* where examinees spend double the amount of time at a station. How this works in practice is described in Chapter 6. Stations can also be arranged as linked stations where the examinee's competence in relation to a patient is assessed over two stations.

Uniform examination

A key feature of an OSCE is that all **examinees are assessed on the same set of stations**. In one circuit of 20 stations, 20 candidates can be assessed in an examination. Where more than 20 candidates have to be assessed, two or more circuits with matched stations can be run in parallel. Alternatively, the same circuit can be repeated sequentially with a further set of candidates examined after the first circuit has been completed (Box 1.1).

Specification of what is assessed

Another key feature of an OSCE is that **what is to be assessed** at each station is agreed upon in advance of the examination. The examinee may be assessed carrying out a practical procedure, such as the measurement of a patient's blood pressure. Decisions need to be taken in advance of the examination as to what is to be assessed at the station (Box 1.2). Should the examinee's attitude and communication with the patient be taken into account or is the assessment to be based only on the examiner's observation of the technical aspect of how the candidate undertakes the procedure? Is the accuracy of the blood pressure measurement arrived at by the examinee and his/her interpretation of the results also to be taken into consideration? What is to be assessed will be reflected in the checklist and rating scale to be used by the examiner at the station, and this is described in Chapter 11.

Box 1.1

When the OSCE was introduced as the final medical examination in Dundee, more than 120 students were examined in one morning. Three circuits, each with 20 stations, were used simultaneously. Stations were identical in terms of the tasks expected of the student and the scoring sheets. Patients or simulated patients (SPs) were carefully matched across different circuits. Following a short break, another group of 60 students was assessed later in the morning on the same three circuits. To ensure that the matched stations were comparable, an analysis of students' performance at each of the matched stations in different circuits was undertaken.

Box 1.2

In a study carried out by RMH and co-workers at Glasgow University, a significant variation was found between the marks awarded by different examiners to students in a traditional clinical examination (Wilson et al. 1969). One of the reasons for the variations was that there had been no decision in advance as to what was to be assessed in the examination. Some examiners took into account the student's dress, how the students presented themselves and their attitudes towards the patient whilst others restricted their assessment of the student to the technique demonstrated by the student.

A number of examiners

During the examination each candidate sees a **number of examiners**. This is a key feature of an OSCE. With a 20-station OSCE there may be 10 examiners or more at one circuit. Each examiner is carefully briefed as to what is expected of them at the station and training is given in advance of the OSCE with regard to what the examiner should be looking for and how the checklist and rating scale should be interpreted. This is discussed further in Chapter 9.

Specification of standards required

The **standard expected** of the examinee in the overall examination and in individual stations is specified. This can be determined by using an established approach to standard setting, as described in Chapter 11. The minimum requirements for a pass can be set and excellence can also be recognised.

Structured

What was assessed in a traditional clinical examination was often opportunistic and depended on the patients available in the hospital or as outpatients. In contrast, a key feature of the OSCE is that what is to be assessed during the examination is carefully planned and agreed upon before the examination is implemented.

OSCE blueprint

A blueprint or a grid for the OSCE is prepared in advance. This outlines the learning outcomes and core tasks to be assessed at each station in the OSCE, for example in the domains of communication skills, physical examination, practical procedures and analysis and reflection. This important feature of an OSCE is discussed further in Chapter 6.

The grid maps on one axis the key learning outcome domains and on the other axis the elements of the course, e.g. the body systems or context in which the learning outcomes are to be assessed. For example, patient education skills may be assessed in the endocrine system with a diabetic patient, history taking in the cardiovascular system in a patient with chest pain, and physical examination in the respiratory system in a patient with asthma (Table 1.3).

Table 1.3 Section of a blueprint showing content of an OSCE as tested at Stations 1, 2, 3, 4, 6, 8, 10 and 12

Learning outcome	Body system				
	CVS	RS	NS	AS	ENDO
History taking	(2) Chest pain			(10) Diarrhoea	
Patient education					(1) Diabetes
Physical examination		(4) Asthma	(6) Hemiplegia		
Practical procedures	(8) BP	(12) FEV			
Problem solving			(3) Headache		

AS, Alimentary system; BP, Blood pressure; CVS, Cardiovascular system; ENDO, Endocrine system; FEV, Forced expiratory volume; NS, Nervous system; RS, Respiratory system.

Box 1.3

A common and important comment from students following an OSCE is that the examination is perceived as 'fair'. One reason for this is that students in general see that the OSCE reflects the teaching and learning programme and the stations overall address the learning outcomes of the course.

What is assessed in the OSCE should reflect the content covered in the teaching and learning programme (Box 1.3). The learning outcomes assessed can be related on a curriculum map to the relevant learning opportunities for the examinee, for example a session in the clinical skills unit, a simulator, a ward-based experience, a video available online or even a lecture.

Clinical

The OSCE is a clinical or performance-based examination. It tests not only what examinees know, but also their clinical skills and how they put their knowledge into practice. Think outside medicine for a moment. If we were to design a test to assess students' ability to tie their shoelaces, it would not be sensible to assess their knowledge relating to the task as shown in Table 1.4, rather than their technical skill. To assess students' competence what we need is to observe their skill as they tie their shoelaces.

Whilst this may seem obvious, all too often in medicine we fall into the trap and rely on testing the students' knowledge with written assessments when what we are interested in is their clinical competence. This represents the bottom of Miller's Pyramid (Miller 1990) at the 'knows' and 'knows how' levels rather than the 'shows

Table 1.4 The assessment of a student's competence in tying shoelaces

Objective: The student should be able to tie his/her shoelaces

Assessment options

- Write short notes on the origin of shoelaces.
- Describe the materials from which shoelaces are made.
- Write an essay to explain how shoelaces are tied.
- Answer an MCQ relating to tying a shoelace.
- Observe an individual tying his/her shoelaces.

how' level, as described in Chapter 5. The OSCE is a performance measure of what the individual would do in a clinical context. Examples of the range of clinical skills that can be assessed in an OSCE are given in Table 1.5.

In an OSCE, it is the examinee's clinical skills and what he/she does when faced with a patient or clinical situation and the competence demonstrated that are assessed – not simply what he/she knows as tested by a written or theoretical question on the subject. It is the application of the knowledge to practice that is assessed in an OSCE.

In 'procedure' stations, examinees are watched and assessed by the examiner as they take a history, examine a patient, or carry out a practical procedure. In a history taking station, for example, the history taking techniques used by the examinees and the questions they ask as well as their approach to the patient are taken into consideration. A 'procedure' station may be followed by a 'question' station, where the examinee is asked about their findings at the previous station and the conclusions they have reached based on their findings. The examinee's response may be in the form of:

- a multiple-choice question (MCQ).

- a short constructed response to a question.

- a note about the patient they have seen – sometimes called a 'post-encounter note'.

- a letter referring the patient for further investigation or treatment; or

- an oral report to an examiner.

In addition to the use of real patients, **simulated or standardised patients** may be used to provide examinees with a standardised experience. This is discussed further in Chapter 8. The emphasis placed on the use of standardised patients varies. In the USA the OSCE is often equated with a standardised patient examination.

Table 1.5 Examples of clinical skills assessed in an OSCE (Harden 1988)

Skill	Action	Example
History taking	History taking from a patient who presents a problem	Abdominal pain
	History taking to elucidate a diagnosis	Hypothyroidism
Patient education	Provision of patient advice	Discharge from hospital following a myocardial infarction
	Educating a patient about management	Use of an inhaler for asthma
	Provision of patient advice about tests and procedures	Endoscopy
Communication	Communication with other members of healthcare teams	Brief to nurse with regard to a terminally ill patient
	Communication with relatives	Informing a wife that her husband has bronchial carcinoma
	Writing a letter	Referral or discharge letter
Physical examination	Physical examination of a system or part of the body	Hands of a patient with rheumatoid arthritis
	Physical examination to follow up a problem	Congestive cardiac failure
	Physical examination to help confirm or to help confirm or refute a diagnosis	Thyrotoxicosis
Diagnostic procedure	Diagnostic procedure	Ophthalmoscopy
Interpretation	Interpretation of findings	Charts, laboratory reports or findings documented in patient's records
Patient management	Patient management	Writing a prescription
Critical appraisal	Critical appraisal	Review of a published article or pharmaceutical advertisement
Problem solving	Problem solving	Approach adopted in a case where a patient complains that her weight as recorded in the hospital was not her correct weight

A flexible format

The OSCE is not a rigid prescription for how a candidate is examined. One is unlikely to see two OSCEs which are identical in the skills tested and the ways in which they are assessed. Within the principles set out above, there is the opportunity to adapt the process to a particular context and to suit the needs associated with:

- a particular discipline or specialty whether this is general practice, surgery or psychiatry.

- a phase of education (undergraduate, postgraduate or continuing education).

- a different educational purpose (summative or formative assessment, etc. as described in Chapter 4); and

- the resources available (number of examiners, patients and accommodation).

Each of the case studies provided in Section D illustrates its own different interpretation of the OSCE concept.

The OSCE and the eight Ps

The features that characterise an OSCE can be highlighted as the 'eight Ps'. At the 5th Ottawa Conference Harden described in a paper, 'The OSCE – a 15 year retrospective', 7 Ps that characterised an OSCE (Harden 1992). An eighth 'P' is added below:

- **Performance assessment:** The OSCE may be identified with a move from theory to practice. Examinees are assessed not just on what they know but also on what they can do.

- **Process and product:** Assessed in the OSCE are the learner's technical skills, for example how they take a history, how a patient is examined or how the learner carries out a practical procedure. The learner's findings, the results and their interpretation can also be assessed.

- **Profile of learner:** The OSCE not only provides a single global rating for the learner but can also present a picture of his/her strengths or weaknesses in the different learning outcome domains.

- **Progress of learner:** The OSCE assesses the learner's progress during the curriculum and training programme and provides feedback to the learner and teacher as to strengths and weaknesses in the learner's performance.

- **Public assessment:** In the OSCE there is transparency as to what is being assessed. A discussion about what is assessed in an OSCE can lead to clarification of aims and expected outcomes relating to the course.

- **Participation of staff:** Examinees are seen by a number of examiners, and staff from different specialties and healthcare professions can participate as examiners in the OSCE.

- **Pressure for change:** The introduction of an OSCE can help to focus the learner's attention on the competencies to be assessed. Poor overall performance in an OSCE by a class of students highlights a need for a change in the education programme or a revision of the assessment.

- **Pre-set standards of competence:** What is expected of a learner and the standard of performance appropriate for a pass in an examination are specified in advance.

OSCE variations

A number of variations to an OSCE have been described, some of which are noted below.

Objective Structured Practical Examination (OSPE)

When first introduced, the OSCE was considered to be essentially a clinical examination for use primarily in the later or clinical years of the course. It was found, however, that the format could be applied also in the early years of the course to assess the student's ability with regard to the application of the basic sciences to clinical medicine. The term 'Objective Structured Practical Examination' was used to refer to this approach (Harden and Cairncross 1980). Malik et al. (1988) described the use of the OSPE to assess students' mastery of physiology in India. Over the years, with the emphasis on vertical integration of clinical skills into the early years of the course, this distinction has become less appropriate, and the term OSCE is now applied to the assessment of students' competence in the early as well as the later years of the course.

Objective Structured Practical Veterinary Examination (OSPVE)

The OSCE approach has been adopted for use in veterinary medicine. May and Head (2010) described its use to assess technical skills required for diagnosis and treatment in veterinary practice. Case Study 11 in Section D provides an example of the use of the OSCE in veterinary nurse education.

Clinical Assessment of Skills and Competencies (CASC)

The examination for membership of the Royal College of Psychiatrists in the UK – the Clinical Assessment of Skills and Competencies (CASC) – uses a 16-station OSCE for the clinical assessment component of the examination in addition to three written papers.

Practical Assessment of Clinical Examination Skills (PACES)

The MRCP(UK) Part 2 Clinical Examination of the Royal College of Physicians in the UK – the Practical Assessment of Clinical Examination Skills (PACES) examination – uses a modified version of the OSCE to test clinical knowledge and skills for entry to higher specialist training (Royal College of Physicians of the United Kingdom 2014).

Objective Structured Assessment of Technical Skill (OSATS)

OSATS was developed at the University of Toronto to meet the need for a reliable and valid method to assess operative technical skills. Surgical trainees perform structured tasks applicable to general surgery in a standardised 'Bench Station' examination consisting of eight 15-minute stations (Martin et al. 1997; Ault et al. 2001). Examinees are rated by direct observation with task-specific checklists and a global rating scale for each station. Feedback is given on performance.

Multiple Mini-Interview (MMI)

The MMI is a type of OSCE used to assess students for admission to medical studies (Eva et al. 2004a,b). Tests of the competencies expected of a student on entry to medical studies are illustrated in Case Study 15 in Section D. The introduction of the MMI is part of the move away from relying solely on academic achievements for selection purposes and is covered in more detail in Chapter 4.

Group Objective Structured Clinical Experience (GOSCE)

The GOSCE assesses individuals in a group setting and was designed for self-assessment and learning in both undergraduate and postgraduate education. It is discussed in more detail in Chapter 6.

Team Objective Structured Clinical Examination (TOSCE)

This has similar characteristics to the GOSCE. Singleton et al. (1999) described a TOSCE for third-year medical students to enhance general practice consultation skills. Teams of five students rotated around five simulated patient (SP) stations as a group, each taking on the role of the General Practitioner, receiving feedback and promoting self-reflection.

Team Observed Structured Clinical Encounter (TOSCE)

This shares the same acronym as the Team Objective Structured Clinical Examination. The McMaster–Ottawa Team Observed Structured Clinical Encounter (TOSCE) is used to assess team skills and interprofessional practice and is discussed further in Chapter 5 when the use of the OSCE to assess team skills is considered.

Team Objective Structured Bedside Assessment (TOSBA)

Miller et al. (2007) described a TOSBA which provides a real patient experience for final-year medical students who spend 30 minutes in groups of five with a hospital in-patient at three different stations, each student performing a clinical task. They receive a grade and individual feedback on performance in a group setting.

Interprofessional Team Objective Structured Clinical Examination (ITOSCE)

The Interprofessional Team Objective Structured Clinical Examination (ITOSCE) was described by Symonds et al. (2003) and Cullen et al. (2003) as a shared learning experience for teams of seven or eight medical students and student midwives, who rotated around five stations presenting different clinical scenarios. Simmons et al.

(2011) described a different initiative, the Interprofessional Objective Structured Clinical Examination (iOSCE) to assess interprofessional competence.

Objective Structured Teaching Encounter (OSTE)

In line with the move to professionalism in medical education and the establishment of faculty development programmes, the OSTE has been introduced as an approach to assessing teaching skills. It has been labelled 'Objective Structured Teaching Encounter', 'Objective Structured Teaching Exercise' and 'Objective Structured Teaching Evaluation'. In the OSTE, students are trained to serve as standardised learners in a scripted teaching scenario, providing feedback to the teacher. Sessions may be observed by faculty members, who also give feedback. This is discussed further in Chapter 4 in the section on faculty development.

Take-home messages

The OSCE is a performance-based examination designed to assess the examinee's clinical competence. Key elements are:

- Examinees rotate around a number of stations with each station focusing on one or more elements of competence.

- The examination is structured and a blueprint or grid is used to plan the learning outcomes to be assessed in the examination.

- Examinees are assessed by a number of examiners who assess their performance at each station using a checklist or rating scale.

- Patients in the examination are real patients, simulated patients or manikins.

- All examinees are assessed in the same set of stations.

A number of variations on the OSCE have been developed for use in specific contexts, including the assessment of surgical skills, interprofessional skills and teaching skills.

 If you have an OSCE in your institution, does it conform to the above features?

The inside story of the development of the OSCE

2

An account of how the OSCE was conceived and developed in the 1970s in response to the assessment challenges facing educators in the healthcare professions.

The traditional clinical examination

The clinical examination conducted at the bedside in the UK was seen traditionally as the keystone, or most important, component in the assessment of a student's competence to qualify and practise as a doctor, or of a trainee doctor's competence to practise as a specialist in their chosen area (Stokes 1974). Whilst a borderline performance in a written examination paper with essays, short answers or multiple-choice questions (MCQs) could be compensated, a clear pass in the clinical component was a requirement in the final qualifying examination in medicine, surgery, obstetrics and gynaecology and paediatrics. A failure to achieve a pass mark in any of these subjects resulted in the student being unable to take up a post as resident house officer and required him or her to re-sit the examination 6 months later. In the traditional clinical examination, the candidate spent about an hour with a single 'long case', and at the end of the time, the student met the examiners and over 20 minutes discussed the details of the history and the physical signs, the possible diagnosis and the management plan. The candidate was then asked to conduct a more focussed examination with several patients for a further 20 minutes and to discuss the findings with the examiners.

Problems with the clinical examination

In the 1960s and 1970s, this established approach to student assessment attracted increasing criticism with regard to its reliability. Moreover, its validity was questioned, as the student was not actively observed communicating with the patient. Stokes, a highly respected clinician and experienced examiner, described the clinical examination as the *'half-hour disaster session'* and the *'sacred cow of British medicine'* (Stokes 1974). He attributed a lack of earlier criticism of the traditional approach to the clinical examination, at least in part, to *'examiners instinctively recognising that this part of the examination provides them with the best chance of preserving the traditional species by making appropriate phenotype judgements'*

(p. 2.3). In the assessment of the student's ability to obtain a relevant history, elicit any abnormal physical signs, synthesise the information into a differential diagnosis, devise an investigation plan and suggest the treatment and prognosis, the examiner also took into account:

'... whether the candidate is clean, gentle, assured or over-confident, talkative or taciturn, whether his hands are more often in his pockets than on the patient's pulse, whether his tie indicates membership of an acceptable club and, in the case of a female, whether she is neatly or ostentatiously clad. Some examiners fail wholly to control the atavistic feelings which come to the surface when confronted with a woman at their mercy, others act out deep-seated Galahad complexes of which they remain blissfully unaware.' (Stokes 1974, p. 2.4)

Stokes also highlighted the 'luck of the draw' nature of the examination with the candidate meeting only one 'long case' and the power that the patient could have over the student by suppressing or providing key information for the student (as illustrated in the 1954 film *Doctor in the House*). As Petrusa (2002) noted:

'The time-honored method of oral examination after a single patient suffers from several measurement shortcomings. Too little sampling, low reliability, partial validity and potential for evaluator bias undermine the oral examination.'

In a World Health Organisation (WHO) publication 'A review of the nature and uses of examinations in medical education' by Charvat et al. (1968, p. 7), it was reported:

'Those responsible for the health services of a country are concerned above all with the quantity and quality of the young physicians who graduate from the medical schools. One of the most effective methods of measuring quality is the evaluation of the students' academic performance by means of examination techniques. The older examination systems suffered from the disadvantages that they were not sufficiently objective and often conditioned the student to memorize only those facts that he believed would best satisfy the examiner.'

In North America, as in the UK, concern was also being expressed about the problems and the unreliability associated with the assessment of the candidate's clinical skills at the bedside. In 1963, the bedside examination was finally abandoned by the National Board of Medical Examiners (Hubbard et al. 1965). In the chapter on the evaluation of clinical competencies in his book *Measuring Medical Education: The Tests and Experience of the National Board of Medical Examiners*, Hubbard (1978) dismisses the use of a bedside clinical examination because of its unreliability. Written, paper-based tests were developed as a substitute to test students' accuracy of observation, their recognition of abnormalities in the pictures of patients and their investigation, clinical reasoning and clinical judgement skills. Graham (1971) working in the New Mexico School of Medicine argued, to no avail, for a systematic evaluation of a student's clinical competence. Decisions about the approach to assessment to be adopted were dictated by the psychometrics, and written examinations in the USA dominated as the tool to assess a student's competence to practise.

Evidence of the unreliability of the clinical examination

Stokes had recognised that in the UK, greater prestige was attached to clinical skills. The General Medical Council, which was responsible for the standard of medical education in the UK, included in its 1967 report the recommendation that the *clinical knowledge and skills* attained by the student should be tested in the final qualifying examinations. The deficiencies in the traditional clinical examinations had become apparent to me (RMH), working as a senior lecturer in the University of Glasgow with responsibility for the organisation of the clinical examinations. With co-workers, I carried out a study in which we explored the reliability (or rather the unreliability) of the marks awarded by clinical examiners (Wilson et al. 1969). Twenty-eight students were assessed independently by two examiners and subsequently by a further 12 examiners, who watched a videotape of the students' performance. The videotape performance was also marked by the two original examiners 2 weeks and 2 months later. As illustrated in Figure 2.1, a wide variation in the marks awarded by the different examiners was noted, with variations between examiners for an individual student as great as 25 marks, the difference between 'excellent' and a 'bad fail', and with all the candidates having a score that varied between examiners by at least 10 marks. It was estimated that to have a 99% chance of scoring a pass mark of 50% in the examination, the student would need to achieve

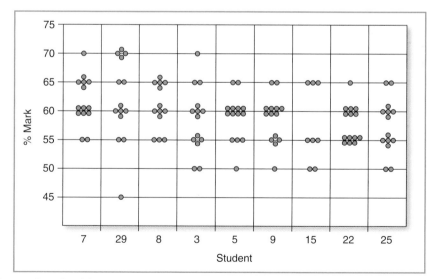

Figure 2.1 A wide variation in the marks awarded by the different examiners was noted, with variations between examiners for an individual student as great as 25 marks. Each dot represents one examiner's score for a student (Wilson et al. 1969).

a mark of 62%. Even the same examiner awarded different scores on repeat marking. This study confirmed for me (RMH) the problems associated with the traditional clinical examination.

The development of the OSCE

It seemed to me (RMH) wrong to follow the American lead and abandon the assessment of clinical skills at the bedside in favour of a written assessment where the emphasis was on a student's knowledge. The ability to answer correctly a set of MCQs was a poor measure of how a student would interact with a patient, take an appropriate history, carry out a relevant examination and come to a management plan in discussion with the patient. What was required was an alternative approach which preserved the key aims of a clinical examination whilst avoiding the problems relating to the traditional approach. In the clinical examination, the three variables are the examinee, the patient and the examiner. The challenge was to find an approach that controlled, as far as possible, the variables of the patient and examiner. What came to be known as the Objective Structured Clinical Examination, or OSCE, was designed with this in mind. The examination was developed with the following features:

- Students should be assessed on a number of patients, and all students should see the same patients. It was important to remove the 'luck of the draw' that characterised the traditional examination.

- A large sample of the required competencies should be assessed to allow a more reliable inference to be made as to the student's competence.

- A combination of real patients and simulated patients should be used to create an authentic assessment.

- To avoid the possibility of examiner bias, with a candidate being examined by a 'hawk' or a 'dove', each student should be assessed by multiple examiners.

- A blueprint for the examination should serve as a basis for the design of the examination, and the competencies to be tested should be agreed upon in advance. Checklists or rating scales should specify the examiners' expectations of the examinee and the learning outcomes to be assessed at each station.

- The approach adopted has to be practical and feasible and capable of adaptation to meet the needs in different contexts and situations.

The outcome was the development of an examination built round a series of stations – initially about 20 – with an aspect of competence assessed at each station, for example history taking in a patient with dyspnoea, examination of the leg in a patient with a hemiplegia or advising a patient on discharge from hospital following admission because of a myocardial infarction. During the examination, the student rotated round the stations spending a standard specified time – initially 5 minutes – at each station. On an agreed audible signal, the student moved to the next station. In this way, 20 students could be assessed simultaneously in one circuit. An examiner stayed at the same station for the duration of the examination. This approach, combining the above features, was subsequently named the *Objective Structured Clinical Examination*, or *OSCE* (Harden et al. 1975; Harden and Gleeson 1979).

Two types of station were included. The first type was a 'procedure' station, where students, watched by an examiner, undertook an activity, e.g. history taking or physical examination. This observation of the student by the examiner was seen as a key feature of the approach. The student's findings and conclusions were also seen as important, and these were assessed at a 'question' station that followed the 'procedure' station. The response of the student was in the form of an MCQ, a constructed response question, or a case history note or a referral letter prepared by the student.

Early work on the OSCE was undertaken in the Department of Medicine in the Western Infirmary at the University of Glasgow. When first introduced in Glasgow, the examination was conducted in a hospital ward and was used as an in-course assessment.

The OSCE as the final qualifying examination

My (RMH) move to Dundee, in 1972, provided an opportunity to develop further the approach and, working with Sir Alfred Cuschieri and James Crooks, to introduce it as part of the final qualifying examination for students, replacing the traditional clinical examination.* Alfred Cuschieri had been recently appointed as Professor of Surgery in Dundee, and he, with his two senior lecturers Robert Wood and Paul Preece, was enthusiastic to replace the traditional final qualifying examination in surgery with an OSCE. In the UK, there is no national examination, and the responsibility for the final examination is left to each school, with external examiners from other schools involved and the process monitored by the General Medical Council. The senior professors in the Faculty of Medicine at Dundee, not unexpectedly, were reluctant to change from the traditional approach to clinical examinations with which they had become familiar. However, the Faculty Board agreed to a pilot study where a final surgery OSCE was run alongside the traditional final surgery examination with students and examiners volunteering to participate in the pilot. This allowed the OSCE to be introduced quickly. All students agreed to take part, and junior and senior members of staff agreed to participate as examiners, some because of their concerns with the traditional clinical examination and others from a curiosity about the new approach.

The result was a major success. The pilot examination proceeded smoothly with no significant problems. Positive feedback was received from students and examiners.

*An interview with RMH discussing the development of the OSCE is available at https://vimeo.com/67224904.

Students noted advantages over the traditional long case, including the wide range of knowledge and skills tested, the provision of a comparable test for all students, a reduction in examiner bias and the opportunity for feedback. Encouraging comments received from students were *'realistic'*, *'helped me to think I was learning to be a doctor'*, *'tested what I had been taught in my clinical attachments'*, *'a fair test'*, *'I liked having a number of examiners'*, *'showed that being a doctor is much more than learning from the books'*, *'to my surprise I enjoyed the experience'*, *'helped me to see gaps in my abilities'*, *'made me think on my feet'*. The advantages as noted by the examiners included the wide range of competencies tested, including the minor specialties, efficient use of the examiner's time and greater reliability compared to the traditional long case (Cuschieri et al. 1979). There was no hesitation on the part of the Faculty Board to formally approve the adoption for subsequent years of the OSCE as the final qualifying examination in surgery. Fifteen years' experience using the surgery OSCE in Dundee was reported by Preece et al. (1992).

The use of the OSCE as the final examination in other disciplines quickly followed the lead given by surgery, and by the 1980s, medicine, therapeutics, obstetrics and gynaecology, and psychiatry had all adopted the OSCE (Peden et al. 1985; Davis 2003). With the introduction in Dundee of an integrated systems-based curriculum, in addition to its use as a final examination, the OSCE was used during Year 2, Year 3 and Year 4 to assess the development in the students of the clinical skills as they related to the cardiovascular, the respiratory and other body systems.

I was joined in Dundee by Fergus Gleeson, a clinician and enthusiastic teacher from Ireland. He contributed to the development of the OSCE and together we co-authored the Association for the Study of Medical Education (ASME) Guide on the OSCE (Harden and Gleeson 1979). The recollections of members of the faculty concerned with the development of the OSCE in Dundee over this period of time are recorded by Brian Hodges (2009) in his book *The Objective Structured Clinical Examination: A Socio-History*. This provides a valuable insight into the development of the OSCE, including how, in the 1970s, the UK and the USA went in different directions in the assessment of students, with examinations in the USA focussing on the use of MCQs.

Dissemination of the OSCE approach

Following its successful adoption in Dundee, the OSCE approach became adopted widely as an examination tool to assess students' clinical competence. Teachers became aware of the approach through the publication of papers on the OSCE and presentations on the subject at meetings and conferences. The staff in Dundee with a commitment to the OSCE who transferred to other schools and the external examiners from other schools who participated in the Dundee initiative made a significant contribution to the spread of the approach to their schools. Ian Hart, a leading Canadian physician with an interest in medical education, spent a sabbatical in Dundee. During this time, he became an important OSCE convert and masterminded the organisation of a conference held in Ottawa in 1985, which had the aim

> **Box 2.1   An ode to clinical assessment**
>
> From Lagos to Sweden
> From McMaster to Dundee
> It seems as if everyone's
> Using an OSCE.
> For Family Practice
> And Obstetrics – Gyn
> Is definitely 'in'.
> Short stations, long stations
> For knowledge, affect, and skills
> Is the OSCE the cure?
> For our measurement ills?
> SAs and PMPs
> MCQs and O-S-C-Es
> Rs and Ps and significant Ts
> Are any letters missing after all these?
> If one more was in it
> The tool kit, I'd buy
> We know all the others
> Now let us hear 'Y'.
>
> Reproduced from Berner, E.S., 1985. Newer developments in assessing clinical competence. Proceedings of the First Ottawa Conference. Heal Publications Ltd.

of sharing across the Atlantic approaches to the assessment of clinical competence, including the OSCE. At the conference in 1985 (Box 2.1), 23 papers described the use in five countries of an OSCE in medicine, physiotherapy and nursing.

The conference proved successful and aroused much interest in the OSCE. Since then, a conference on the theme of assessing competence, now referred to as the Ottawa Conference, has been held biennially (www.ottawaconference.org). The 2012 conference took place in Kuala Lumpur, and in 2014 it returned to its roots in Ottawa. An interesting development presented at the second Ottawa Conference in 1987 was the adoption of the OSCE approach in the UK by the police as a promotion examination to replace a written examination previously used for this purpose. This acknowledged that the general competencies required in the police of observing, examining, communicating, problem solving and investigating – were similar to the general competencies required in medicine. The OSPRE (the Objective Structured Performance Related Exam), as it became known in the police force, featured in an episode of a British television drama *Inspector Morse* (see page 46).

Increasing popularity of the OSCE

Since the OSCE was first described in 1975, the importance of student assessment has become increasingly recognised, as highlighted by Wass et al. (2001):

> *'Assessment drives learning. Many people argue that this statement is incorrect and that the curriculum is the key in any clinical course. In*

reality, students feel overloaded by work and respond by studying only for the parts of the course that are assessed. To promote learning, assessment should be educational and formative – students should learn from tests and receive feedback on which to build their knowledge and skills. Pragmatically, assessment is the most appropriate engine on which to harness the curriculum.'

The need to assess a student's clinical skills was widely recognised, and during the 1980s and 1990s, the OSCE resonated with an increasing number of practitioners around the world as the answer to the challenge of finding a practical solution to the assessment of a student's clinical competence. Its allure in offering something different from the MCQ-based examination in an authentic voice was appreciated. In South Africa, for example, at least 20 departments in six of the seven South African Medical Schools had implemented an OSCE into their school in the 2 years to 1983 (Lazarus and Harden 1985). The OSCE was seen as a factor that *'enhanced a paradigm shift from the assessment of knowledge to the assessment of physicians' performance'* (Friedman Ben-David 2000a). As Hodges (2003) noted, *'Because of the intense focus on performance, OSCEs have had a powerful influence on doctor training and practice.'*

Evidence for the growing interest in the OSCE is the increase in the number of papers published each year since 1975. The number of papers retrieved through PubMed is illustrated in Figure 2.2. This is an underestimate of the number of papers published. For example, in 1998, 28 papers were noted in PubMed, but 55 references could be found with a more detailed search of the literature, with an additional 70 papers published in the grey literature. Since 2011, in excess of 400 papers have been published on the topic – almost one new paper every 3 days (Figure 2.2)! The figures also underestimate the use made of the approach, as not all schools adopting the technique have published their experiences. In the chapter that follows, the uses made of the OSCE since its inception are illustrated in dif-

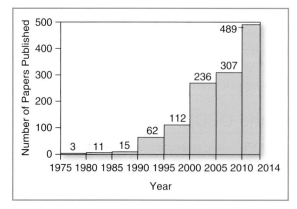

Figure 2.2 The increasing popularity of the OSCE is shown. The number of papers listed in PubMed (http://www.ncbi.nlm.nih.gov/pubmed) on the topic is an indicator.

ferent countries, in different subjects, in different professions and for different purposes.

Regional variations

Whilst the basic principles remained the same, fundamental variations appeared in different countries. In most countries, patients were represented by both real patients and simulated or standardised patients (Harden and Gleeson 1979). As described by Hodges (2009), in the USA the OSCE became identified widely as a standardised patient examination. This is discussed further in Chapter 8. Regional variations also appeared as to who should observe and rate the students' performance in the OSCE – a clinician or trained standardised patient – and this is discussed further in Chapter 9.

Why the OSCE has been adopted widely

How education ideas and results of research are adopted in teaching practice was examined by Schneider (2014). Using examples, Schneider showed how penetration of an innovation into the world of practice is determined less by scholarly merit of the innovation than by its particular set of traits. The examples he studied were Bloom's taxonomy, Howard Gardner's theory of multiple intelligences, the project method and Direct Instruction. He found common to all of the developments were four characteristics crucial to the adoption of the initiative by teachers – perceived significance, philosophical compatibility, occupational realism and inference portability.

The same analysis when applied to the OSCE can explain its wide adoption as an assessment tool. The first characteristic is perceived significance. Schneider argues that ideas that are adopted stand out not because they *are* but rather because they *seem* significant. The OSCE was seen by teachers as addressing an important problem – the assessment of a learner's clinical competence. Schneider's second characteristic was philosophical compatibility. He argued that for education research to gain traction in practice, teachers must view it as reasonable and appropriate for use. Research must not be perceived as the work of outsiders and must not clash with teachers' values and commitments. In the case of the OSCE, clinical teachers and examiners could easily identify with the approach and the principles underpinning it. Schneider's third crucial characteristic was occupational realism. Ideas must be practical and easy to put into immediate use. This was certainly true of the OSCE. Its application in practice required neither extensive training nor the overhaul of existing practices. The fourth characteristic described by Schneider was transportability. He argues that for an educational approach to be widely adopted it should have simple principles that can be explained easily to a busy colleague and can be adapted for use in different situations relatively easily. The OSCE is a user-friendly tool and, as shown in this book, can be adapted for use in many different contexts.

2

Take-home messages

The OSCE was introduced in the 1970s as a tool to assess a student's clinical competence. It was recognised that:

- How a student is assessed is key to the success of an education programme.

- The reliability (consistency) of an assessment tool is important and so also is its validity – is it measuring what we want it to measure? It is essential to have an assessment tool that tests not only knowledge but also the clinical competence of the student.

- The OSCE was developed as a valid, reliable and practical approach to assessing a student's clinical competence.

- The OSCE has been widely adopted worldwide, partly because of its perceived significance, philosophical compatibility, occupational realism and transportability.

How has an OSCE been promoted in your institution?

The OSCE as the gold standard for performance assessment

3

The OSCE with its multiple samples of performance has come to dominate performance assessment and merits a place in every assessor's toolkit.

The gold standard

Over the last 40 years, the OSCE has been widely adopted as the recommended approach to the assessment of clinical competence in different phases of education, in different specialties and in different parts of the world. Indeed, it has been recognised as the gold standard for performance assessment (Sloan et al. 1995; Medical Council of Canada 2011; Humphrey-Murto et al. 2013), and its impact on education has been immense.

In this chapter, we examine the characteristics of a 'good' assessment and how the OSCE matches each of these features. Some of the concepts were introduced in Chapter 1.

Characteristics of a good assessment

A decade ago the established criteria for a good assessment emphasised:

- Reliability – was it consistent?

- Validity – did it measure what should be measured?

- Feasibility – was it practical?

Today an assessment method is also judged on its educational qualities:

- What impact does it have on the students' learning and on the curriculum?

- Is it perceived as fair, and is it acceptable to staff and students?

- Is the approach flexible, and can it be adapted to local needs?

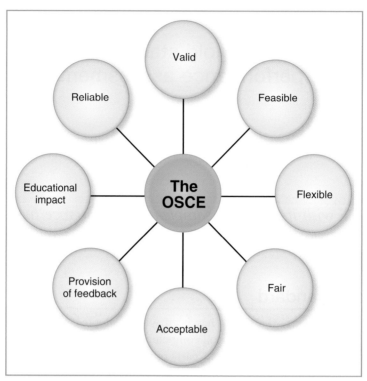

Figure 3.1 **The OSCE is the gold standard for performance assessment.**

- Is it cost effective?

- Can it be used to provide students with feedback as to their strengths and weaknesses?

This expanded view of what should be looked for in an assessment tool, as summarised in Figure 3.1, has been highlighted by van der Vleuten (1996), Norcini et al. (2011), the General Medical Council (2011) and others.

Reliability and the OSCE

The *reliability* of an assessment is the extent to which the results are considered consistent, dependable and free from error. The reliability of the OSCE has been extensively studied and well established (Walters et al. 2005; Pell et al. 2010; Boursicot et al. 2014). Measures used to assess the reliability of the OSCE are discussed in Chapter 14.

The OSCE was initially introduced, as described in Chapter 2, as a response to the problem of poor reliability in the traditional clinical examination. Features of the OSCE contributing to its greater reliability include:

- Students rotate around a series of stations, where multiple samples of competence are assessed.

- Every student is assessed on the same competencies.

- Each student is seen by a number of trained examiners, who observe the students' performances at the stations.

- What is tested in the examination is defined in advance, and this is reflected in the scoring sheet for each station.

- Simulated patients (SPs), when used, present a standardised patient simulation.

Validity and the OSCE

For an examination to be valid, the content and form of the assessment needs to be aligned with the purpose of the examination and the desired learning outcomes. The examination is valid if it measures what it is intended to measure. To be valid, the test needs to assess the learning outcome domains as defined in the curriculum and to do this through a realistic test. The sample tested in the examination should be representative of the learning outcome domains. This is illustrated in Figure 14.1, p. 175.

The OSCE assesses student competence at a higher level than the 'knows' and 'knows how' levels in the Miller Pyramid (Miller 1990) and requires the student or trainee to 'show how' and demonstrate their competence in practice. It is what is described as a performance test and as such is part of the movement to more authentic assessment.

Validity in the OSCE is promoted by:

- The use of a blueprint to structure the examination. This relates what is assessed at the stations to the course learning outcomes and the body systems or other course framework. An example is given in Table 1.3, p. 6.

- The observation by the examiner of examinees in a realistic setting performing a clinical task, such as communicating with a patient, examining a patient or carrying out a procedure.

- The assessment of both the examinee's technique and approach to the patient as well as the examinee's findings and conclusions.

The OSCE was introduced in the 1970s at a time when there was a risk that validity was being sacrificed in response to pressures for greater reliability (Figure 3.2). In the OSCE, much of the focus was on communication skills, physical examination,

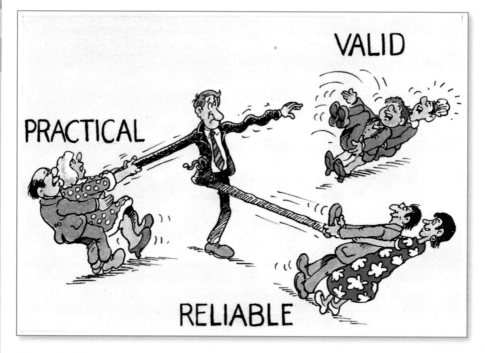

Figure 3.2 In an assessment instrument, validity should not be sacrificed for reliability and feasibility.

practical procedures and data interpretation. Learning outcomes reflecting current medical practice now addressed in an OSCE include professionalism, patient safety and interprofessional skills.

Validity has been widely acclaimed as a feature of the OSCE and almost certainly has been an important reason for its wide adoption. At the University of the West Indies (Jamaica), for example, students considered that the OSCE in Paediatrics provided a true measure of their essential clinical skills (Pierre et al. 2004); and with regard to the OSCE implemented at the University of Sherbrooke Department of Gynaecology and Obstetrics, teachers and students agreed that content validity of the OSCE was high (Grand'Maison et al. 1985).

Feasibility and the OSCE

Feasibility can be defined as the degree of practicality of the assessment instrument. Feasibility can be looked at from:

- A technical perspective: Are the necessary elements/conditions present to conduct an examination?

- An economic perspective: Can the costs of running an OSCE be met?

Evidence from more than 1600 papers published on the OSCE demonstrates the feasibility of the approach in a wide range of situations (Patricio et al. 2013). No record was reported of a situation where the OSCE was found not to be a feasible approach to the assessment of a student's or trainee's clinical competence. It has to be accepted, however, that publication bias may have prevented the report of unsuccessful attempts to administer an OSCE.

The OSCE can be adapted for use in different contexts through the use of various formats, as described in Chapters 4 and 6. The OSCE has been used:

- in geographical locations around the world.

- with a range of professions and specialties.

- at different stages of education, including undergraduate, postgraduate and continuing education.

- for educational purposes including formative or summative assessment of a student/trainee and evaluation of a course.

- with the numbers of students/trainees assessed from fewer than 10 to more than 1000.

- to assess different learning outcome domains; and

- where the clinical encounter is focussed on real patients or SPs.

Concerns have been expressed as to the cost of administering an OSCE. In considering whether an approach justifies the associated costs, Kenkel et al. (2004) argued that the justification of an implementation decision must be related to the likelihood of success of the initiative. The likely benefits resulting from an OSCE are many, and the benefits greatly outweigh the costs, as described in Chapters 15 and 17. The use of the OSCE is feasible even in situations where resources are limited, and this is discussed in Chapter 15.

Flexibility and the OSCE

The *flexibility* of an examination approach is the extent to which it can be adapted in different situations. The flexibility of the OSCE is another important reason why the approach has been widely adopted in different contexts (Chapter 4).

As demonstrated in the case studies in Section D and as described in Chapter 6, teachers/trainers can adapt the OSCE approach to suit their own needs in terms of:

- the numbers and duration of stations and the length of the examination.

- the role of examiners and their briefing and training.

- the role of patients, including real patients, SPs and manikins.

- the tasks assessed at each station and the format of the required response from examinees.

- the use of paper or electronic recording of examiners' scores and examinees' responses.

- the examination venue; and

- the feedback given to examinees.

Fairness and the OSCE

Fairness is the quality of making judgements that are free from bias and discrimination. Fairness requires conformity with a set of rules and standards.

A problem with the traditional approach to clinical assessment, as described by Stokes (1974) in Chapter 2, was that it was not fair due to examiner bias and the fact that the 'long case' examination was conducted on a single patient. The OSCE can be described as a 'fair examination', and contributing to fairness of the OSCE are:

- All examinees have a number of tasks to perform, and these are the same for all students.

- Examinees are assessed by a number of examiners who are briefed in advance and score the examinee's performance on an agreed checklist and ratings scale.

- SPs give a standardised presentation and are selected by gender, age and ethnic background.

- The rules for the OSCE are decided in advance with regard to the format, scoring approach and the standard setting procedure to be adopted.

- What is assessed in the OSCE is closely matched with the curriculum and the expected learning outcomes.

Fairness was implicit in Newble et al.'s (1994) description of the OSCE: *'It clarifies the purpose of the exam, it defines what is to be tested, it selects appropriate tasks, it addresses practical and technical issues of administration/scoring and it sets standards for performance.'* Fairness is perceived by students and teachers as an important characteristic of the OSCE (Box 3.1). In the adoption of the OSCE by the police in the UK (p. 46), fairness was seen as an important factor (Box 3.2).

Box 3.1 The OSCE as a 'fair' examination

A survey of students and examiners in a final-year OSCE at the University of Adelaide, reported a *'remarkable level of acceptance and support by both students and examiners. This positive reaction has been maintained over the 8-year period. The main reasons seem to be its perceived relevance and fairness'* (Newble 1988).

Students participating in an OSCE at the University of Texas Medical School Branch at Galveston to evaluate skills on data gathering and synthesis, oral presentation, differential diagnosis, problem solving and patient interaction, perceived the OSCE as *'a fair exam appropriated to assess students' skills'* (Ainsworth et al. 1995).

Students participating in a multimodality objective structured clinical examination (OSCE) in undergraduate psychiatry consistently appraised the OSCE as a *'fair assessment, as it reflects their course and curriculum, being well organized and clinically relevant'* (Walters et al. 2005).

The impact on study behaviours of an OSCE was investigated by looking at how fifth-year medical students identify what to learn for a summative OSCE. Students perceived the OSCE as *'fair and appropriate in assessing clinical ability'* (Rudland et al. 2008).

Box 3.2 The OSPRE as a 'fair' examination

The OSPRE (Objective Structured Performance Related Examination) was introduced as the promotion examination by the Police Training Council for England and Wales (1987). The following were identified as attractive features of the OSCE approach:

- *Predictive validity* – research shows that those who pass OSPRE Part II go on to perform successfully in the next rank.
- *Reliability* – all candidates go through the same exercises and are assessed against the same set of performance criteria by highly trained assessors.
- *Fairness* – the whole examination process is developed in close consultation with many representative groups and is monitored at each stage by Equal Opportunities/ Community & Race Relations advisors and key stakeholders.
- *Marking process* – OSPRE uses well-established techniques to identify better candidates and provides both candidates and their parent organisations with feedback on performance across each exercise and each competency.

Acceptability and the OSCE

The Consensus Report from the 2010 Ottawa Conference (Norcini et al. 2011) highlighted an examination was acceptable when stakeholders find the process and results to be credible. According to the GMC Criteria for Assessment (General Medical Council 2011), the *acceptability* of an assessment tool relates to two important dimensions, namely the relevance of the examination and the satisfaction of stakeholders. Boursicot et al. (2014) noted, *'The increased reliability of the OSCE format over other formats of clinical testing and its perceived fairness by candidates has helped to engender the widespread acceptability of OSCEs among test takers and testing bodies.'* The increasing use that has been made of the OSCE for different purposes around the world is testimony to its acceptability (Figure 4.2, p. 47).

Students find the examination acceptable because of its perceived fairness, in particular the sample of competencies assessed, the number of examiners and the transparency of the process. Students value the experience not only as an assessment of their competence but also as a valuable form of feedback. Teachers find the approach acceptable, in particular the authentic nature of the assessment and its validity. Comments from staff and students supporting the approach when it was first introduced in Dundee are reported in Chapter 2. When compared with other assessment formats the OSCE approach is almost universally reported as being preferable. Students and examiners have a remarkable degree of confidence in the OSCE as a fair examination in contrast with ward ratings (Newble 1988).

In an OSCE implemented in Paediatrics at the University of the West Indies (Jamaica), the students saw the OSCE as the fairest examination when compared to other methods (Pierre et al. 2004). McFaul and Howie (1993) reported that students, after their first experience with the OSCE, considered it a fairer examination, and they preferred the OSCE when compared to the traditional 'long case' examination. Examiners considered the OSCE a major improvement on traditional methods with many advantages, including the range of skills and knowledge tested and standardisation of testing.

Feedback and the OSCE

The provision of *feedback* to a learner about their clinical competence, including their strengths and weaknesses, is an important attribute of an assessment tool, particularly, but not exclusively, when the assessment is formative. The provision of feedback to students both during and following the examination is a powerful element in the OSCE. This is discussed further in Chapter 12.

The OSCE and educational impact

It is a well-recognised phenomenon that students focus their attention on assessments rather than on the learning objectives of the course (Boursicot et al. 2014). *Educational impact* is now recognised as one of the most valuable characteristics of any assessment tool (van der Vleuten 1996; Roediger et al. 2011; McDaniel et al. 2011). The assessment can steer and influence the students' learning in a desirable or undesirable way. It can influence the curriculum and what is taught (Figure 3.3). Sometimes referred to as *consequential validity*, assessment can help or hinder learning. An assessment should have, as described by the General Medical Council (2011), a catalytic effect by enhancing and supporting the educational programme.

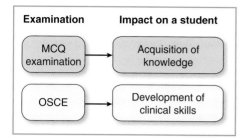

Figure 3.3 The impact of an assessment.

Box 3.3

Concern was expressed in the Dundee Medical School that students were not paying sufficient attention to Ear, Nose and Throat (ENT), which was seen as an important subject, particularly in general practice. Time specifically allocated in the curriculum to an ENT clerkship and the introduction of a new problem-based learning course made little difference. Students recognised that they were not examined on the subject in the formal clinical assessment. The answer was to incorporate an ENT station into the final qualifying OSCE, where every student met an ENT examiner. This brought about a significant change in students' attitude to the subject. What was examined was recognised by the students as important.

The impact of the OSCE and the effect it has on learning is well documented. The examination motivates a student to acquire necessary clinical skills and creates an environment which favours this. As a diagnostic tool, the OSCE can identify weaknesses in both the student and in the curriculum, both of which can be remedied. The increasingly close relationship between the OSCE and the curriculum and the concept of assessment *for* learning and assessment *as* learning (Earl and Katz 2006; Schuwirth and van der Vleuten 2011) is explored further in Chapter 17. Experience has shown that introducing an OSCE can increase students' attention to their clinical experience (Newble and Jaeger 1983; Newble 1988). Testing clinical skills leads students to seek opportunities to practise these skills (Box 3.3).

What an educational assessment must do

The Gordon Commission on the Future of Assessment explored the features required of an assessment programme if it is to remain relevant to the changing educational needs (Bennett 2013). These are described in Box 3.4. Many of these aspirations are addressed in the criteria for a good assessment, as described above, and are met by the use of the OSCE as an assessment tool.

How an OSCE meets the features of a good assessment tool is also highlighted by Salvatori and Brown (1995) (Box 3.5).

Box 3.4 What educational assessment must do

Bennett (2013) described in the Gordon Commission Report what we should look for in the future in an assessment instrument:

- Provide meaningful information
- Satisfy multiple purposes
- Use modern conceptions of competency as a design basis
- Align test and task designs, scoring and interpretation with those modern conceptions
- Adopt modern methods for designing and interpreting complex assessments
- Account for context
- Design for fairness and accessibility
- Design for positive impact
- Design for engagement
- Incorporate information from multiple sources
- Respect privacy
- Gather and share validity evidence
- Use technology to achieve substantive goals

Box 3.5 Advantages of an OSCE (Salvatori and Brown 1995)

1. Face validity (i.e. seductive appeal of the reality of the clinical setting).
2. A wide range of skills for a large number of students can be evaluated in a relatively short period of time.
3. Pre-set standards of competence can be established using an objective checklist format.
4. Patient and examiner variability are reduced.
5. The format allows for immediate and meaningful feedback for students.
6. A bank of OSCE stations can be developed which serves to reduce preparation time.
7. Can be used for formative and summative purposes.
8. The format is flexible (e.g. number of stations, duration of stations, parallel circuits, mix of examiner and marker stations, range of competencies to be tested).
9. Student performance may indicate deficits in the skills training curriculum.
10. Can be used to evaluate performance at all levels of professional education (undergraduate, graduate, continuing education, licensure, certification, etc.).

Take-home messages

The OSCE is the gold standard for performance assessment:

- The OSCE is a reliable assessment tool – it provides consistent results.

- The OSCE is a valid assessment tool – it measures what should be measured in terms of clinical competence.

- The OSCE is a feasible tool which can be used to assess learners in a range of situations.

- The OSCE is a flexible tool which can be adapted to local needs.

- The OSCE is perceived as being fair by both students and examiners.

- Both students and staff find the OSCE an acceptable tool to assess clinical competence.

- Feedback to students is a powerful feature of the OSCE.

- Importantly, the OSCE has an impact on student learning and the curriculum.

Does the OSCE as implemented by you meet these criteria?

How the OSCE can contribute to the education programme

4

The OSCE can be adopted as an assessment tool in any situation or phase of education where an assessment of the learner's clinical or practical skills is important.

Uses of the OSCE

The OSCE has an important role to play in an education programme. As an assessment tool it serves a number of different functions and can be used in a wide range of contexts (Figure 4.1). It can be used to certify a student's or trainee's clinical competence and can contribute to a teaching and learning programme by influencing the student's learning and by guiding and providing feedback to the learner. Many competencies and learning outcomes can be assessed in an OSCE, including skills in communication, physical examination, practical procedures, problem solving, health promotion, attitudes, ethics and teamwork. These are discussed further in Chapter 5.

Nevo (2006) proposed a distinction between the primary and secondary functions of a student evaluation. In its primary use, the student is the object of the evaluation which has a diagnostic or certifying function. In a secondary use, the education programme, rather than the student, is the object of the evaluation. The primary aim of the OSCE is the evaluation of the student. The OSCE also serves as a useful tool for evaluating a curriculum or a new approach to teaching and learning and in so doing can serve as a tool for research in medical education.

The OSCE can be used on a small scale at the level of an individual course or department or on a larger scale as a final medical school or national qualifying examination or as a postgraduate specialty examination.

Evaluating the learner

The OSCE was initially introduced as an instrument to evaluate students' clinical competence. This can be looked at from a number of perspectives, as discussed below.

35

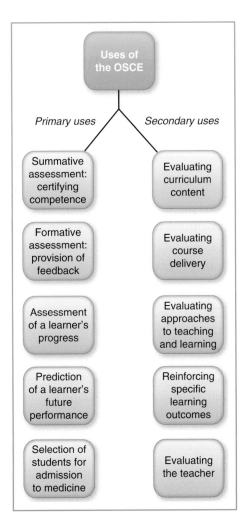

Figure 4.1 Uses of the OSCE.

Summative assessment

The OSCE can be used as a high-stakes barrier examination (summative examination) designed to certify that students have achieved the level of competence necessary to pass from one phase of the undergraduate programme to the next phase. Students may have to demonstrate, for example, that they have mastered the basic clinical skills before progressing to the clerkship year as illustrated in both Case Studies 1 and 2. On completion of the basic undergraduate training programme, students may be assessed in an OSCE as to whether they have the clinical skills necessary to practise as healthcare professionals. An example is given in Case Study 5.

In 2004, the United States Medical Licensing Examination (USMLE®) adopted the Clinical Skills Assessment Program previously developed by the Educational

Commission for Foreign Medical Graduates (ECFMG®) for their Step 2 Examination involving 12 standardised patient encounters, each lasting 15 minutes, followed by 10 minutes to write a note. More than 35,000 examinees are tested each year. A final summative examination incorporating an OSCE is common in many medical schools around the world (Grand'Maison et al. 1996; Boulet et al. 2009; Kim 2010). In the USA, Barzansky and Etzel reported that 101 out of 130 Liaison Committee on Medical Education–accredited schools used a final comprehensive OSCE and OSCEs in one or more clerkships in the 2009–10 academic year (Barzansky and Etzel 2011).

In postgraduate training, the OSCE is used to certify that the trainee doctor has completed, to the specified standard, a period of general or specialist training (Reznick et al. 1993a). Examples of the use of the OSCE as summative examination include the Medical Council of Canada Part II examination (Case Study 7) and the examination for membership of the Royal Colleges in the UK, including the Royal College of Paediatrics and Child Health (Webb et al. 2012). The MRCP(UK) Part 2 Clinical Examination of the Royal College of Physicians in the UK – the Practical Assessment of Clinical Examination Skills (PACES) examination – uses a modified version of the OSCE to test clinical knowledge and skills for entry to higher specialist training (Royal College of Physicians of the United Kingdom 2014).

Formative or diagnostic assessment

An attractive feature of the OSCE is that detailed feedback can be given to the learner about areas where they have achieved the standard necessary and areas where further study is required. A learner may demonstrate mastery of the required skills of physical examination and in practical procedures at the appropriate level whilst remaining deficient with regard to communication skills. Poorly performing students can be identified and appropriate remediation offered (Pell et al. 2012). The formative role of the OSCE and the different approaches to the provision of feedback to the learner are discussed in more detail in Chapter 12.

In practice, many OSCEs fulfil both summative and formative functions, as shown in Case Studies 1 and 14.

Assessment of the learner's progress

An OSCE may be administered at different times during the curriculum to assess and monitor a student's progress and to provide personalised guidance to the student about their progress. Stations are designed recognising the expected learning outcomes of the specific stage of the curriculum. Communication skills stations, for example, may be developed to assess the increasing level of competence expected in a student from basic communication skills in first-year students to more complex skills, such as breaking bad news, in graduating students and other skills, such as communicating about errors in practice and dealing with the difficult patient, in postgraduate trainees. At the University of Hertfordshire School of Pharmacy, students complete a 15-station OSCE administered in all 4 years of the programme.

Each 5-minute station assesses a distinct learning outcome and the complexity and content of the assessment reflects the year of the student's study (Kirton and Kravitz 2011).

A learner's progress can be assessed in OSCEs on four progression dimensions (Harden 2007):

- *Increased breadth of competence* – At the history taking station, for example, the problems addressed may be extended from the cardiovascular and respiratory systems to other body systems. At the OSCE station on cardiac auscultation, students may be assessed on different cardiac murmurs.

- *Increased difficulty* – At the history taking station, the patient may be programmed to be more aggressive. The task at the communication station may be a more difficult one (e.g. breaking bad news). The cardiac murmur presented at the auscultation station may be less typical and more difficult to interpret.

- *Increased utility* and application to practice – Students demonstrate their skills in a situation more closely resembling clinical practice. At an OSCE station on catheterisation, for example, students will be expected to be assessed on their communication skills as well as their procedural skills. This is discussed in the section on hybrid simulators in Chapter 8.

- *Increased proficiency* – Students may demonstrate in the OSCE increased proficiency through a more effective and efficient performance with less time required to complete a task at a station and a higher standard expected.

Progress tests that use multiple-choice questions to assess students' knowledge acquisition and understanding over time have been described (Freeman et al. 2010; Friedman Ben-David et al. 2001b). On a yearly or twice-yearly basis, students in every year of the course are given a written examination paper that comprises the same questions. Students are expected to increase their performance on the questions as they progress through the curriculum. Greater use can be made of the OSCE as a progress test to assess a student's progression not only with knowledge and understanding but also with regard to clinical and practical skills.

The potential of the OSCE as a progress test to assess clinical skills in postgraduate education has also been demonstrated (Pugh et al. 2014). Ten stations, each of 9 minutes' duration, were used to assess ethics, communication, procedural, oral and physical examination skills. As expected, senior residents scored higher than junior residents.

Predicting a learner's future performance

The OSCE can be used to predict the learner's future performance in practice. It provides a more valid assessment of the different clinical domains than a traditional final examination and predicts better clinical performance, for example, of junior doctors after graduation (Probert et al. 2003). Performance in an OSCE early in a clinical course was found by Martin and Jolly (2002) to strongly predict later clinical performance. Students in the lowest three deciles of OSCE performance were six times more likely to fail another clinical examination.

Wallenstein et al. (2010) found that a five-station OSCE administered early in residents' training predicted the trainees' future overall performance and their performance in some specific core competencies, particularly patient care, medical knowledge and practice-based learning and improvement. Poor initial performance can be used to alert the residents and their supervisors to remedial action that may need to be taken.

In dentistry, Graham et al. (2013) looked at the transition from pre-clinical to clinical education and administered a 35-station OSCE with the aim of assessing preparedness for practice of students embarking on their first clinical year. Moderately high correlations were found between performance on the pre-clinical OSCE and performance during the first year of clinical training. The OSCE results were of value in that they provided an early indication of students who may find the clinical year challenging and also identified high performers who should be stimulated and challenged further.

Selecting students for admission to medical studies

In recent years, increasing attention has been paid to methods used to select students for admission to medical studies. Traditionally, emphasis has been placed on academic ability and achievement. It is now recognised that academic qualities on their own do not necessarily identify those students who have the attributes required to serve as doctors and who will meet the needs of the community they will serve in the future. Interpersonal skills, problem solving, motivation, empathy, creativity and an ethical stance are necessary qualities alongside academic ability. Traditional admission tools, including the personal interview, measures of academic achievement, references and personal statements, have proved unreliable in terms of assessing for non-cognitive skills (Kreiter et al. 2004; Turner and Nicholson 2011).

A modified version of an OSCE – a Multiple Mini-Interview (MMI) – has been designed to assess a broader range of attributes deemed to be relevant in the future doctor (Eva et al. 2004a,b). Applicants rotate around a series of stations designed to test both cognitive and non-cognitive skills, including critical thinking, ethical decision-making and communication skills. Imaginative and challenging stations have been developed for this purpose. An example of stations in an MMI introduced at the University of Dundee Medical School is given in Case Study 15.

There is now a significant body of evidence in support of the MMI as a method of selecting medical students. It has been shown to be feasible and reliable and to have predictive validity (Eva et al. 2004a; Lemay et al. 2007) and can predict performance during clerkship and on the Canadian national licensing examinations (Reiter et al.

2007). The MMI over a 2-year period was the most consistent predictor of success in medical school examinations at the University of Dundee Medical School (Husbands and Dowell 2013). A systematic review of the use of the MMI found it to be valid, reliable and feasible as a selection tool (Pau et al. 2013).

Evaluating the curriculum

The OSCE can be used to evaluate the content of a curriculum or course; education strategies, such as community-based education; new teaching methods, such as simulation; and an education instrument, such as the explanation and planning instrument – EPSCALE – designed to assess shared decision making and the skills of planning and explanation in consultations with patients (Edgcumbe et al. 2012). The OSCE also has been used in undergraduate education to evaluate courses, for example longitudinal clinical clerkships (Zink et al. 2010; Hirsh et al. 2012), courses in clinical skills (Smith et al. 2009), the introduction of a new curriculum (Peeraer et al. 2009) and the training of students in a primary healthcare centre (Widyandana et al. 2011). In postgraduate education, the OSCE has been used to evaluate the training programme and methods employed. Innovative continuing education programmes have also been evaluated using an OSCE (Castel et al. 2011; Nieman and Cheng 2011).

The OSCE described in Case Study 8 for PGY1 residents from 10 specialties implemented at the beginning and end of the year was used to assess the education programme and the extent to which it addressed the six Accreditation Council for Graduate Medical Education (ACGME) core competencies. The data were fed back to the curriculum committee, and the courses where the competencies were taught were evaluated. Information about where a significant improvement in the residents' scores was not achieved was used to improve the courses. In dental education, Zartman et al. (2002) recognised that the OSCE has applications beyond grading student performance and that analysis of OSCEs can provide valuable information to determine whether the curriculum is meeting its remit, that is, to produce competent practitioners.

The OSCE has an important role to play not only in curriculum evaluation and quality assurance but also in research in medical education. An example can be seen in the GULiVer project, which examined video recordings of students' performance in a final-year OSCE to assess how the lay public in different European countries evaluates a doctor's communication skills and whether the lay public's perceptions of good communication differ from those of the experts (Moretti et al. 2012).

Reinforcing the specified learning outcomes and directing learning

The OSCE has an important influence on learning and can encourage students to prioritise their learning experience in an applied clinical context (Newble and Jaeger 1983). Stations in an OSCE can have instructional traction, influencing students'

Box 4.1

When the OSCE was first introduced in Dundee, the medical librarian commented that she normally expected to see an influx of students into the library in the weeks before the final graduation examination, this had not happened. She asked why. The explanation was that with the introduction of an OSCE as the main component of the final examination, students appreciated that hospital wards were a better context for them to learn the necessary skills rather than reading books in the library! This is an example of how a change in assessment can change students' behaviour.

behaviour before the examination. This was found when the OSCE was introduced in the final examination in medicine in Dundee (Box 4.1). An OSCE was demonstrated by Duvivier et al. (2012) to be one of the factors influencing students' learning strategies. In nursing education, Meechan et al. (2011) found that the early introduction of an OSCE stimulated student nurses to improve their skills in drug administration.

Students' mastery of a subject was found to be increased when they were involved in the development of an OSCE. German students developed and tested their own Emergency Medicine OSCE stations and assessed each other in a simulated OSCE. In the end-of-year OSCE, the students involved in developing the OSCE performed significantly better than those in the control groups at all stations (Heinke et al. 2013). The authors attribute the enhanced performance to the longer period that the students spent actively learning the principles of emergency medicine compared to the control groups.

Faculty development

Increasing emphasis is being placed on healthcare professions' education on faculty development. An OSCE incorporating teaching tasks designed to assess a teacher's teaching competence – an Objective Structured Teaching Encounter (OSTE) (also referred to as a Teaching Objective Structured Clinical Examination [TOSCE]) – can make a useful contribution to a staff development programme. Standardised students trained to portray learners may take part. Lu et al. (2014) created eight OSTE cases to help faculty develop and evaluate their skills in teaching professionalism and medical ethics using standardised students and standardised patients. An overview of the cases is given in the paper, together with a detailed case scenario and checklists. The resulting workshops were well evaluated, and the standardised students additionally reported a sense of empowerment and motivation from taking part in the workshops. Some schools offer students the opportunity to participate in an OSTE as an elective which attracts credits (Morrison et al. 2003).

At the University of Chicago, the OSTE is used to train residents and some faculty members in the skills of the 'One Minute Preceptor' (Fromme 2013) and in geriatrics the four-station G-OSTE is used to improve the geriatric medicine teaching skills of non-geriatricians (Scott et al. 2013). The annual Resident-as-Teacher OSTE at

Harvard Medical School uses videotaped teaching encounters with trained medical students to help residents improve their teaching skills. The faculty and self-evaluations form part of their resident portfolios (Ricciotti 2013).

Further evidence of the effectiveness of the OSTE comes from a systematic review of 22 published reports, as documented by Trowbridge et al. (2011). These authors concluded that the OSTE was *a promising and innovative means of assessing and improving the teaching performance of clinical educators* whilst recognising that more evidence is needed to support its validity. Siddiqui and Ahmed (2013) found the OSTE to be a reliable and valid assessment tool in Pakistan. Ottolini et al. (2011) described the use of Objective Structured Teaching Exercises and how, when incorporated into a faculty development programme they proved to be effective in improving teaching behaviour. We will see in the years ahead greater use made of the OSTE in faculty development.

Subjects and disciplines assessed

The OSCE has been used as an assessment instrument in a wide range of subjects and disciplines. These include major areas and disciplines, such as medicine, surgery, gynaecology, psychiatry, ophthalmology and radiology. More specialised subject areas can also be assessed, such as abdominal ultrasound, management of abdominal pain, patient safety and marriage and family therapy. A list of some subjects commonly assessed is given in Table 4.1.

Phases of education

Undergraduate education

The OSCE was originally described in the context of undergraduate medical education and has been widely used in both the early and later years of basic medical training (Townsend et al. 2001; Davis 2003; Newble 2004). Case Studies 1–4 provide examples of OSCEs in the early years of the medical curriculum, and Case Study 5 is a final examination. The term Objective Structured Practical Examination (OSPE) was used with respect to an OSCE-type examination in the early years where the emphasis was on the basic medical sciences (Harden and Cairncross 1980; Malik et al. 1988). With an increasing emphasis on vertical integration in the medical curriculum and the inclusion of clinical skills in the early years of the programme, the distinction between an OSCE and an OSPE has become blurred. Learning outcomes relating to communication skills and practical procedures, such as measurement of blood pressure, are now expected of first-year students in many schools and can be tested at the stations in an OSCE. The term 'OSCE' is now commonly used to cover assessment in both the early and later years of the undergraduate curriculum.

The OSCE is routinely used to assess students' progress in the later years of the medical course and in the final graduating examination as described above. The OSCE may be an integrated examination across the different disciplines or a series

Table 4.1 Examples of subjects where the OSCE has been used as an assessment tool

Accident/Emergency Medicine/Trauma (Shih et al. 2013)

Anaesthesiology (Berkenstadt et al. 2006)

Dermatology (Gormley et al. 2013; Langley et al. 2009)

Environmental Medicine (Shanahan et al. 2000)

Gastroenterology (Chander et al. 2009)

Geriatrics (Scott et al. 2013)

Obstetrics and Gynaecology (Casey et al. 2009; Rymer 2001)

Ophthalmology (Bhatnagar et al. 2011)

Orthopaedics (Griesser et al. 2012; Phillips et al. 2013)

Paediatrics (Waterston et al. 1980)

Patient Safety (Singh et al. 2009; Wagner et al. 2009; Daud-Gallotti et al. 2011)

Physical/Rehabilitation Medicine (Garstang et al. 2012)

Primary Care/Community Medicine (Townsend et al. 2001)

Psychiatry (Wallace et al. 2002; Hodges et al. 2014)

Radiology (van den Berk et al. 2011)

Surgery (Brauer et al. 2013)

Ultrasound (Hofer et al. 2011)

This list is not comprehensive, and some areas where the OSCE has been used may not be included. The references are also not comprehensive and are intended only as an indication of the use of the OSCE in the area.

of OSCEs designed to assess competency in the different disciplines as reflected in the range of clerkships, including surgery and medicine.

Postgraduate education

From its initial use in undergraduate education, the OSCE rapidly expanded as an assessment tool into postgraduate education, where it is now recognised as a reliable and valid method of assessing the required competencies (Sloan et al. 1995). Some examples of the use of the OSCE in postgraduate education are given below:

- The OSCE cited as best practice when used as a tool to assess the six competencies described by the Accreditation Council for Graduate Medical Education (ACGME) (Yang et al. 2010; Falcone et al. 2011).

- The use of the OSCE to assess the incoming baseline ACGME competencies of junior doctors and to evaluate the effectiveness of the postgraduate training programme (Short et al. 2009).

- Integration of the OSCE into fellowship training programmes, for example in gastroenterology to fulfil ACGME mandates (Chander et al. 2009).

- To probe key competencies desired in first-year postgraduate students relating to specific skills, including patient safety (Wagner et al. 2009).

- Yearly assessment of residents in New Jersey with a nine-station OSCE, allowing 27 key areas expected of the junior doctor to be assessed over the 3-year period (Garstang et al. 2012).

- The assessment of complex skills, such as handoff communication (Stojan et al. 2014) and telephone management (Williams et al. 2011).

- A test before and after a 7-day induction programme for new first-year surgical residents (Pandya et al. 2010).

- As a basis for tailoring an induction programme for new residents to their individual needs in Queensland, Australia.

- As a summative assessment for the membership examinations of the Royal Colleges in the UK (Rymer 2001).

Continuing education

Less use has been made of the OSCE in continuing education compared to under-graduate and postgraduate phases. Its main use has been as a tool to evaluate continuing medical education (CME) programmes.

In the UK, an OSCE has been adopted as part of the re-validation process of doctors in whom potential difficulties have been identified. The Professional and Linguistics Assessment Board (PLAB) test, organised by the General Medical Council in the UK, is an assessment to ensure that international medical graduates have the necessary knowledge and skills to practise in the UK. Part 2 of the PLAB is an OSCE with 14 clinical stations (General Medical Council 2007).

Use in healthcare professions and other fields of practice

Whilst originally described and applied to medicine, the use of the OSCE has extended to a range of other healthcare professions and in other fields where performance assessment is relevant.

Nursing and midwifery

The OSCE has been found to be a valid, reliable and feasible method of assessing the competence of student nurses and midwives. It provides an effective tool to assess safe practice in terms of performance of psychomotor skills as well as the declarative and schematic knowledge associated with their application (Watson et al. 2002; Bartfay et al. 2004; Ward and Barratt 2005; Mitchell et al. 2009; McWilliam and Botwinski 2010). The OSCE has been used in nursing in different countries around the world, such as Spain (Sola Pola et al. 2011) and Iran (Erfanian and Khadivzadeh 2011). Case Study 9 describes a summative examination to assess essential foundation skills, techniques and practices in first-year undergraduate nursing students in Dundee, UK.

Barry et al. (2012) found the OSCE to be a valuable learning tool in midwifery education. An Australian study reported that the OSCE improved student confidence and prepared student midwives for practice (Mitchell et al. 2014).

Dentistry
The OSCE has been shown to be a reliable and valid test in dentistry, a field where mastery of practical skills is important (Schoonheim-Klein, et al. 2006; Eberhard et al. 2011; Ratzmann et al. 2012). Graham et al. (2013) reported student perceptions that the OSCE was an authentic assessment requiring integration and application of knowledge. Case Study 10 provides a list of typical stations included in a dental OSCE.

Veterinary medicine
The OSCE has been used increasingly in veterinary medicine to test a range of practical procedures (Davis et al. 2006; Hecker et al. 2010). Real animals and animal simulators have been used along with simulated clients/owners. In veterinary nursing, the OSCE is now the established qualifying examination recognised for the UK Diploma in Veterinary Nursing, and an example is given in Case Study 11.

Pharmacy
In pharmacy education, the OSCE is used both as a formative and as a summative assessment. The Royal Pharmaceutical Society of Great Britain advocates the inclusion of the OSCE as a performance assessment tool in pharmacy (Kirton and Kravitz 2011). Case Study 12 describes a final-year undergraduate Pharmacy OSCE with a focus on patient education and communication, clinical pharmacokinetics, identification and resolution of drug-related problems and critical appraisal of the literature.

Other healthcare professions
Other healthcare professions, as noted in Table 4.2, where the OSCE has been adopted as a performance assessment tool include physical/occupational therapy and dietetics. The College of Optometrists has introduced a 16-station OSCE as a final examination (College of Optometrists 2010). Since 1996, the National Board of Chiropractic Examiners (NBCE) has used an OSCE as part of their Part IV Examination to assess more than 60,300 chiropractic students (NBCE 2014).

HOW THE OSCE CAN CONTRIBUTE TO THE EDUCATION PROGRAMME

Table 4.2 Other healthcare professions where the OSCE has been adopted as a performance assessment

Chiropractic (Kobrossi and Schut 1987; NBCE 2014)

Dentistry (Graham et al. 2013)

Dietetic (Lambert et al. 2010)

Marriage and Family Therapy (Miller 2010)

Massage Therapy (College of Massage Therapists of Ontario 2014)

Midwifery (Govaerts et al. 2002)

Nursing (Rushforth 2007; Walsh et al. 2009)

Optometry (College of Optometrists 2010)

Osteopathy (Vaughan and Florentine 2013)

Pharmacy (Awaisu and Nik Mohamed 2010)

Physical/Occupational Therapy (Sakurai et al. 2013; Silva et al. 2011; Wessel et al. 2003)

Physiotherapy (Nayer 1993)

Podiatry (Woodburn and Sutcliffe 1996)

Clinical Psychology (Yap et al. 2012)

Psychotherapy (Manring et al. 2003)

Radiography (Marshall and Harris 2000)

Veterinary Medicine (Davis et al. 2006; Artemiou et al. 2014)

Box 4.2

The Objective Structured Performance Related Examination (OSPRE), developed by the police force as a national examination in England for promotion to police sergeant or inspector, was modelled on the OSCE, as it was considered that the types of competencies expected in a police inspector were similar to those required in a doctor. Stations were designed to assess communication skills, observation and examination skills, priority setting, problem solving and decision making as well as the application of theory to practice. Context for the stations in the examination was seen as important, and the stations were presented as being located in one geographical area; Dundee, with the names of streets changed, was selected. From the advance information provided before the examination, candidates were expected to become familiar with facts about the area being policed. The examination was featured in an episode of the British TV police drama *Inspector Morse*.

Fields outside the healthcare professions

Some fields outside the healthcare professions where performance assessment is seen as important have adopted the OSCE. An interesting example is the Objective Structured Performance Related Examination (OSPRE), adopted as the national promotion examination by the Police Force in England and Wales (Police Training Council for England and Wales 1987). Stations were designed to assess communication skills, observation skills, examination, investigation, problem-solving, and decision-making in the context of police work (Box 4.2).

Use around the world

The OSCE is now widely used internationally (Box 4.3), and its use has been reported in countries around the world as illustrated in Figure 4.2. The figure under-estimates its spread geographically, as countries which have adopted the OSCE may not yet have described their approach in a published paper. The case studies in Section D give examples of its use in a number of countries, including the UK, the USA, Canada, Germany, Malaysia and Saudi Arabia. Its use in India was described by Gupta et al. (2010).

How the OSCE is implemented may be influenced by local, cultural and financial circumstances. Real patients are seldom used in the USA, with patients most commonly represented by standardised patients. In the UK, a variety of patient representations is commonly used, including real and standardised patients and models, and in other countries, such as India, even greater reliance is placed on the use of real patients.

Box 4.3

Brian Hodges (2003), in a paper where he used the metaphor of a drama performance, referred to the widespread use made of the OSCE internationally.

'Harden's OSCE, performed again and again the world over, is a tightly scripted event that requires a concerted effort by a large cast of players. After much rehearsal, the OSCE begins with the signal of a director and is performed in a series of "scenes". From India to Indiana, from Trinidad to Toronto, OSCE performances that hardly differ from Harden's original are mounted. There are also many variations, new roles and new settings. There are very short OSCEs and very long OSCEs. Some involve a small cast of actors while others employ a legion. In fact, one enormous, national OSCE involves over 4000 people in 14 different Canadian cities at the same time!'

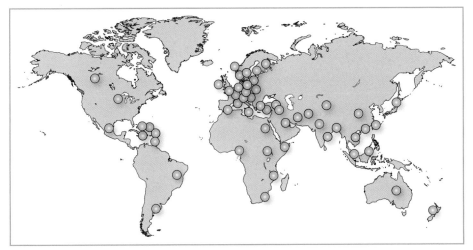

Figure 4.2 Geographical spread of the OSCE.

In Chapter 16, we describe how the OSCE may be used in circumstances where resources are limited.

Take-home messages

The OSCE is widely used as a performance assessment tool for the following reasons:

- Because of its flexibility, it can be used in a variety of contexts for a range of educational purposes. Its use is limited only by the innovativeness and imagination of the user.

- The OSCE can be used across undergraduate, postgraduate and continuing education programmes for formative and summative assessment purposes in the healthcare professions and other fields.

- The OSCE can be used to monitor and guide the progress of the learner with regard to a wide range of learning outcomes and to provide feedback as to required further learning.

- The OSCE can be used as a tool for curriculum evaluation and education research.

- The OSCE can be implemented as a sophisticated tool that requires significant resources or as a simple tool where available resources are more limited.

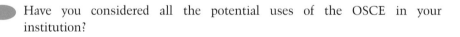 Have you considered all the potential uses of the OSCE in your institution?

What is assessed in an OSCE? 5

The OSCE can be used to assess a range of learning outcomes, including communication skills, physical examination, practical procedures, problem solving, clinical reasoning, decision making, attitudes and ethics and other competencies or abilities.

In earlier chapters in this book, we look at how the OSCE has been widely adopted as a tool to assess an individual's clinical competence and we explore the uses for the OSCE in different disciplines and phases of education. In later chapters, we look in more detail at how an OSCE can be implemented in practice. In this chapter, we consider the learning outcomes or competencies that can be assessed in an OSCE. Some examples of what can be assessed have already been presented in Chapter 1, Tables 1.1, 1.3 and 1.5, pp. 3–8.

An assessment of clinical competence

What sets the OSCE aside from other assessment tools, such as the frequently used multiple-choice question (MCQ), is that the OSCE focusses on what a student can do and not just what they know. The need to assess more than knowledge was highlighted by George Miller (1990):

> *'There are many who appear to believe that this knowledge base is all that needs to be measured. And it is unquestionably measurement of knowledge, largely through objective test methods, that dominates current institutional and specialty Board examination systems. But as Alfred North Whitehead pointed out many years ago, there is nothing more useless than a merely well informed man. Tests of knowledge are surely important, but they are also incomplete tools in this appraisal if we really believe there is more to the practice of medicine than knowing.'*

Miller went on to describe an assessment framework which has been widely referred to as 'Miller's Pyramid' (Figure 5.1). This represents a hierarchy of assessment approaches of increased authenticity (van der Vleuten and Schuwirth 2005). At the base of the pyramid is what the student or doctor *'knows'*. The next level is whether the student or doctor *'knows how'* to apply the knowledge in practice. The level

49

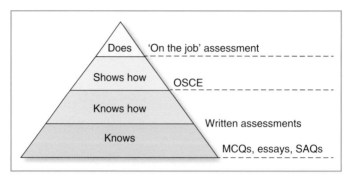

Figure 5.1 Miller's Pyramid with related assessment approaches. MCQs, multiple-choice questions; SAQs, self-assessment questions.

above is *'shows how'*, and here the student or doctor needs to be able to demonstrate in an assessment when faced with a patient that they have the necessary clinical skills and competencies in practice. For such a judgement to be made, they need to be observed directly communicating with a patient, undertaking a physical examination of the patient or carrying out a procedure, such as cardiopulmonary resuscitation. It is not sufficient that, as in the traditional clinical examination described in Chapter 2, the examinee simply reports to the examiner the history they have taken from the patient and the results of the physical examination. In the OSCE, both process and product are assessed. How the student or doctor behaves in an OSCE setting may, however, be different from their performance in practice. At the top of the pyramid, *'does'* can be seen as representing the doctor's (student's) performance in their day-to-day practice or activities. This is more difficult to assess, but tools such as multisource feedback (Wood et al. 2006), the mini-CEX (Norcini et al. 2003), and other on-the-job assessment tools have been described.

Learning outcomes and competencies

An important trend in medical education has been the move to an outcome- or competency-based model, where the learning outcomes are defined and decisions about the curriculum are based on these (Harden et al. 1999a,b; Harden and Laidlaw 2012). Indeed, it has been suggested that this move to outcome-based education (OBE) has been the most significant development in medical education in the past one or two decades (Harden 2013, p. 151).

Assessment is an intrinsic component of competency-based education (Davis and Harden 2003; Shumway and Harden 2003; Holmboe et al. 2010). Miriam Friedman Ben-David (1999) argued that OBE and performance assessment are closely related paradigms and that in OBE assessment techniques are needed to capture a broad range of activities. The OSCE is of value in this respect.

The five Scottish medical schools adopted the same framework for learning outcomes (Simpson et al. 2002) based on the three-circle model devised to classify the learning outcomes (Harden et al. 1999a,b). The inner circle addresses the learning outcomes relating to technical abilities expected of a doctor, the middle circle how the doctor approaches their practice and the outer circle the professionalism of the doctor (Figure 5.2).

The 12 learning outcomes addressed in the three circles are listed in Table 5.1. A survey of the published literature up to 2003 (Harden et al. 2003) showed that the OSCE has been used at least on several occasions as a tool to assess each of the 12 learning outcomes.

The Accreditation Council for Graduate Medical Education (ACGME) in the USA also provided a framework of six learning outcome domains (Swing 2007) (Table 5.2). The ACGME/ABMS Toolbox of Assessment Methods developed in September 2000 explored these competencies and suggested that the OSCE was the best method of assessing interviewing skills, patient education and counselling, performance of routine physical examination, preventive health services, creation of a therapeutic relationship with patients, listening skills, respect/altruism, and sensitivity to culture, age, gender and disability issues.

There are various reports in the literature of the OSCE being used to assess the ACGME competencies. Casey et al. (2009) related this in the specialty of obstetrics and gynaecology, and Chan (2011) used the OSCE as a reliable instrument to assess postgraduate first-year residents' attainment of the ACGME core competencies. Short et al. (2009) concurred that the OSCE was a valuable tool (as described in

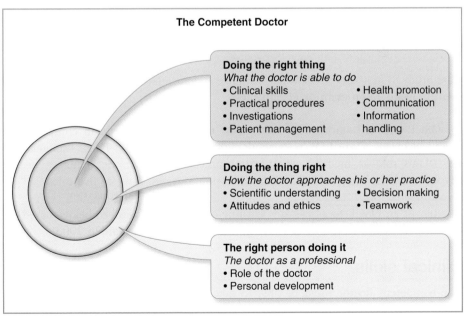

Figure 5.2 Three circle model of outcome-based education.

Table 5.1 The use of an OSCE to assess the 12 learning outcomes described in the three-circle model (Harden et al. 2003)

Learning outcome	References to the OSCE	%
Clinical Skills	381	54
Practical Procedures	95	13
Patient Investigation	107	15
Patient Management	152	22
Health Promotion and Disease Prevention	43	6
Communication	275	39
Information Handling	31	4
Understanding of Basic and Clinical Sciences	56	8
Attitudes and Ethics	72	10
Decision Making/Clinical Reasoning	102	14
Role of the Doctor	2	0.3
Personal Development	7	1

Table 5.2 The six learning outcome domains specified by the Accreditation Council for Graduate Medical Education (ACGME)

- Patient care – what you do
- Medical knowledge – what you know
- Practice-based learning and improvement – how you act
- Interpersonal and communication skills – how you interact with others
- Professionalism – how you get better
- Systems-based practice – how you work within the system

Case Study 8) to assess resident performance and also used the results of the assessment to evaluate programme effectiveness.

An OSCE with 10 stations has been used to assess the physician competencies described in the CanMEDS framework (Jefferies et al. 2007). These included the physician's role as medical expert, communicator, collaborator, manager, health advocate, scholar and professional. Each station assessed three to five roles.

The use of an OSCE to assess key learning outcomes is described below, based on domains identified in the three-circle model (Shumway and Harden 2003).

Clinical skills

The competent doctor must be able to take a history from a patient, perform a physical examination, interpret findings, and formulate an action plan to characterise the problem and reach a diagnosis. These are the key learning outcomes that the

OSCE was designed to assess as described in Chapter 2. At a station in the OSCE, examinees are assessed as they take history or examine a patient, and their findings are assessed at the same station or, more commonly, at the following station.

In the time normally allocated to a station in an OSCE, it is not possible for the examinee to take a full, comprehensive history and to conduct a systematic physical examination. As described in the case studies in Section D, the task presented to the examinee has to be focussed in one area, such as taking the history of a patient who presents with chest pain. An examiner's checklist identifies what is expected of the examinee in terms of his/her performance in the time available when confronted with the task. The examiner may also be required to complete a global rating scale where the examinee's performance is scored on several dimensions, such as their relationship with the patient, their technique and the key points addressed. The use of checklists and global rating scales are discussed further in Chapter 11.

A patient presenting with chest pain is the subject of Station 1 in the undergraduate OSCE Case Study 4. A checklist with 20 key points that the student is expected to address is scored by the examiner who also selects a global rating which best describes the student's overall competence at the station.

At Station 2 in Case Study 1, the undergraduate medical student is asked to examine a patient's hip. The examiner is asked to grade the student on a five-point scale in each of five domains: accuracy, skilfulness, supportiveness, efficiency/structure and safety. The global score ranges from 'clear fail' to 'excellent'.

Practical procedures

The competent doctor should be able to carry out a range of procedures on a patient for diagnostic or therapeutic purposes. This usually involves some instrument or device. Simple procedures (e.g. suturing a wound or catheterisation) or more complex procedures (e.g. cardiopulmonary resuscitation) can be assessed in an OSCE.

Examples of practical procedures that can be assessed are given in the case studies. These include venepuncture, venous cannulation, management of acute collapse, catheterisation, suturing and aseptic technique. Applying a bandage and a splint to immobilise the leg of a model dog is the subject of a station in Case Study 11, which details the end-of-year examination for the Diploma in Veterinary Nursing Course. A 27-step checklist is scored by the examiner. Practical procedures in the stations for the dental OSCE (Case Study 10), include tooth extraction, suturing and prosthodontics.

Investigation of a patient

The doctor should be competent to arrange appropriate investigations for a patient and, where necessary, to interpret them. The examinee may be shown X-rays, ECGs or other laboratory results and asked to interpret these or be asked to carry out an investigation, such as measurement of the peak expiratory flow rate, charting the field of vision or examination of the urine. Patient investigation can be assessed in an OSCE at a 'linked station' (see Chapter 6), where the examinee is asked in the second of the two linked stations to order investigations for the patient whose history they have taken or who they have examined at the previous station. In Case Study 14, an OSCE is used to explore in more depth the examinee's competence in one type of investigation – abdominal ultrasound. The assessment includes the theoretical underpinnings of how to differentiate lymph nodes from tubular structures, handling of the transducer and scanning performance and communication with the patient.

Health promotion and disease prevention

Doctors should be competent in the promotion of health and the prevention of disease. The OSCE can contribute to the assessment of the learner's competence in this domain. The linked station shown in Figure 6.7 in Chapter 6 is an example of a station designed to assess an examinee's understanding of health promotion. Box 5.1 describes a station where the examinee's knowledge was assessed relating to the appropriate advice to be given to a patient following a myocardial infarction with regard to issues such as diet, smoking and exercise. In addition, the students' attitudes to the importance of health promotion was measured by the time they chose to devote to the subject compared with the time spent discussing drug treatment and the physical aspects of myocardial infarction in the interview with the patient and his wife (Box 5.1).

In another example of the assessment of health promotion in an OSCE, Roseby et al. (2003) used a summative OSCE station to assess fifth-year medical students' ability to take a smoking history and counsel an adolescent with asthma on the links between smoking and health.

Communication skills

The good healthcare professional is competent in a range of communication skills, both oral and written. The delivery of care is only as good as the professional's ability to communicate clearly with patients and their families and with fellow healthcare

---

Box 5.1

Students' understanding and attitudes to health promotion were assessed at an OSCE station where they had to advise a patient on discharge from hospital following a myocardial infarction. Students had demonstrated in a written paper their knowledge of the features relating to lifestyle management, such as smoking cessation, an appropriate diet, and exercise. In the OSCE, however, many chose to ignore this and used the time at their disposal to discuss with the patient the physical aspects of myocardial infarction as it related to the patient and the drugs prescribed. Attitudes are, at least in part, reflected in what people do, and the failure of the students to address in the station the promotion of the patient's health suggested that they attributed less importance to this than to other aspects of the patient's management.

professionals. A measure of a learner's communication skills can tell much about a learner's potential skills and their ability to become a competent and caring health-care professional. Communication skills that can be assessed in an OSCE include:

- history taking from a patient with a specific problem.

- communication with other members of the healthcare team either orally or in writing.

- communication with the patient's family, including breaking bad news.

- acting as a patient's advocate to defend a patient's interests.

- appearance in a court of law as an expert witness.

- public interviews, such as at local meetings or on television or radio; and

- teaching students or colleagues.

The OSCE is well suited to the assessment of communication skills. The examinee's face-to-face communication with a patient, a patient's relative, or another member of the healthcare team can be assessed at a station in an OSCE. Telephone communication or communication in writing, such as a referral letter, can also be assessed.

In the OSCE described in Case Study 3, the student is asked to take a medication history and write a prescription for a newly admitted surgical patient. The examiner is asked to rate the student's overall conduct of the consultation, his/her history-taking and prescribing skills, and non-verbal communication with the patient. Patient education and counselling is the subject of Station 7 in Case Study 12. Final-year undergraduate pharmacy students are assessed on their competence to counsel a type 2 diabetic patient on insulin delivery.

One of the most challenging communication tasks the doctor may face is to inform a relative of the death of a close family member. Case Study 8, Station 1, gives details of an OSCE station that forms part of a first-year postgraduate resident examination to assess competence in this area.

The examiner may rate an examinee's performance in a communication station on the basis of:

- the elicitation or addressing of key points in the communication.

- the relationship with the patient (e.g. establishment of rapport with patient; empathy towards the patient; use of patient's name; and consideration of patient's feelings); and

- the communication technique (e.g. correct phrasing of questions; correct pace of communication; attention paid to patient's answers; answers followed up appropriately; and dates established).

Handling and retrieving information

The healthcare professional should be competent in retrieving, recording and analysing information using a range of methods. This is of increasing importance in an age of 'ubiquitous information', a phrase coined by Charles Friedman from the University of Michigan in the USA, recognising the wealth of information available in the 'knowledge cloud'. Such skills need to be developed in students and trainees. In addition to knowing how to access information, they also need to be able to determine its relevance in individual patients and apply evidence-based judgement. Information handling skills can be assessed in an OSCE, for example at a station where a student has to find online the advantages of a particular therapeutic regimen or recommend a website for a patient with a disability.

Evidence-based Medicine (EBM), introduced into the literature in the early 1990s,

> '...de-emphasizes intuition, unsystematic clinical experience, and
> pathophysiologic rationale as sufficient grounds for clinical decision
> making and stresses the examination of evidence from clinical research.
> Evidence-based medicine requires new skills of the physician, including
> efficient literature searching and the application of formal rules of
> evidence evaluating the clinical literature.' (Evidence-based Medicine
> Working Group 1992).

EBM skills can be assessed in an OSCE. They are recognised by the ACGME as part of its medical knowledge and practice-based learning and improvement competencies. Whilst EBM is included in the curricula of many medical schools (Meats et al. 2009; Hosny and Ghaly 2014), there are few studies that report how to assess this competency. Tudiver et al. (2009) set out to design and test an OSCE station to measure four EBM skills with an eight-item checklist and a two-item global rating scale. Frohna et al. (2006) developed a computer-based station for inclusion in a fourth-year OSCE, and Bradley and Humphris (1999) reported on linked stations, where students read at the first station two *British Medical Journal* abstracts about the management of sore throats, followed by a station where they meet a patient presenting with a sore throat. The instruments used were found to have good validity and inter-rater reliability.

Creative problem solving and decision making

The importance of these different skills in a healthcare professional has now been recognised. They were examined in an OSCE introduced by Sean Lavelle at the National University of Ireland in Galway to assess students on an experimental

Box 5.2

I (RMH) had the good fortune to be invited by Sean Lavelle when he was Professor of Experimental Medicine at the National University of Ireland, in Galway, to serve as an external examiner in the end-of-course OSCE. I observed students' performance at the 'railway track' and at the 'letter of complaint' stations.

At the 'railway track' station, some students attempted to estimate the speed of the train over too short a time interval (one rail on the track), others took an excessive amount of time and used inappropriate instruments to measure the length of the rail track and some failed to follow the simple instruction on the engine as to how to start the motor. Others lacked the manual dexterity to place the engine on the track or, once they had the necessary data, failed to use the calculator provided to determine the speed of the train.

Students demonstrated a huge range of responses to the 'letter of complaint' station (Figure 5.3). Many failed to consider the possibility of an error in conversion of pounds to kilograms, a transcription error, an observer error, an error in the standard used (the chemist scale) or variations in the control. Two students indicated that they would refer the patient who had complained to a psychiatrist.

Having observed students' performance at both of these stations, I came to the conclusion that if I were to appoint one of the students as a future house officer, I would choose a student based on their performance at these stations rather than on their performance in a more traditional MCQ examination paper.

medicine course (Lavelle and Harden 1986) (Box 5.2). An example of the stations incorporated into the OSCE is given in Table 5.3. At one station where students were presented with a model railway engine, a figure-of-eight railway track and a range of measuring and timing devices, they were asked to determine the average speed of the train. Many students failed to complete this simple experiment for a number of reasons (Box 5.2). At another station, the students were informed that they were to assume the role of the hospital administrator and investigate a complaint from a patient, as shown in a copy of the patient's letter (Figure 5.3), that her weight had been noted incorrectly in the hospital records. Rather than answer a theoretical question on the reasons for the experimental error, the student had to consider and explore the possible explanations in this practical example. Both of these stations recognise that problem solving is important in medicine and that it is best assessed in practice rather than on paper.

Problem solving and decision making are major components of the Multiple Mini-Interview (MMI) OSCE described in Chapter 4. At one station in the example in Case Study 15, the candidate is asked to work with a young person with learning difficulties to sort cards into piles based on specific criteria. Competencies assessed include critical thinking, teamwork and communication skills. The MMI is now used in some schools as one of a series of measures for selecting students for admission.

Table 5.3 Examples of stations used in an OSCE to assess students' achievement of the learning outcomes in a course on experimental medicine (Lavelle and Harden 1986)

Learning outcome	Task	Resources
Literature analysis	Abstract and comment	Reprint of a medical article
Objective pattern of disease	Find the combination of symptoms which optimises the probability of a specified disease	A diagnostic programme on a computer with a database of 10 symptoms in each of six diseases
Perception of body language	Describe and interpret each gesture	Video of a doctor–patient consultation, which pauses at points where the patient gestures or moves
Sampling procedures	Estimate the ratio of red blood cells to white blood cells in each smear and determine the significance of any difference using a suitable statistical test	Drawings of two blood smears of several hundred cells and statistical tables and rulers
Randomisation of sampling	Put into other containers by random allocation a specified and equal number of counters	A bag containing a number of black and white counters and a table of random numbers
Assembly of instruments	Assemble the items into an apparatus which will make a propeller fly	Seven items: wire, rubber band, spool, etc.
Dosage quantitation	Decant the fluid as necessary so as to leave a specified amount in the largest one	Three beakers of specified, but unequal volumes; the largest filled with water and the others are empty

Attitudes and professionalism

Professionalism, appropriate attitudes, ethical behaviour and legal approaches to the practice of medicine are all fundamental to the practice of medicine and are high on today's public and professional agenda in medical education. Theodore Roosevelt is thought to have first said, *'People don't care how much you know until they know how much you care.'* An inappropriate attitude is a common criticism by patients of healthcare professionals. Unprofessional behaviour in medical school has been shown to increase the incidence of subsequent disciplinary action by US state medical boards on doctors in practice (Papadakis et al. 2004). It is important to identify such behaviours at an early stage in training. However, whilst most people instinctively know what is 'unprofessional', defining professional behaviour is less easy, and the assessment of such competencies in a student or doctor is challenging.

Simulated patients (SPs) can be used for the assessment of professional attributes (van Zanten et al. 2005). Larkin (1999) used an OSCE to assess clinical ethical

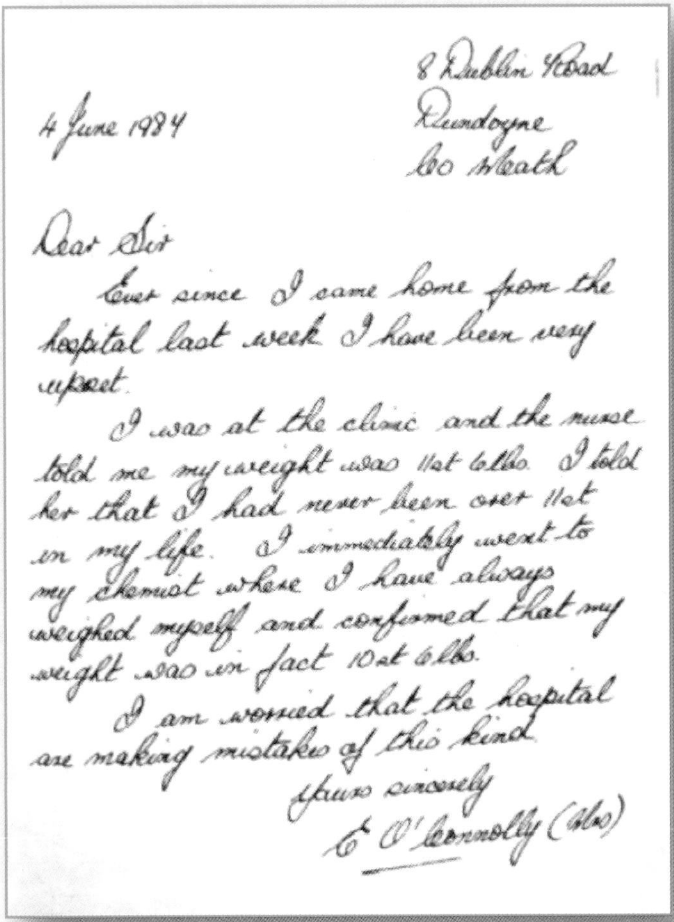

8 Dublin Road
Dundoyne
Co Meath

4 June 1984

Dear Sir

Ever since I came home from the hospital last week I have been very upset.

I was at the clinic and the nurse told me my weight was 11st 6lbs. I told her that I had never been over 11st in my life. I immediately went to my chemist where I have always weighed myself and confirmed that my weight was in fact 10st 6lbs.

I am worried that the hospital are making mistakes of this kind.

Yours sincerely

E O'Connolly (Mrs)

Figure 5.3 **A patient's letter of complaint.**

competence in emergency medicine and developed a blueprint for an advanced trauma life support OSCE station designed to assess ethical competence.

Station 16 of Case Study 5 assesses not only the final-year medical student's competence in communicating with the daughter of a chronically ill older woman but also assesses the student's knowledge and understanding of legal and professional guidance relating to end-of-life care. This final-year OSCE demonstrates how it is possible to assess in an OSCE a broad range of competencies expected of the junior doctor on graduation, from history taking and procedure stations to complex communication and prioritisation of activities on the ward.

A formative examination to assess and improve second-year residents' cultural competence on a range of very challenging issues, including ethnicity, language, race, religion and sexual orientation, is described in Case Study 6. Station 1 assesses the resident's cultural competence in communicating with the mother of a 17-year-old boy recently diagnosed with leukaemia, and the conflict between the wishes of the mother and the rights of the child. A 'culture' OSCE was described by Altshuler and Kachur (2001).

When asked to evaluate the professionalism of medical students in an OSCE, doctors, patients and SPs consider a wide range of verbal and non-verbal behaviours, and different observers may attend to different behaviours even with the same rating forms (Mazor et al. 2007). It has been suggested that ethics OSCEs are more suited to formative assessment than summative assessment, as to achieve on their own the necessary high-stakes reliability, the number of stations required could be prohibitively expensive (Stern 2006, p. 49). The OSCE has a contribution to make to the assessment of professionalism, and some aspects can be observed and assessed during an OSCE. A range of methods can be used in the assessment of the student's competence, and evidence about ethics obtained in an OSCE can be used alongside evidence from other assessments (Singer et al. 1996). These can include multisource feedback (Wood et al. 2006) and the use of portfolios (Friedman Ben-David et al. 2001a). O'Sullivan et al. (2012) highlighted that in the assessment of professionalism, the evidence from different sources needs to be triangulated before an overall judgement can be made. The evidence can be collated in a portfolio and can include the student's performance in OSCEs, multisource feedback and attendance records. The challenges implicit in the assessment of professionalism were highlighted by Hodges et al. (2011) in the Ottawa conference consensus statements.

Despite the difficulties, there is merit in including professionalism as a learning outcome to be assessed in an OSCE. As Stern (2006, p. 50) suggests:

> 'A comprehensive OSCE ... that covers domains of professionalism sends
> a powerful message to physician and the public that our medical
> educational system values ethical reasoning and communication skills
> on the same level as scientific knowledge and technical abilities.'

Competence as a member of a team

For the most part, healthcare workers no longer work in isolation, but instead play their part in the delivery of healthcare as members of a team. There is a wealth of information available relating to training interprofessional teams and their importance in the delivery of safe patient care (Institute of Medicine 2000; Lerner et al. 2009; Reader et al. 2009; Manser 2009; Weller et al. 2014). There is a need also to assess in the student and healthcare professional the competencies necessary for interprofessional collaborative practice. As with professionalism, this can be achieved by using a range of approaches, including an OSCE.

One or more stations may be introduced into an OSCE to assess interprofessional skills. This may be in the context of patient safety as illustrated in Case Study 13, which addresses the issue of patient safety in an OSCE for first-year postgraduate residents. Station 7 assesses the resident's team skills in interacting with the nurse to ask about the patient's condition and to communicate any further actions necessary.

As mentioned in Chapter 1, the Team Observed Structured Clinical Encounter (TOSCE) was developed by McMaster University and the University of Ottawa in Canada to assess a team approach to patient care (Marshall et al. 2008). The TOSCE was initially used in undergraduate education, with both uniprofessional groups of medical students and interprofessional groups comprising medical, nursing, social work, chaplaincy and occupational therapy students, and was found to be valid, reliable and acceptable to students as a formative assessment tool (Hall et al. 2011). Use of the TOSCE has been extended to healthcare teams in several specialty areas. The phrase *'clinical encounter'* rather than *'clinical examination'* was introduced in an attempt to reduce any stress associated with the OSCE and to emphasise the formative nature of TOSCE in giving feedback to teams as to how they can work together more productively (Solomon et al. 2011). Use of the TOSCE has been reported in postgraduate education, where scenario-based encounters have been developed for learning and formative feedback for groups of nurses and midwives (Gordon et al. 2012).

Murray Davis et al. (2013) reported on the development of the TOSCE for use with family physicians, midwives and obstetricians to provide better maternity care. The OSCE consisted of seven stations, each of 20 minutes plus 10 minutes for feedback, and included participation from three professions. The focus was on team skills rather than clinical knowledge and aimed to assess changes in knowledge and behaviour.

Work has also been reported to develop interprofessional OSCEs (iOSCEs) through collaborative interprofessional projects (Morison and Stewart 2005; Simmons et al. 2011).

The OSCE and core tasks

As described above, the OSCE can be used to assess the different learning outcome domains as they relate to the different body systems. The OSCE can also be used to assess the core tasks facing a healthcare professional. Examples of the tasks which form the basis of an undergraduate curriculum are shown in Table 5.4. At an OSCE station, the students' competence may be assessed in relation to a core task in respect of history taking, physical examination, further investigations, practical procedures, management or health promotion.

Take-home messages

- The OSCE can be used to assess a wide range of learning outcomes not tested in written examinations.

Table 5.4 Examples of core clinical tasks that can be the basis for an OSCE station (Harden et al. 2000)

1. **Pain**
   Pain in the leg while walking
   Acute abdominal pain
   Loin pain and dysuria
   Chest pain
   Joint pain
   Back and neck pain
   Indigestion
   Headache
   Cancer pain
   Earache

2. **Bleeding and bruising**
   Bruising easily
   Pallor
   Haemoptysis
   Vomiting blood
   Rectal bleeding
   Blood in urine
   Anaemia
   Post-operative bleeding

3. **Fever and infection**
   Chest infection
   Rash and fever
   Urethral discharge
   Pyrexia of unknown origin
   Immunisation
   Sweating
   Hypothermia
   Sepsis

4. **Altered consciousness**
   Immobility
   Falls
   Collapse
   Confusion
   Dizziness
   Fits

5. **Paralysis and impaired mobility**
   Loss of power on one side
   Tremor
   Peripheral neuropathy
   Muscle weakness
   Immobility
   Falling over

6. **Lumps, bumps and swelling**
   Lump in the neck
   Lump in groin
   Lump in breast
   Swollen scrotum
   Joint swelling
   Swollen ankles
   Skin lump

7. **Nutrition/weight**
   Thirsty and losing weight
   Difficulty swallowing
   Weight loss
   Seriously overweight

8. **Change in body function**
   Wheezing
   Pleural effusion
   Shortness of breath
   Cough
   Change in bowel habit
   Inability to pass urine
   Incontinence
   Raised blood pressure
   Palpitations

9. **Skin problems**
   Skin rash
   Itching
   Psoriasis
   Mole growing bigger/bleeding
   Blistering
   Photosensitivity
   Bedsore
   Jaundice
   Burn
   Wound

10. **Life threatening/accident and emergency**
    Shock
    Involvement in accident
    Fracture

11. **Eyes**
    Loss of vision
    Painful red eyes
    Squinting in child
    Foreign body in child's eyes

12. **Ear, nose and throat**
    Ringing in ear
    Going deaf
    Earache
    Sore throat
    Hoarseness
    Stuffy nose

Table 5.4 Examples of core clinical tasks that can be the basis for an OSCE station (Harden et al. 2000)—cont'd

13. Behaviour
Anger
Anxiety
Phobias
Drug addiction
Suicide
Sleep problems
Bereavement
Alcohol dependence
Schizophrenia
Tiredness
Depression
Adolescence

14. Reproductive problems
Pre-menstrual syndrome
Infertility
Normal pregnancy
Menstrual problems
Contraception
Sterilisation
Smear results
Painful intercourse

15. The child
Child abuse
Down syndrome
Prematurity
Poor feeding
Failure to thrive
Respiratory distress syndrome
Developmental delay
Sudden infant death syndrome/near
    miss

16. Priority setting, decision making and audit
Dying patient
Population screening
Waiting lists
Triage
Acute versus chronic

- What is assessed in an OSCE will vary, depending on the stage of the learner and the purpose of the examination.

- Most commonly, the examination has been used to test clinical skills in history taking, physical examination, practical procedures and data interpretation.

- The OSCE can also contribute alongside other assessment approaches to an assessment of other outcomes, including ethics, attitudes, professionalism and teamwork skills.

 Are you assessing what should be assessed in terms of clinical competence?

Choosing a format for an OSCE | 6

Flexibility is a major advantage of the OSCE. Many factors influence the choice of format. These include the number of examinees, the purpose of the examination, the learning outcomes to be assessed, the resources available and the context of the local situation.

Factors influencing the format

A major advantage of the OSCE is that with the adoption of different formats, the approach can be adapted to suit local needs. Indeed, this flexibility is one of the reasons for the popularity and widespread use of the OSCE as a tool to assess the clinical competence of students and trainees.

Whilst the general principles that underpin an OSCE, as set out in Chapter 1, should be adopted, the details of the design of the examination in terms of what is tested and how it is tested can be decided locally. Factors that impact the format of an OSCE include:

- The number of examinees to be assessed – fewer than 20, or hundreds of examinees?

- The purpose of the examination – a summative examination to assess the competence of the examinee at a key point in training, a formative examination to provide feedback to the examinee or an examination with the results used to evaluate a course or a particular aspect of a course?

- The breadth of focus of the examination – an integrated overall assessment of competence or an examination of competence in a specific area, such as surgery?

- The learning outcomes to be assessed – physical examination or interprofessional skills?

- The resources available – examiners, real patients, simulated patients (SPs) or simulators?

- The options with regard to the venue.

- The stage in training or seniority of the examinee.

Variables in designing an OSCE

The variables to be considered in the design of the OSCE format include:

- number of stations.

- length of time allocated for each station.

- number of circuits.

- use of 'procedure' and 'question' stations.

- use of 'double' and 'linked' stations.

- organisation of the stations in a circuit; and

- provision of feedback to the examinee.

Number of stations

The number of stations used in an OSCE varies considerably. It is reported as ranging from less than 10 to more than 30. Figure 6.1 illustrates the number of

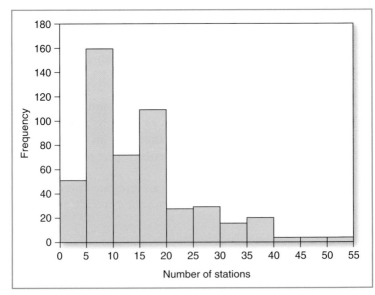

Figure 6.1 The number of stations incorporated in an OSCE as reported in a review of published papers (Harden et al. 2003).

OSCE stations documented in published reports, with as many as 40 stations reported.

In the original design plan for an OSCE and in its use in Dundee, 20 to 25 stations were incorporated. The reasons for choosing this number of stations were:

- Students could be assessed in groups of 20–25 in one circuit of the examination. With three simultaneous parallel circuits and with the circuits repeated later in the morning 120–150 students could be assessed in one morning (Figure 6.2).

- A range of competencies, such as history taking, physical examination and practical procedures, could be assessed, with each competency tested at several stations. Communication skills, for example, could be assessed in patients presenting with respiratory, cardiovascular and alimentary problems.

- The reliability of the OSCE correlates with the number of stations – the greater the number of stations, the greater the reliability. This is discussed further in Chapter 3.

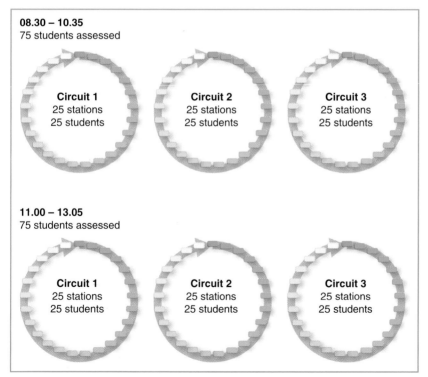

08.30 – 10.35
75 students assessed

Circuit 1
25 stations
25 students

Circuit 2
25 stations
25 students

Circuit 3
25 stations
25 students

11.00 – 13.05
75 students assessed

Circuit 1
25 stations
25 students

Circuit 2
25 stations
25 students

Circuit 3
25 stations
25 students

Figure 6.2 With this design, 150 students are assessed in one morning. Three circuits, each with 25 stations, are used, with the circuits repeated later in the morning. The duration of each station is 5 minutes.

- The logistics in relation to the organisation of a 20- to 25-station OSCE were not too onerous, provided that there was appropriate advance planning, as discussed in Chapter 10.

Local circumstances and requirements will vary and will influence the number of stations to be included in the OSCE. Related to a decision about the number of stations to be included is the time allocated to a station and the total time planned for the examination. For example, for a 100-minute examination, one option is 20 stations each of 5 minutes and another is 10 stations each of 10 minutes. For the reasons above, we preferred a 20-station OSCE with 5-minute stations.

Sequential testing

One approach that has attracted less attention than it deserves is sequential testing (Miller 1990; Smee et al. 2003; Cookson et al. 2011; Pell et al. 2013). Here the OSCE is organised in such a way that the number of stations at which a candidate is examined varies, depending on the performance of the candidate and the number of stations required to make a reliable decision about him/her. Candidates who have performed well or poorly complete their assessment in a short screening OSCE that consists of a range of stations that assess different competencies. A longer, more detailed examination is used for borderline candidates, where a question about their performance is raised in the earlier shorter examination. Poorly performing students may also be assessed further in the more detailed examination. The candidate may be examined on a full range of competencies or specifically on those where there was concern about their performance in the shorter OSCE. In Dundee, for example, all final-year students undertook a 24-station summative OSCE in the morning. Over lunch, the results of their performance were processed and profiles produced for each student in terms of their performance in the major areas of competence, including history taking, physical examination and practical procedures. Immediately after lunch, the examiners met to review the results. Students whose performance was borderline in one or more of the areas were identified, and they were then examined on a series of OSCE stations in the afternoon to assess further their performance in these areas.

Whilst in principle and psychometrically the approach is attractive, it has not been widely adopted because of the logistics required to set up a two-stage examination. It is also important to be able to identify with adequate reliability after fewer stations, those examinees who would perform to an appropriate standard throughout the remaining stations if they were asked to continue with the second stage of the examination. An attempt to introduce sequential testing by the Medical Council of Canada in 1997 was not well received, even though costs were significantly reduced, reliability was higher than expected and the format directed attention towards the borderline group whose performance was in doubt (Smee et al. 2003). Cookson et al. (2011) reported on the two-stage 2009 final examination at Hull York Medical School. The first stage comprised Objective Structured Long Examination Record (OSLER) and OSCE stations that had acceptable reliability. This was highly predictive of the results of the second stage, with the potential for significant cost saving. Like Smee et al. (2003), Cookson et al. (2011) highlighted the advantage of the format in that *'it concentrates resources where they are needed, at the pass/fail interface, to make this judgement more reliable'*. With increased awareness of the need for cost effectiveness of medical education processes and with greater understanding of psychometrics, station design and more sophisticated marking technology in recent years, it may be that sequential testing is worth revisiting. Costs of the OSCE are examined in more detail in Chapter 16.

Time allocated to a station

The time allocated to a station in an OSCE varies widely, as shown in Figure 6.3. The most common time for a station was 5 to 10 minutes, although many reports described stations of up to 25 minutes.

As the total time available for an OSCE is relatively fixed, there is an inverse relationship between the number of stations and the time allocated to each station. OSCEs with more stations tend to allow less time at each station, whereas OSCEs with a smaller number of stations allow more time at each station. The advantages of the former are noted above. The relation between number of stations, time allocated to each station and the total examination time is given in Table 6.1. Three options for a 120-minute examination, for example, are:

- 8 stations, each of 15 minutes.

- 12 stations, each of 10 minutes; or

- 24 stations, each of 5 minutes.

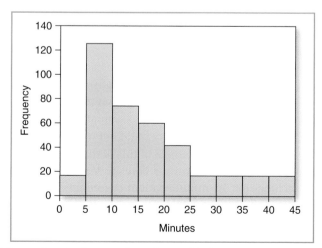

Figure 6.3 Time allocated to stations in an OSCE, as reported in a review of published papers (Harden et al. 2003).

Table 6.1 Relation between the number of stations, duration of stations, duration of examination and number of students examined in one to six circuits. The circuits may be scheduled simultaneously, sequentially, or both (Figure 6.2)

No. of stations	Duration of station (minutes)	Duration of examination (minutes)	Number of students examined					
			1 Circuit	2 Circuits	3 Circuits	4 Circuits	5 Circuits	6 Circuits
24	5	120	24	48	72	96	120	144
12	10	120	12	24	36	48	60	72
10	15	150	10	20	30	40	50	60
8	20	160	8	16	24	32	40	48

The case studies in Section D vary considerably in the duration of each station. In general, OSCEs for formative purposes have fewer but longer stations than those used for summative purposes, with stations ranging from 8 to 20 minutes in length. The two OSCE case studies with the longest time allocated for a station were those addressing challenging issues for residents, including patient safety and cultural issues. Three of the formative OSCE case studies incorporate a period of between 1.5 and 5 minutes at the end of the station for feedback to the candidate from the assessor and/or the SP before the candidate moves on to the next station. This adds to the length of the station.

The summative OSCE case studies have a larger number of shorter stations of between 5 and 15 minutes. Case Study 5, which forms part of the University College London final examination, has 18 stations, each of 5 minutes, and is a classic final-year OSCE sampling a wide range of competencies in order to achieve high reliability.

The Medical Council of Canada Part II Qualifying Examination (Case Study 7) comprises 12 stations, eight of 10 minutes and four of 15 minutes, reduced from the original 20 stations in the late 1990s, as high reliability and validity has been demonstrated with a lower number of stations.

Whilst some examinations favour longer stations (e.g. 20 minutes), what is sacrificed is that a smaller sample of competencies can be assessed with an associated decrease in reliability. The longer station time does, however, allow the examinee to take a more comprehensive history or to test the candidates' history taking and examination skills on the same patient. An example of this is the Clinical Skills Assessment (CSA) of the Educational Commission for Foreign Medical Graduates (ECFMG). This assessment includes ten 15-minute patient encounters, during which the candidates take a history and conduct a physical examination. Chambers et al. (2000) found that the average time examinees spent with the standardised patient was 13.3 minutes and concluded that the 15-minute time allocation was sufficient to cover both history taking and physical examination.

Including both history taking and physical examination in one station has the advantage that it represents a more holistic approach to the patient. However, competencies relating to history taking and physical examination may be better tested in an OSCE in different contexts at two stations. History taking, for example, may be assessed in a patient with chest pain and physical examination in a patient complaining of weakness in a leg. The shorter stations also allow more candidates to be examined in a circuit at the same time. There may well be situations, however, where 5 minutes is too short for a focussed history. In this case, a 'double' station can be included as described below. 'Linked' stations also allow clinical problems to be assessed over two or more stations.

Number of circuits

One circuit of OSCE stations is all that is required when the number of students is equal to the number of stations or where different groups of students can be assessed sequentially on the same circuit over a period of time, either later in the day or on a following day. An example is given in Case Study 8 of an 8-station (12 minutes each) OSCE, where one circuit is repeated four times per day over 2 days to assess 106 residents. In many situations, however, more than one circuit is required, either because of the large number of students to be examined or the need to complete the examination in the course of 1 day or one morning. As we have described, 150 students in Dundee had to be examined in one morning. This was achieved through the organisation of three parallel, simultaneous circuits with identical OSCE stations. Two groups of 25 students were assessed at each circuit in the course of a morning (Figure 6.2). In Case Study 2, two parallel circuits are used to examine 100 students in 1 day, in an OSCE with ten 7-minute stations.

Circuits may be at the same location or at different sites. In New Zealand, for example, an identical OSCE is administered simultaneously at three different school sites – Christchurch, Dunedin and Wellington. It was shown that it is possible to implement a multicentre OSCE that is psychometrically sound, simultaneous and identical at each site (Wilkinson et al. 2000). In Case Study 7, more than 4,000 candidates for the Medical Council of Canada's Qualifying Examination Part II are assessed at 18 sites over 2 days, each site running between two and eight circuits, and three administrations per day. Case Study 5 reports on a summative OSCE with 400 students being assessed at three sites, with the OSCE repeated up to four times a day over 2 days.

If 100 students are to be assessed on a 25-station OSCE, with each station allocated 5 minutes, a number of options are available (Figure 6.4):

- one circuit with four groups of 25 students assessed at the circuit, two groups in the morning and two in the afternoon (or on the following day).

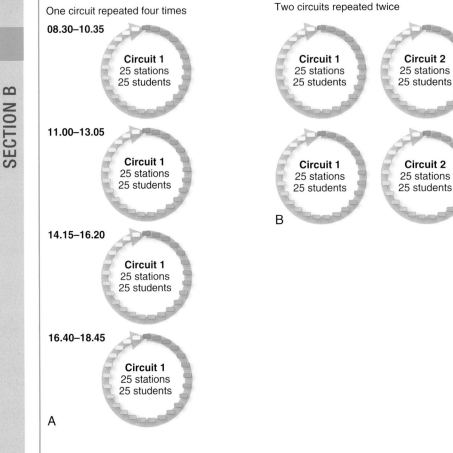

Figure 6.4 Three options for examining 100 students in a 25 × 5-minute station OSCE.

- two identical, simultaneous circuits organised with two groups of 25 students assessed at each circuit in the course of the morning.

- four circuits with identical OSCE stations and with each group of 25 students assessed at a different circuit in the course of the morning.

The best option will be determined by local circumstances.

Test security

Where different groups of candidates are assessed on the same examination over a period of time, for example over 2 days, questions have been raised about confidentiality and the prompting of later groups by candidates who have already completed the examination. In Dundee, the examination is completed over one morning, and the second group of students to be assessed at each of the three circuits assembles before the first group of students leaves the examination area. Where examinations are conducted over a period of time, 'quarantining' or 'corralling' of students may be implemented in an attempt to ensure the integrity of the OSCE stations, for example as in Case Study 2 and Case Study 3. The use of mobile phones and other forms of communication are closely controlled. For OSCEs that extend over more than 1 day, quarantining is impractical. Whilst students who are assessed later may appear to have an advantage if they can be briefed by students who completed the OSCE earlier, in practice this does not appear to be a significant problem. Minor changes may be made to a station, such as revisions to the patient's history. In this case, prior knowledge of the station may even put the student at a disadvantage. An example is given in Case Study 5, where students are also required to sign a statement that they will not discuss station content with other students.

The general consensus appears to be that the briefing of students who are assessed at repeat administrations of a circuit by students who had been assessed at an earlier administration does not put the later students at a significant advantage (Colliver et al. 1991). As the OSCE assesses a student's performance at the 'shows how' rather than 'knows' level (Miller 1990), the time available to a student for further preparation is probably insufficient for advance warning to make a difference (Swanson et al. 1999). However, there remains the perception amongst students that those who complete the OSCE later may have an advantage (Whelan et al. 2005). A student survey found that the majority of students considered the sharing of information amongst other candidates unprofessional, and they were in favour of corralling, as it avoided the dilemma some faced as to whether or not to share information about the examination (McCourt et al. 2012).

Humphrey-Murto et al. (2013) reviewed the question of test security in an OSCE and came to the following conclusions:

> 'Two general interpretations that can be drawn from the research to date are that foreknowledge of the OSCE content is not sufficient to allow for significant changes in one's clinical performance and that such knowledge may even be detrimental to clinical performance. While these studies suggest no significant concern about re-use of stations in summative settings, the potential advantage or disadvantage to those whose performance is close to the pass mark and for whom even a small change in performance may change their result is still unclear.' (p. 529)

It is desirable to complete the OSCE over one morning or in 1 day with corralling of the students. This, however, may not be possible.

'Procedure' and 'question' stations

Stations in an OSCE can be classified into two types (Figure 6.5) – 'procedure' stations, where the candidate has a task to perform, such as examination of the abdomen or taking a history from a patient complaining of chest pain; and 'question' stations, where the candidate has to answer open-ended or multiple-choice questions (MCQs), write a letter based on the information obtained at the previous station or complete a post-encounter note describing their findings at the previous station and possibly their interpretation of the findings and a management plan for the patient. Durning et al. (2012) described the use of a free text 'post-encounter form' (PEF) to assess clinical reasoning in second-year medical students. No examiner is present, and student responses are on paper or on a computer or tablet. They can be marked by an examiner at the time of the examination or subsequently with one examiner marking student responses at several question stations.

At the procedure stations, the examinee is observed and assessed by an examiner. The procedure stations are sometimes referred to as 'manned stations' and question stations are referred to as 'unmanned stations'.

Some OSCE developers have chosen to combine the procedure and question stations into one longer station. This may be effective as in Case Study 7, where the time allocated for questions is relatively short. In this case the candidate has 9 minutes to assess and manage a patient with chest pain, and in the final minute the examiner asks a related question. Where the procedure and question elements require approximately the same amount of time, it is more efficient to organise them as separate stations. This is more cost effective in relation to the examiner and the SP. When the procedure and question elements are combined, the patient does not have a part to play whilst the examinee is responding to the questions, and the examiner's time may be more effectively spent observing the next candidate rather than questioning the previous candidate (Figure 6.6). More accommodation is also required if the

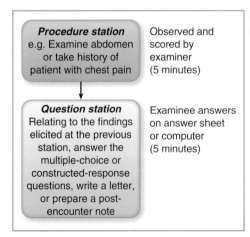

Procedure station
e.g. Examine abdomen
or take history of
patient with chest pain

Observed and
scored by
examiner
(5 minutes)

Question station
Relating to the findings
elicited at the previous
station, answer the
multiple-choice or
constructed-response
questions, write a letter,
or prepare a post-
encounter note

Examinee answers
on answer sheet
or computer
(5 minutes)

Figure 6.5 Stations in the OSCE are of two types.

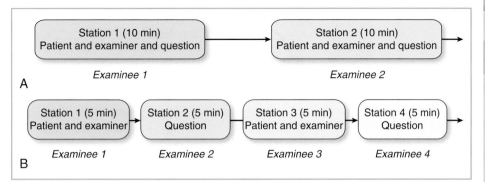

Figure 6.6 'Procedure' and 'question' stations: (A) combined or (B) separate.

question and procedure stations are combined, because if they are designed as separate stations, the question station may be located in a corridor as described in Chapter 7.

Double stations

In the OSCE, a standard time has to be set for all stations, and the task with which the examinee is faced should be achievable within this time. Occasionally, particularly when the time allocated to stations is 5 minutes, a longer period of time is required to assess one aspect of competence, such as history taking in a particular area. In this case a double station may be arranged. The station is duplicated with the 'A' and 'B' versions each having their own examiner and the patients carefully matched. Candidates are assessed alternately, as shown in Figure 6.7, at the 'A' or the 'B' station. When the first time signal is given, the candidate does not move on to the next station, and spends10 minutes at the station. This can be made to work well but needs careful signposting and management on the day of the examination. Case Study 5 includes a 10-minute double station on explaining a medical condition and treatment to a relative as part of the final-year OSCE with 'A' and 'B' stations running in parallel.

An alternative, less frequently adopted option is to have candidates complete two circuits, the first circuit with stations with a shorter duration of 4 minutes and the second circuit with stations with longer duration of 8 minutes (Ruesseler et al. 2010). This approach is illustrated in Figure 6.8. It has merit and is less confusing with the rotation of students where there are a number of double stations in an OSCE.

Linked stations

Each station in the OSCE can stand on its own, or two stations can be linked in one of a number of ways. The most frequent use of linked stations is where a process, such as a physical examination of a patient, is tested at one station (described above as 'procedure' stations) and at the second of the two linked stations (the 'question'

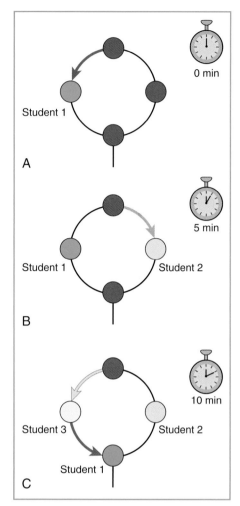

Figure 6.7 Organisation of a 10-minute double station in an examination with 5-minute stations.

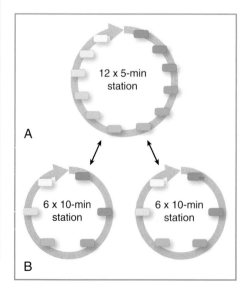

Figure 6.8 Students complete (A) a circuit of 12 × 5-minute stations followed by (B) 6 × 10-minute stations. Other students start with (B) followed by (A).

station), the examinee answers questions or prepares a report on what was found at the previous station. Linked stations may also be known as 'couplet' stations. In Case Study 13, the resident is asked to examine a patient in respiratory distress and at the following station to write an admission order for the patient seen at the previous station. In Case Study 5, the examinee is asked at the following station to complete a handover of the patient examined at the previous station. Several stations in Case Study 7 follow a similar format where the examinee sees a patient at an 'A' station and at the following 'B' station is asked to complete short answer or extended matching questions.

A second type of linked station is where an examinee is asked to undertake part of a procedure, for example preparing a slide for microscopy at the first station, and has to complete the procedure, perhaps being given the slide already prepared for examination under the microscope at the second station.

Another use of linked stations is to present the examinee with information at the first station about the patient to be seen at the next station and the task to be completed at that station. The first station is sometimes termed a 'preparation station'. This allows the examinee to assimilate the information from the patient's case records and to plan actions. The examinee may be shown the case sheet of a patient with a myocardial infarction (Figure 6.9A) and then asked to interview the patient at the next station (Figure 6.9B).

A fourth type of linked station is one where the examinee undertakes some activity or observes an activity, for example a recorded interview with a psychiatric patient at the first station, and discusses this with the examiner at the second station.

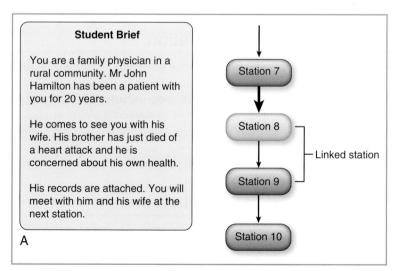

Student Brief

You are a family physician in a rural community. Mr John Hamilton has been a patient with you for 20 years.

He comes to see you with his wife. His brother has just died of a heart attack and he is concerned about his own health.

His records are attached. You will meet with him and his wife at the next station.

A

Station 7

Station 8

Station 9 — Linked station

Station 10

Figure 6.9A The first of two linked stations in an OSCE.

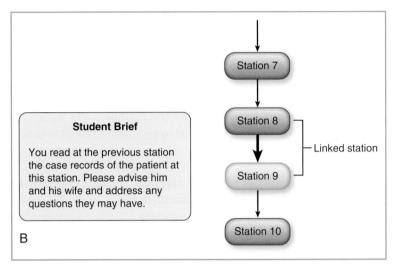

Figure 6.9B The second of two linked stations in an OSCE.

As described in Chapter 10, examinees cannot start the OSCE at the second of two linked stations. They can start at the second linked station as a rest station and complete the examination one station length after the other candidates. An alternative is for the examinee to start one station length ahead of the other candidates at the first of two linked stations. This is the method used in Case Study 12, where the examinee is asked to review a patient's records before meeting the patient at the next station. However, the former method is usually favoured, since there are advantages in starting the examination with all the examinees, assessors and SPs in place at the beginning of the OSCE. Whilst more than two stations can be linked, for practical reasons this is best avoided unless there are special circumstances that make it necessary.

Feedback during the examination

The OSCE is widely recognised for its value in providing examinees with feedback on their performance. This is discussed in more detail in Chapter 12. Feedback may be provided during or after an OSCE. If provided during an OSCE, the time allocated to stations may be lengthened, as described in several of the case studies, to allow for feedback to the candidate from the examiner and/or the patient. Alternatively, additional stations may be included where the aim is to provide feedback to the learners on their performance at the previous station.

The organisation of stations in a circuit

Examinees rotate in an OSCE around a circuit with a series of stations, as shown in Figure 6.10, and as illustrated in the MFDS Part 2 OSCE (http://vimeo .com/46687101). Less usually, as described above, students may be required to complete two circuits with stations of a different duration (Figure 6.8). In the

UK Royal College of Psychiatrists OSCE, one circuit consists of eight 7-minute stations and a second four pairs of linked stations each of 10 minutes' duration. A long-station OSCE and a short-station OSCE are described in Case Study 1.

In some circumstances where the number of candidates is few and examiners are limited, as in the Veterinary Nursing Case Study 11, examinees can complete three different circuits with a short break between the circuits (Figure 6.11). The same examiners may act as assessors in the second and third circuits.

More unusually, the OSCE may be organised such that the learner is assessed at the OSCE stations in no set order and the time allocated for each station may vary. This procedure has been adopted at induction courses for newly qualified doctors and only works where the number of examinees is limited (Figure 6.12) and the purpose of the OSCE is formative.

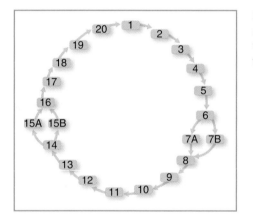

Figure 6.10 Organisation of two double stations (Stations 7 and 15) with alternate students passing through each version of the station.

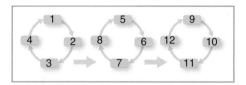

Figure 6.11 Students complete 12 stations arranged in three circuits each with four stations with a break between each circuit.

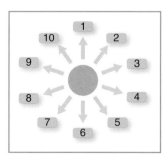

Figure 6.12 Examinees complete the stations in an OSCE in no set order.

Group OSCE (GOSCE)

The standard practice in an OSCE is for examinees to rotate individually around the stations. Examinees can also participate as a member of a group. There are two circumstances where this may be appropriate:

- *The McMaster–Ottawa Team Observed Structured Clinical Encounter (TOSCE).* This is used to assess team skills and interprofessional practice. This is described in Chapter 5, where the assessment of interprofessional and team skills is discussed.

- *As a team experience where learners learn from each other.* Biran (1991) described a Group Objective Structured Clinical Examination (GOSCE), where doctors, as part of a refresher course for General Practitioners, rotated around the OSCE stations in groups, were assessed and reflected on their competence.

A GOSCE has been used with groups of four or five students to one SP as a cost-effective means of assessing large numbers of students (Elliot et al. 1994). It has been used to combine teaching of communication skills using SPs with clinical reasoning exercises in paediatrics and medicine clerkships (Konopasek et al. 2014). Students assess their own competence and in addition receive feedback on their communication skills from SPs, faculty and peers.

The term TOSCE, has been used to describe a similar OSCE experience, as reported by Singleton et al. (1999). To enhance their general practice consultation skills, teams of five third-year medical students rotated around five SP stations as a group, each taking on the role of the General Practitioner, receiving feedback and promoting self-reflection.

Take-home messages

- The OSCE should be designed taking into account the purpose of the examination, the numbers of examinees to be assessed, the breadth of focus of the examination, the learning outcomes to be assessed and the resources, including SPs and examiners available.

- A major advantage of the OSCE is that the format can be adjusted to meet local needs.

- In the development of an OSCE, consideration should be given to:

  - the number of stations.

  - the time allocated to each station and the overall duration of the OSCE.

- the use of 'procedure' and 'question' stations.

- the use of 'double' and 'linked' stations.

- the number of circuits to be organised; and

- the inclusion of feedback as part of the examination.

Does the format adopted for the OSCE best meet the needs of your institution?

The setting for an OSCE 7

The OSCE can be located in a range of settings. The selection of a venue will depend on the nature of the examination and the local circumstances.

The venue

In observing the OSCE in action, we have seen the examination located in a wide range of venues from permanent, custom-designed locations to improvised, temporary settings created specifically to host the examination. We cannot recall ever having encountered a situation where a lack of an appropriate location prevented the organisation of an OSCE. The choice of a location may, however, occasionally test the imagination and organisation skills of those responsible. We were impressed, for example, by the organisation of an OSCE outside in a village in Africa. Only in a few situations will a location be devoted exclusively to the running of OSCEs. Examples include test centres used by The Educational Commission for Foreign Medical Graduates (ECFMG), and the purpose-built assessment centre in Manchester, UK, used for the General Medical Council Professional and Linguistic Assessments Board (PLAB) Part 2 OSCE and the Future Health Care Scientists' Objective Structured Final Assessments (OSFAs). The choice of venue will, to a large extent, be determined by local circumstances.

Choosing a location

In choosing a location, the following points should be taken into account:

- The location needs to be able to accommodate the required number of stations. Twenty or more stations may be needed at one venue. Where more than one circuit has to be run in parallel to cope with the number of examinees, stations from a number of circuits must be accommodated, although circuits can be located at different venues.

- The stations should be located in reasonable proximity so that time is not wasted by the examinee in moving from one station to the next. This is easier if the stations are located as in a circuit shown in Figure 7.1. The location may dictate a more linear arrangement of the stations as in Figure 7.2. In this

83

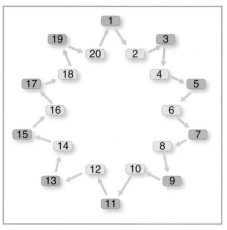

Figure 7.1 Twenty OSCE stations arranged in a circle with alternate procedure stations and questions stations where students are expected to answer a written question, make a note or write a letter.

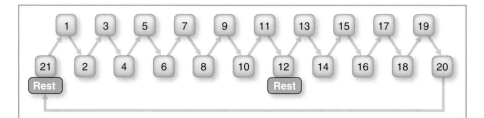

Figure 7.2 Stations are located in rooms 1, 3, 5, 7, 9, 11, 13, 15, 17 and 19. The stations 2, 4, 6, 8, 10, 12, 14, 16, 18, 20 and 21 may be located in the corridor. They may be linked to the preceding or following station, may be data interpretation or problem solving stations, or may be rest stations.

situation, it is helpful to have a rest station at the beginning of the sequence to allow the examinee time to move from the last station to the first station in the circuit. Examinees should be informed about this in the briefing.

- The requirement of process stations where the examinee is observed taking a history, examining a patient or carrying out a procedure are different from the requirements of a station where the examinee has to answer questions, make notes on the previous station or prepare for a process station that follows, for example by reading a patient's case notes. Whilst the former require a measure of privacy and soundproofing, the latter may be located in a corridor outside the room that housed the previous station (Figures 7.1 and 7.2).

- Accommodation at the venue also has to be found for rooms where the examinees assemble and are briefed and the simulated patients (SPs) and examiners assemble.

Multisite OSCEs

OSCEs where large numbers of candidates are to be examined at the same time may be run over several sites. The Manchester Medical School Phase 2 Formative OSCE (Case Study 3) uses education centres at four teaching hospitals simultaneously, with seven or eight circuits at each of the four locations. National licensing examinations, for example in the USA and Canada, are run over multiple sites and across several time zones. Where this is the case, there are several important issues to consider:

- Each venue should, as far as possible, provide a similar experience for candidates in terms of accommodation and equipment for the examination.

- Selection and training of SPs should be coordinated across different sites.

- Selection and training of examiners should be coordinated across the sites.

- Examinee performance across the different sites should be evaluated to confirm the comparability of venues.

Options for an OSCE venue

The most common options for accommodating an OSCE are described below.

A custom-designed suite in a clinical skills unit or simulation centre

Clinical skills suites or centres are now a well-established feature in medical schools and hospitals, and several of the case studies in Section D report the use of clinical skills centres as a location for their OSCEs. Some have been designed with OSCEs in mind and include a number of rooms, each with a couch and a chair. The rooms may have one-way glass windows which allow the performance in the rooms to be observed from an adjacent room. Alternatively, the rooms may be equipped with video recording facilities with the performance monitored from a central room (Box 7.1).

Box 7.1

In the OSCE at the medical school in Groningen, the student was seated in a room with the patient and a video camera. The examiner located elsewhere in the medical school watched and marked the performance of the student. This had the advantages that the examiner was less obtrusive and could not interfere with the examination process. A telephone in the student's room rang when it was time for the student to move to the next station.

In the 1970s, when we first introduced the OSCE, the setting used was the traditional hospital ward. This required close collaboration with the medical and nursing staff. Patients in some bays in the wards and side rooms to the wards served as patients for stations in the OSCE, and other bays were used to house outpatients or SPs. Patients who could not be moved easily from the ward on a temporary basis whilst the examination was in progress remained in their own bays.

Patient care areas

Patient care areas can be adapted to house an OSCE, provided the examination does not interfere with services to patients and ongoing patient activities do not interfere with the examination (Box 7.2). Clinic examination rooms were used for 13 years for the Culture OSCE detailed in Case Study 6 before a hospital simulation centre became available.

With the greater intensity of care and rapid turnover of patients, the hospital ward is now a less likely home for the examination. Newly commissioned hospital wards or wards temporarily out of use for some reason, such as refurbishment, provide useful and attractive venues. Where the majority of patients used are ambulatory patients or SPs, the hospital ward is less appropriate as a venue.

Outpatient clinics or ambulatory care centres can offer a useful venue for an OSCE as in the large-scale Medical Council of Canada's Part II Qualifying Examination, described in Case Study 7. During the working week, these venues are normally fully committed to patient care. However, it is often possible for arrangements to be made so that the facilities are available for use as an OSCE venue outside the normal clinical hours, for example during the weekend.

Teaching accommodations

Accommodations designed primarily for teaching activities may be adapted for use as a venue for the OSCE. A classic example is where there is a series of small rooms available which would normally be used for tutorials or problem-based learning.

Larger rooms and halls can be divided with temporary partitions or screens to provide a venue. This was the practice for the OSCE in experimental medicine organised by Sean Lavelle in Galway, Ireland (Lavelle and Harden 1986, pp. 78–86). In Case Study 5, dividers are brought in to convert teaching rooms into individual OSCE stations. The veterinary nursing OSCE (Case Study 11) utilises teaching accommodation for weekend OSCEs, with minimal changes necessary apart from moving tables and chairs out of the rooms. On Monday the rooms revert to teaching accommodation.

Enhancing realism in an OSCE venue

In a clinical encounter OSCE station, in order to enhance realism, the portrayal of the patient and the environment in which the encounter takes place are important. Even if the OSCE cannot take place in a purpose-built venue or a clinical skills centre or a hospital ward, steps can be taken to make the setting as realistic as possible.

In addition to the station essentials of bed or couch/examination table, desk and chairs, there are other ways to enhance the reality of the encounter in order that the examinee feels he/she is in a real clinical situation. Some measures may be inexpensive to implement; others may not be warranted unless it is a high-stakes examination. For example:

- If the patient is an inpatient, he/she should be dressed either in a hospital gown or night clothes and have a hospital wristband. If in bed, appropriate hospital-issue sheets, pillows and blankets should be used, and an authentic hospital chart should be in place.

- Additional staff, such as nurses, should be dressed in uniform.

- A box of tissues can be provided at a 'breaking bad news' station.

- A stretcher with a covered manikin can be present if the station involves the death of a relative in the emergency room, as in Case Study 8.

- The venue for a ward-based scenario or an emergency room can be enhanced with the use of fake blood and urine; sounds, such as a computer replicating a cardiac monitor; and the smell of alcohol to stimulate the senses (Gormley et al. 2012a). Moulage kits may be purchased to simulate blood and other body fluids, and several YouTube videos are available online to demonstrate their use (website: http://www.youtube.com/). Gormley et al. (2012a) caution, however, that *'it is important that such methods are driven more by pedagogy than by novelty'*, with the aim of stimulating examinees to perform to the best of their ability.

If a station involves a patient encounter, the placement of the bed, couch/examination table, desk, chairs and the position of the patient and the assessor should be arranged such that the assessor has a clear line of sight to the actions and facial expressions of the examinee, the patient and any other participants in the station.

Online OSCE

Recent technological advances have led to the development of online OSCE stations. Mucklow et al. (2012) described an online OSCE designed to assess medical student competence in prescribing. It has 12 stations which assess the student's competence in different aspects of prescribing (Table 7.1).

Table 7.1 Stations in an online OSCE to assess prescribing skills (Mucklow et al. 2012)

1. Deciding on the most appropriate prescription drug to write on a variety of charts
2. Reviewing a prescription; deciding which components are most appropriate
3. Planning management in a particular clinical situation
4. Communicating information to a patient about a newly-prescribed medicine
5. Calculating drug dosage
6. Identifying adverse reactions of specific drugs
7. Drug monitoring
8. Data interpretation of the results of investigations as they relate to decisions

The use of virtual patients to assess clinical reasoning in an OSCE has received support (Cook and Triola 2009). Courteille et al. (2008) used a virtual patient case to assess clinical reasoning and problem solving, including history taking, laboratory tests, physical examinations and a preliminary diagnosis. Oliven et al. (2011) described a computerised OSCE using virtual patients as a reliable tool to assess students' competence in history taking, physical examination and ordering laboratory and imaging tests.

The Drexel University College of Medicine has pioneered web-based OSCEs where the examinees interact with a series of SPs in real time via a teleconferencing programme. This allows students to take the examination at a distance without coming into the academic centre (Novack et al. 2002).

Such online and web-based OSCEs offer possible convenience and cost savings, particularly when the campuses are widely dispersed. They do have limitations associated with the absence of physical interaction in terms of the competencies that can be assessed at a distance.

The use of OSCEs where the examiner, not the examinee, is at a distance has been explored by Chan et al. (2014). Examiners located remotely were able to participate in an OSCE by observing the performance of students at history taking and physical examination stations through a webcam. Ratings by local and remote examiners were found to be reasonably comparable.

Take-home messages

- The OSCE may be located in a custom-designed venue or may be in an area such as a hospital ward or outpatient clinic normally used for patient care, or accommodation used at other times for teaching purposes.

- Not everyone is fortunate to have a custom-designed suite to house an OSCE. Those responsible for organising an OSCE may need to be imaginative and innovative in how they adapt existing accommodation.

- The identification of a venue for an OSCE, which in some circumstances may pose a challenge, should not be seen as an obstacle that cannot be overcome. With imagination and creativity, a solution can be found.

- Attention should be paid to creating a realistic clinical setting for stations in the OSCE.

- Online and web-based OSCEs offer the potential to supplement face-to-face OSCEs.

Have you created an authentic setting for your OSCE?

The patient

8

Patients in an OSCE may be represented by real or simulated patients, computer representations, video recordings, medical records and investigation results or a combination of all these. Each has a specific role to play.

The patient as a variable in the clinical examination

The clinical examination has three variables: the examinee, the examiner and the patient (Figure 8.1). In a clinical examination, the examiner and the patient should be standardised so that the assessment of the examinee's performance is a true measure of his/her clinical competence. In Chapter 9 we look at the role of the examiner. The role of the patient is addressed in this chapter.

We have already highlighted in Chapter 1 a key feature of an OSCE is that the examinee's performance is assessed not just on one but on a number of patients. An examinee's performance with one patient, as in the traditional clinical examination, is simply too limited a sample for a prediction to be made of their performance with other patients. It is also desirable that every examinee is assessed on the same or similar patients and that each patient presents in the same way for every examinee.

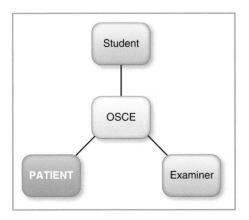

Figure 8.1 The three variables in a clinical examination.

Representation of patients in an OSCE

If patients are a key element in an OSCE, how can they be represented? A number of approaches may be adopted:

- real patients with or without training or briefing.

- simulated or standardised patients (SPs) and their families.

- models or manikins.

- hybrid representations incorporating a simulated patient (SP) and a model.

- video recordings of a patient.

- results of investigations, such as X-rays or ECGs.

- patient medical records.

- text description of a patient.

A station in an OSCE may include interaction with a member of the healthcare team in addition to an interaction with a patient, for example, a nurse as in Case Study 7.

There is no one best approach as to how a patient should be represented in an OSCE. If the OSCE is to achieve its full potential as a tool to assess a candidate's clinical competence, a number of approaches should be adopted, including the use of both real patients and SPs and manikins (Collins and Harden 1998).

In the mid-1980s in the USA, the term *simulated patient* was replaced with *standardised patient* to recognise the importance of keeping constant and not varying how the patient presented to the candidate. We prefer the use of *simulated patient*, however, as it distinguishes an actor portraying a patient from a real patient. 'Real' patients may be rehearsed so that to some extent they can also be standardised.

The decision as to how patients can be best represented in an OSCE will be influenced by local contexts and logistics. For example, the use of SPs dominates OSCEs in the USA to the extent that the OSCE has been referred to as 'a standardised patient examination'. In other countries, only real patients or a mixture of real and standardised patients are used (Figure 8.2). However, this position is changing. Where on the real patient/SP continuum an OSCE is placed depends mainly on three factors:

- *The availability of real patients for use in an OSCE:* Difficulties in recruiting real patients to take part in an OSCE have encouraged the use of SPs as a substitute.

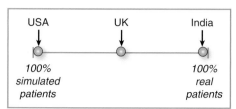

Figure 8.2 **The real patient/SP continuum. The use of real and SPs in an OSCE varies in different contexts. This is changing, however, with real patients used in some situations in the USA, and in countries where only real patients were formerly used, SPs have been introduced in their examinations.**

- *The learning outcomes and clinical skills to be assessed:* Whilst an actor may simulate a real patient in a communication station or some physical examination stations, a real patient is required for physical examination stations where the patient has a finding, such as a hernia or rheumatoid arthritis.

- *The emphasis placed on standardisation is such that all examinees should have an almost identical experience.* This can be more easily achieved with standardised patients. Real patients, however, can also be standardised and carefully matched in terms of their physical findings with their history rehearsed so that examinees have a similar experience.

In this chapter, we look at each of the different approaches to representing a patient in an OSCE.

The real patient

Real patients have an important role to play in an OSCE, particularly where examinees are to be assessed on their approach to a patient with abnormal clinical signs and their interpretation of the signs, for example, in a patient with a goitre or hernia. Smith et al. (2009) described an OSCE used to assess the competence of third-year students in bedside clinical examinations. Patients were selected according to availability, and the examination included those with physical findings that the students were expected to be able to identify at the end of the medicine clerkship, including wheezing, thyroid nodules, exophthalmos, rheumatoid arthritis, mitral regurgitation, ascites, ventral hernia, peripheral neuropathy and muscle wasting. Case Study 3 provides another example of the use of real patients in an OSCE.

In many situations, real patients are readily available and require no rehearsing or training if they are used simply to exhibit their personal signs. If the examination is explained to patients and their permission sought, they are usually willing to participate and frequently appreciate the opportunity to take part in the OSCE. If many examinees are to be assessed, it is advisable to have available for each station two patients matched as far as possible and the patients can be used with alternate candidates. Following the examination, the marks awarded to candidates can be checked to ensure that there are no differences in standards where more than one patient was used. The same applies when patients are used at different circuits of the examination.

When using real patients in an OSCE, it is important to ensure that:

- What is required is carefully explained to the patient and the patient has given his/her consent.

- The patient is not subjected to pain or discomfort, and his/her condition is not exacerbated in any way by repeated examinations.

- The patient's condition is appropriate for him/her to be asked to take part in the examination.

- Any physical findings are checked, as they may have changed with time.

- Patients who may be interrupted during the examination are not selected (e.g. patients on diuretics).

- Tea and refreshments are available for the patient.

- If the patient is an outpatient, travel arrangements have been made.

- The patient is thanked at the end of the examination.

If a real patient is used at a history taking station, the patient may be instructed to:

- Respond to questions asked according to their own experience.

- Modify his/her story in some rehearsed way in order to standardise the history provided.

The inclusion of real patients in an OSCE, even if used alongside standardised patients, has a fundamental effect on the examinee's perception of the OSCE and on the credibility of the examination. Where real patients are used, the examinees' willing suspension of belief is less necessary, as in the case of an examination where the patients are all simulated. Even if examinees know that some of the patients they encounter are SPs, they can never be sure who is the real patient and who is the SP. This can affect their approach to the OSCE and their attitude to the patients they meet in the examination. The use of real patients adds to the validity of the OSCE. Students focus more on the clinical condition when they meet real patients and report a feeling of responsibility to the patient (Bokken et al. 2009).

Simulated patients

A simulated or standardised patient, first established by Howard Barrows in 1963, has been defined as:

> 'a person who is carefully trained to accurately, repeatedly, and realistically re-create the history, physical findings, and psychological and emotional responses of the actual patient on whom the case is based so that anyone encountering that 'patient' experiences the same challenge from the SP, no matter when the case is performed or which of the SPs trained to portray the case is encountered.' (Wallace 2007, p. xvi)

Since the first description of the OSCE in 1975, increasing attention has been paid to the use of SPs in the OSCE, and much research has been undertaken about their role in the examination; their selection, including issues of gender, ethnicity and socio-economic background; their training and briefing; and the possible impact on the SP of acting the role of a patient (Petrusa 2002; Adamo 2003). An SP is an individual who has undergone training to provide a realistic and consistent representation of a clinical encounter. The SP may be a lay person or an actor. In Dundee, SPs were recruited through an advertisement in the local newspaper.

In the OSCE, examinees interact with the SP as though they were taking a history or carrying out a physical examination on a real patient. If appropriately trained and used correctly, the SP should be indistinguishable from a real patient by an expert clinician (see Box 8.1).

Use of simulated patients

SPs can be used to test a broad range of skills, including history taking, physical examination, demonstration of practical procedures and counselling. Most commonly, SPs are used to assess communication skills or physical examinations where no abnormality is found. A range of findings, however, can be simulated (Barrows 1993). Some are more demanding of the patient than others. One case is reported of an SP who developed a skin pathology following an attempt to simulate a dermatology lesion.

SPs can be used in OSCEs to assess the examinee's competence in different fields. The use of SPs in a psychiatric nursing OSCE was described by Selim et al. (2012).

Box 8.1

At a station in a final OSCE in Dundee, medical students had to advise a patient with gastric carcinoma. The patient was accompanied by his wife. At the end of the examination, the external examiner at the station, an experienced surgeon, complained that it was ethically wrong to subject a patient with gastric carcinoma and his wife to the ordeal of the examination. He found it difficult to believe that the patient and his wife at the station were, in fact, simulated and only when he met and talked with them did he accept that this was the case.

This highlighted that the design of scenarios was critical in this particularly challenging area. The scenarios were based on real clinical cases, and psychiatric nurses received intense training in order to act as SPs. The author of each station along with senior faculty watched the SP in training to ensure realism and consistency.

Reliability of simulated patients

In an early study, Tamblyn et al. (1991) reported on variability in the accuracy of patient representation by SPs trained at different institutions. It has been demonstrated since then, however, that an appropriately trained SP can present a consistent portrayal of a patient's history over multiple encounters in an OSCE and that there is also a high level of consistency where different SPs in parallel circuits portray the same encounters. Portrayal of physical findings may be less accurate, but this may be corrected with additional training.

Overall, the gender or ethnicity of the SP has little, if any, effect on the student's performance in the OSCE (Petrusa 2002). Male students may perform marginally better with male SPs and female students with female SPs.

Realism and the simulated patient

It is important to make the SPs portrayal of the patient as realistic as possible in order to trigger more authentic conscious responses from examinees (Gormley et al. 2012a). There is considerable evidence from the psychology literature to support the importance of context in relation to learning and assessment. Godden and Baddeley (1975) found that scuba divers who learned and recalled lists of words under water performed better when asked to recall in the environment in which they learned the words. As the OSCE can be a powerful learning experience as well as an assessment tool, the closer the patient representation relates to clinical practice, the better.

There are a number of measures that can be taken to facilitate a realistic portrayal of a patient in an OSCE, as discussed below.

The patient narrative

In preparing for an OSCE, Nestel et al. (2008) interviewed real patients in the emergency department shortly after a procedure. They used these interviews to create a more realistic simulation. In the training of SPs, their use of 'verbatim statements from patients provided authentic language for actors, offering a richness and consistency of character sometimes lacking in roles crafted by our team'. The authors acknowledge this approach is time consuming and is not appropriate for all SP encounters. SPs have found that meeting and talking with a patient whose condition they are simulating helps them to enact the role better in the context of the OSCE.

Patient characteristics

Realism and credibility is important in terms of SP portrayal. A SP selected to play the role of a young person with anorexia would be more believable if she were a teenager and underweight. Conversely, an obese SP might be used to portray a patient with cardiovascular disease or diabetes or a patient being counselled on the need to lose weight at a health promotion station. However, when the student is aware that the overweight patient they are meeting is an SP, they may experience conflict and not want to hurt the SP's feelings by advising him/her to lose weight (Yazbeck-Karam et al. 2014).

Prosthetics and makeup may be used, for example, to add realism to SPs who do not have physical manifestations of the condition they are portraying, such as wounds and other skin conditions. Water or glycerine may be used to simulate perspiration, as in Case Study 7 in a patient with acute chest pain. Dermatology as a specialty has not, until recently, used SPs to any great extent because of the difficulty in replicating skin lesions, but a novel, temporary tattoo to simulate malignant melanoma was found to be valid, easy to use and replicable across many simultaneous OSCE administrations (Langley et al. 2009), and with the potential to extend to other lesions (Gormley et al. 2012a).

Faculty and students as simulated patients

Members of staff may act both as SP and as examiners in an OSCE and it has been claimed that students are able to think of the staff SP as a real patient (Abdelkhalek et al. 2009). However, if there is a possibility that the student may identify the SP as a member of staff, this is not to be recommended as it does make it more difficult for the student to relate to the patient as they would relate to a real patient. Faculty SPs were found by Mavis et al. (2006) to be more intimidating than actors or student peers acting as SPs. Students did find, however, that the feedback they received from faculty about their performance was more helpful. It may be that where feedback to students is the main purpose of the OSCE, the use of faculty as SPs should be considered.

Students can successfully serve as SPs, and this offers a number of advantages. Students usually require less training than actors in portraying a patient case, and they are a low-cost option. Probably most importantly, students regard acting as an SP as a valuable learning experience and gain significant benefit from acting out the role and from watching their peers perform at an OSCE station. Third-year students were used as SPs and fourth-year students as examiners in a practice formative OSCE at Sydney Medical School, consisting of two history taking stations and one physical examination, one procedural skills and one communication skills stations (Burgess et al. 2013). The student SPs reported a very positive learning experience, allowing them to identify common mistakes. The experience helped their feedback technique and also enhanced their understanding of the patient's perspective.

As in the above example, students usually serve as SPs in the context of a formative OSCE, but they may also act as SPs in a summative examination, as described in Case Study 14. Here students take turns at acting as sonographer and patient at each of the three stations in the abdominal ultrasound OSCE.

Simulated patient as examiner

In addition to simulating the role of a patient, the SP can also be used in an OSCE to assess the examinee's performance. Research suggests that they can assess the examinee more reliably in respect of well-defined technical skills such as history taking and physical examination rather than on social skills, such as empathy and teamwork (Berg et al. 2011). The combination of acting as an SP whilst at the same time assessing the examinee, however, can be extremely challenging, and Newlin-Canzone et al. (2013) suggested: *'The attentional demands of the portrayal task may impact the ability of standardized patients to notice and/or recall important aspects of a learner's nonverbal behaviour that could potentially affect how they rate the learner's communication skills.'* The role of the SP as an examiner is discussed further in Chapter 9.

Level of interaction with simulated patients

The level of interaction between the examinee and the SP should be specified, as it can vary widely. Examples are given below, starting with little or no interaction and increasing to more complex interactions:

- No response is expected from the SP, and no rehearsal or training is necessary in stations where, for example, the student simply has to measure the blood pressure or auscultate the heart.

- The SP is rehearsed on the basic key elements of a history and left to respond to other questions from their own perspective. The SP is expected to replicate his/her portrayal as consistently as possible for each candidate.

- The SP is rehearsed not only in the key points in the patient's history but also in more detail about the patient they are simulating and in the words to be used in response to specific questions. The SP is given a detailed scenario and background to the character they are to portray, scripts to learn, and very detailed instructions as to how to respond to examinees' questions. They may be told what information may be volunteered, what should be said in response to a specific question, and what should not be said. Some of the case studies give very specific instructions to SPs as to the patient they are simulating and what to say and what not to say, as in Case Study 3.

- SPs are trained to respond both verbally and non-verbally with gestures, facial expressions and eye contact to convey emotion. They may be asked to behave in a particular way towards the doctor, for example 'respectful and polite' and 'soft-spoken', to nod when the doctor speaks or to look down rather than making eye contact, as in Case Study 6. They may be asked to be 'a co-operative and friendly patient', as in Case Study 9. In Case Study 8, the SP who is portraying a woman anticipating bad news about her mother is asked to pace the room as the resident arrives and to become emotional and inconsolable. The SP may be briefed also as to the extent to which they should be helpful or obstructive in their responses to questions from the examinee.

- The scenario is rehearsed to evolve according to a strict schedule, with the SP asked to change his/her behaviour at a previously agreed time in the consultation. In Case Study 7 the patient with chest pain simulates differing intensity of pain and fear at each stage of the examination. The mother in Case Study 6 becomes more amenable to the doctor's suggestion for action as the interview proceeds.

- In addition to responding to questions from the examinee, the SP is instructed to ask questions at various stages in the interview. The daughter of a chronically ill patient in Case Study 5 is asked to prompt the student if he/she does not suggest the use of bilevel positive airway pressure (BiPAP) ventilation, or the patient presenting with chest pain in Case Study 2. In Case Study 3, the SP is rehearsed to ask the meaning of any jargon used by the student.

The simulation may involve more than one person. Relatives of the patient may be involved, including a husband, wife, or the parent of a child. Other members of the healthcare team may also be involved, for example the simulated nurse in Case Study 6, who is given clear instructions as to how to respond to the candidate and how to avoid influencing the candidate's decisions. The SP and the simulated nurse need to coordinate their actions according to the candidate's responses and need to devise signals for communication.

SPs should be asked to complete a form expressing satisfaction or dissatisfaction with the simulation, their preparation for it and any recommendations for action. An example is given in Case Study 6.

Training programmes and quality assurance

The situation has moved on from when the SP was an untrained volunteer receiving the minimum of training to a more formal recognition of the role and status of the SP. From the above descriptions, it will be obvious that the extent and forms of SP training required will vary considerably, depending on how the SP is to be used and the extent of their participation in the role play. Extensive resources and advice are now available relating to the training of an SP and facilities may be located through programmes locally in a medical school or centralised regionally or nationally (Adamo 2003). Professional organisations focussing on the SP, such as the Association of Standardised Patient Educators (ASPE), are now established (www.aspeducators.org). Rigorous quality assurance programmes are in place, such as the Clinical Skills Evaluation Collaboration Quality Assurance (CSEC QA) programme, which is responsible for all aspects of the National Board of Medical Examiners Step 2 Clinical Skills examination which includes SPs (Furman 2008).

The advantages of using a simulated patient

As can be deduced from the above descriptions of the role an SP can play in an OSCE, SPs offer many advantages and opportunities to enrich an OSCE station in terms of what is assessed. The use of SPs in an OSCE offers many advantages:

- SPs contribute to the reliability of the OSCE through their training to respond to the examinee consistently and with the response replicated by other SPs at the same station or in other parallel circuits.

- The complexity or difficulty of the presentation can be controlled and modified to the stage of training of the examinee.

- Problems associated with the use of a real patient are avoided, and SPs can be used in a situation where the use of a real patient would be inappropriate (Box 8.1).

- An SP may tolerate more examinee encounters in an OSCE than a real patient would.

- SPs can be trained to assess the examinee's performance and to provide feedback to the learner (see Chapter 9).

- If there is a bank of SPs, an SP may be readily available and can be 'pre-ordered' to meet specific assessment needs.

Simulated patients as a valuable resource

SPs have become widely accepted as a valuable assessment tool in an OSCE. As Adamo (2003) reported, *'We used to hear, "Why would anyone use SPs to test for clinical skills?" Now we hear, "Why would anyone not use SPs to test for clinical skills?"'* The role of the SP can be extremely challenging, and good SPs are a valuable resource to an institution. They need to be looked after and appreciated for the valuable work they do. SPs frequently, as described above, perform three roles – portraying a patient, assessing the examinee and providing feedback on performance – and have become much-respected and valued members of the team. An SP needs to display the same attention to detail with each examinee and may see in excess of 30 examinees in the course of one morning. Whilst they are usually well rehearsed, they may not be working from a script, and their role can be challenging, particularly when asked to respond to an unanticipated question from the student or doctor. Some SPs, particularly when involved in high-stakes examinations, report feeling under pressure to perform to the best of their ability so as to give examinees the best possible chance (Harvey and Radomski 2011).

Issues of potential concern result from portraying psychologically challenging SP roles, such as dementia, mania and schizophrenia, and SPs may report exhaustion, insomnia and short-term depression following the experience (McNaughton et al. 1999).

Simulators

Simulator technology is a powerful educational tool in medicine. Although its use has typically been in formative assessment, simulators are now established in summative high-stakes assessment as well (Damassa and Sitko 2010). Simulators play an important role in an OSCE when either a real patient or an SP is not appropriate at a station designed to assess a practical procedure, such as cystoscopy or cardiopulmonary resuscitation, or when a real patient with the necessary physical findings is not available. Part-task trainers (PTTs) can be used to assess a range of specific competencies in an OSCE, including the insertion of intravenous lines, catheterisation of male and female bladders, pelvic examination, suturing, ring block with local anaesthesia and wedge excision of the nail bed, injection of a joint and anastomotic technique. Information about simulators that can be used for this purpose is available in the catalogues of recognised suppliers. The Ventriloscope, a stethoscope with built-in MP3 player, has been found to provide consistent, abnormal auscultatory signs within an OSCE framework (Verma et al. 2011) and can be controlled by a trained SP to provide hybrid simulation (see below). High-fidelity simulators, such as the Harvey Cardiopulmonary Patient Simulator, have been used in OSCEs to assess competence in auscultation in local and national high-stakes settings, such as the Royal College of Physicians and Surgeons of Canada OSCE (Hatala et al. 2009). Whole body simulators, such as SimMan, can be used to assess a range of anaesthetic and resuscitation activities.

Hybrid simulation

A simulator can be used alongside an SP to provide greater realism or authenticity to the experience (Kneebone et al. 2006). The SP may present, for example, with a simulated wound on the abdomen which requires suturing or may be lying on a bed attached to a simulated pelvis for catheterisation. Such hybrid simulators can be presented to appear authentic and multiple and more complex competencies can be tested. The examinee not only has to catheterise the patient but must also communicate with the patient regarding the procedure. The SP may be programmed to interrupt the catheterisation and ask questions, such as 'Have you done this procedure before?' or 'Will it hurt when the catheter is removed?'

Stations with hybrid simulators allow an assessment to be made not only of the examinee's competence in the practical procedure but also their rapport with the patient and their communication skills. An examinee may be asked to perform an intimate examination whilst at the same time engaging in conversation with an SP trained to be very talkative and friendly, with the aim of simulating what may be perceived as a 'normal' doctor–patient relationship. Posner and Hamstra (2013) found that the communication skills of medical students assessed by using either a PTT or an SP-PTT hybrid to conduct a pelvic examination did not vary; however, if the SP engaged in 'superfluous conversation' students' technical skills were not as good.

The preparation for a hybrid station is demanding and time consuming. Its use should be considered in an OSCE, particularly in a final qualifying or postgraduate examination, where the doctor is expected to communicate with a patient whilst carrying out a procedure.

Video recordings

Video recordings of patients can be incorporated into an OSCE in a number of ways. In a paediatric postgraduate examination, for example, they were used to assess the candidates' decision-making abilities with regard to the management of acutely unwell children and vulnerable infants (Webb et al. 2012). Video recordings are a convenient method of assessing communication skills, particularly in difficult areas, such as paediatrics, geriatrics and psychiatry (Jolly 1981; Fenton and O'Gorman 1984) (Box 8.2).

In a variation of the OSCE – the Objective Structured Video Exam (OSVE) – students watch a series of videos of doctor–patient communications and then answer a set of written questions to assess their ability to identify and understand the communication skills they have seen in the videos (Baribeau et al. 2012; Karabilgin et al. 2012).

Patient medical records and investigations

The patient's records and their investigations may feature in an OSCE, and several of the case studies in Section D include stations where examinees are asked to discuss and interpret the results of an investigation, such as an ECG, abnormal blood results or X-rays.

In the linked station 6.9A and B described in Chapter 6, the patient's medical record is made available to the student at the first station, with the student meeting the patient at the second station.

A letter from a patient was the basis for a station in an examination on experimental medicine described in Chapter 5 (Box 5.2, p. 57).

Box 8.2

In Dundee, video-recorded interviews with patients with psychiatric problems were used at a station in the final-year OSCE. The video recording was programmed to stop at pre-determined points where the examinee was asked to suggest to the examiner what he or she would say next to the patient and why. Whilst the student was not assessed directly on their communication skills with the patient, it was possible with the video recording to assess their understanding of the patient's problem and how they might explore this further in an interview with the patient.

Take-home messages

- Patients may be represented in an OSCE in a number of ways: real patients, SPs, simulators, SPs combined with a simulator, video recordings, case records, and laboratory investigations.

- Each approach has a particular role to play and can assess learning outcomes not easily assessed with other approaches.

- A hybrid SP–simulator should be considered in stations where communication skills and the approach to the patient are to be tested alongside the carrying out of a practical procedure.

- Whilst the selection of approaches will depend on local circumstances, a mixed economy that recognises the stage of the learner and learning outcomes to be assessed is recommended.

Are you getting the most out of your OSCE by using real patients, SPs, manikins and video recordings?

The examiner | 9

Health professionals, simulated patients and students can serve as examiners in an OSCE. Their roles and responsibilities should be defined and training provided.

Examiners and the OSCE

We have discussed in earlier chapters the three variables in the assessment of an examinee's competence – the examinee, the patient and the examiner (Figure 9.1). In this chapter, we look at the examiner. One of the criticisms of the traditional clinical examination, as noted in Chapter 2, was the unreliability of the examiner's judgement, with different examiners awarding a wide range of marks when observing the same performance (Wilson et al. 1969) and with some examiners acting as 'hawks' and others as 'doves' (Stokes 1974).

The OSCE was designed to address these problems, and the examiners have a key role to play. This may include:

- identifying in advance of the examination an overall blueprint for the examination with details of what is to be assessed at each station and an agreed scoring sheet to rate the candidate's performance.

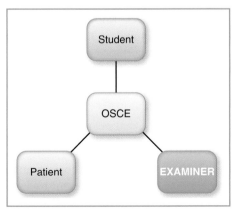

Figure 9.1 The examiner is a key player in the OSCE.

- on the day of the examination, observing and scoring the examinee's performance at the station for which they are responsible. The responsibilities of some examiners may be limited to this role.

- establishing the required standard or pass grade for the OSCE and deciding which students have achieved this, and

- providing feedback to the learner on their performance at the time of the examination or later.

Who is the examiner?

In the traditional clinical examination, the examiner is a senior clinician, with senior physicians taking part in medical examinations, senior surgeons in surgical examinations, and so on, and what is assessed is left to the discretion of the examiner. In the OSCE, the situation is very different. What is assessed at each station, the design of the station, and the marking checklist or global rating scale to be completed at each station are all agreed in advance and a standard setting procedure is in place. On the basis of this it is decided the examinees who are considered to have passed and those who have not passed (Chapter 11). Three things follow from this:

- Advance preparation for the OSCE is essential, with agreement as to what is assessed and how it is to be assessed.

- Briefing and training of the examiner is also essential in advance of the OSCE.

- A wider range of examiners can be used in the OSCE. Examiners can include senior and junior doctors, other healthcare professionals, simulated and real patients and students. The examiners may come from different backgrounds, and this has advantages both from a logistical perspective and from the impact that it has on the examinees. Knowledge, for example, that a student will meet with a family physician and an ENT surgeon in the OSCE highlights for the student the importance of these disciplines. The fact that they will meet a nurse or other healthcare professional recognises the contributions made by these members of the healthcare team and the need for interprofessional teamwork.

Senior and junior doctors

With appropriate training, both senior and junior doctors can play an important role in the OSCE. The examiners may come from different backgrounds and include not only hospital-based, but also community-based specialists. The participation of a qualified healthcare professional as the examiner in an OSCE adds to the validity of the examination and provides a more holistic perspective in the global rating scores for examinees. In some countries, it would need a considerable cultural shift to make it acceptable to rely on assessors who were not qualified healthcare professionals.

Other healthcare professionals

Nurses, dieticians, physiotherapists, chiropodists, health promotion officers and other healthcare workers can all contribute as examiners. For example, a chiropodist may serve as an examiner at a station in a medical OSCE that focuses on a diabetic patient with a problem in his/her foot, and the health promotion officer at a station that focuses on the provision of advice about health promotion.

Simulated patient

We discussed in the previous chapter the important role that simulated patients (SPs) have to play as patients in the OSCE. With suitable training, SPs can also have a role to play in evaluating the learner's performance and in providing feedback to the learner, as described in Chapter 12. The extent of their involvement as an assessor may be confined to rating the examinee's rapport with, and attitude towards, the patient. Alternatively, they may be responsible for rating more generally the examinee's overall performance at the station to complement the professional examiner's rating. They may even serve as the sole examiner at a station, replacing a clinical examiner. In the Educational Commission for Foreign Medical Graduates (ECFMG) Clinical Skills Assessment (CSA), for example, the SP is responsible for assessing the examinee's performance and is considered to be the best assessor of communication skills, particularly non-verbal communication, rather than a third party who is just observing the interaction (Whelan et al. 2005). This is supported by Schwartzman et al. (2011), who noted that, even after identical training, faculty and SPs graded examinees in a communication skills pharmacy OSCE differently, possibly because SPs are directly involved in the interaction with the examinee.

The use of SPs as assessors of the learner's clinical competence in an OSCE is well documented in the literature (Petrusa 2002). Groups including Liew and co-workers (2014) at the International Medical University in Malaysia have demonstrated that SPs can be trained and involved in the assessment of communication skills. In a veterinary OSCE, standardised clients (pet owners) have been used as assessors of a veterinary communication skills OSCE, and the approach was found to be reliable and valid (Artemiou et al. 2014).

Where both an examiner's and an SP's ratings of a student are available, the SP ratings can be considered either separately from the ratings of the clinical examiner, or a method may be devised to combine them (Homer and Pell 2009). There is no general agreement as to the weight that should be attached to the SP rating where both SP and/or health professional rate the examinee.

Real patients have not been used formally as examiners in an OSCE, but their views as to the communication skills and attitude of the examinee may be recorded and taken into account.

Student

Consistent with the move to greater student engagement in the curriculum is a role for students as examiners in an OSCE. For the most part this is in a formative examination with the student working alongside a qualified examiner. There is evidence to support the use of student examiners in a formative capacity, and Moineau et al. (2011) reported moderate to high correlations between fourth-year students and faculty examiners, with a higher correlation on checklist items than on global ratings. Ogden et al. (2000) demonstrated that final-year dental students could be used in an OSCE where basic clinical skills were to be evaluated. Burgess and co-workers (2013) at the University of Sydney, Australia, introduced a practice OSCE where junior students were assessed by senior peers in history taking, physical examination and procedural skills. This peer assessment in a mock OSCE was found to be a useful learning activity, but training of the student examiners was necessary.

Students are notoriously bad at assessing their own competence in examinations and should be encouraged to assess their own performance in an OSCE. Self-assessment should be encouraged, as it is an important competence for the practising doctor and represents one aspect of professionalism – the healthcare worker needs to be an enquirer into his/her own competence. Students may be able to assess their own competence in some areas better than others, but the skills of self-assessment can be improved with practice (Jahan et al. 2011).

Familiarity of examiner and examinee

Familiarity of the examiner with a candidate may be a source of bias in an OSCE (Stroud et al. 2011), but training can help to reduce this. In Case Study 3 where circuits are run concurrently at four teaching hospitals in Manchester, students are assessed at a different site from where they are trained so that they do not meet examiners who know them. This option, however, may not always be possible. In the OSCE administered by the College of Massage Therapists of Ontario (2014), candidates have an opportunity to view a list of examiners and standardised clients and examiners are given a list of candidates. Candidates and examiners are expected to indicate if there is a potential conflict of interest.

The distant examiner

Distributed medical education is now commonplace, with students taught away from a main teaching centre. Examinations including the OSCE are usually organised centrally because of resource and security issues. However, as demonstrated by Chan et al. (2014), examiners from a distant teaching site may take part in an OSCE at a distance.

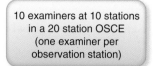

| 10 examiners at 10 stations in a 20 station OSCE (one examiner per observation station) | > | 10 examiners at 5 stations in a 10 station OSCE (two examiners per observation station) |

Figure 9.2 If examiners are available, increasing the number of stations leads to a more reliable and valid examination than having multiple raters at a station (van der Vleuten and Swanson 1990).

Number of examiners

A feature of the OSCE is that examinees are assessed by a number of examiners. Usually one examiner is allocated to each station where the examinee's performance has to be observed and scored. The use of multiple examiners at a station has only a marginal effect on the reliability of the scores (van der Vleuten and Swanson 1990). There is more value in using additional examiners to increase the number of stations rather than using two examiners at one station (Figure 9.2).

Role of the examiner

The examiner has a number of possible roles in an OSCE, but not all examiners are required to fill all of the roles.

Before the OSCE

The examiner's role before the OSCE may include:

- preparing the OSCE blueprint and deciding what learning outcomes, core tasks and subjects should be assessed in the OSCE (Chapter 10).

- designing individual stations in the OSCE, including the preparation of the checklist and rating scale, instructions for candidates, and briefing for SPs, if required.

- determining the standard setting procedures to be adopted; and

- briefing the candidates in advance and, if necessary, familiarising them with the approach through a mock OSCE.

During the OSCE

The examiner's role during the OSCE may include:

- checking resources at the station for which the examiner is responsible, including the patient or SP.

- greeting the examinee and checking his/her name or number.

- observing the examinee and completing the checklist and/or global rating scale.

- providing comments on the scoring sheet with regard to the examinee's performance which will serve later as feedback to the examinee.

- confirming that a SP at a station portrays the clinical condition appropriately throughout the examination and responds to the examinee according to the brief provided.

- ensuring the station keeps to time, particularly when there are several timed elements, as in Case Study 14, and ensuring that examinees move to the next station on the time signal; and

- keeping a record of any problems that arise in the examination.

After the examination

Following the OSCE, the examiner's role may include:

- marking written question stations.

- deciding the outcome for each examinee on the basis of agreed standard setting procedures.

- providing feedback to examinees individually or in a group (see Chapter 12).

- evaluating the stations and the examination process with a view to determining whether any changes are required on a future occasion; and

- reviewing the curriculum or training programme in the light of the examinees' performance in the OSCE.

Instructions for examiners

Written instructions as to what is expected at the station should be given to the examiner in relation to the station for which he/she is responsible. These should include:

- any verbal instructions to be given to the candidate in addition to the written instructions provided at the stations.

- the instructions for the SP and/or others involved in the station, if applicable.

- directions as to the record to be kept of the candidate's performance, including the completion of any checklist or global rating scale, together with the provision of narrative feedback.

- when and under what circumstances, if at all, an examiner should intervene or comment during an examination; and

- what, if any, timekeeping is required relating to the different tasks faced by the examinee at the station.

Examples of examiners' instructions are given in the case studies. Some stations are complex and the examiner receives a detailed briefing. An example is the card sorting task in the multiple mini-interview Case Study 15 where the examiner is asked to read the simulated helper instructions as well as the examiner briefing, and is also given an explanation of the appropriate card sorting strategy and scoring criteria.

In Case Study 3 from Manchester Medical School the examiner is briefed on his/her role, what is expected of the candidate and the marking guidance sheet. In this case, the examiner is asked to read the station instructions to the student only if necessary to help the student to get started and is asked to prompt the student to speed up if he/she is unlikely to complete both parts of the task of taking a history and writing a prescription chart within the time allocated. In other OSCEs, examiners are told not to interact with the student during or after the station, for example the chest pain station in Case Study 2 and the counselling of an insulin-dependent patient in Case Study 12. The station detailed in Case Study 14 gives the examiner a written script for communication with students performing an abdominal ultrasound examination. Instructions to examiners are typed in italics to remind them not to read these out to the student. A precise timeline is included for each stage, with 1 minute for theoretical questions and a suggested response to deal with students with 'verbal diarrhoea'.

Opinions will differ as to whether it is appropriate to prompt candidates in an OSCE, but all examiners should know the agreed policy with regard to prompting in advance in order that all candidates are given the same experience. The policy with regard to intervention by an examiner is likely to depend on the year of the candidate and the purpose of the examination, for example a formative or a summative barrier examination.

Training of the examiner

We have discussed in earlier chapters how the reliability of an OSCE can be enhanced by increasing the number of stations. The reliability of the examination can also be enhanced by investing in the training of the examiners (Box 9.1). Regardless as to who serves as an examiner in an OSCE, it is important that with appropriate training they have sufficient experience and expertise to undertake accurately what is expected of them in the examination.

Box 9.1

At Vienna Medical University, the last hurdle before the 720 students' progress to their first clerkship is an OSCE designed to assess their basic clinical skills. In order to improve the reliability of the examination, it was decided that rather than adding another station to the OSCE, the most valuable approach would be to provide effective training for the 74 examiners involved (Preusche et al. 2012).

It is essential that examiners are briefed in advance of their participation on the day of the OSCE about:

- the philosophy underpinning the OSCE.

- the interpretation and format of the OSCE in the local context.

- the timing and arrangements on the day of the examination.

- their role at a station in the OSCE, including the use of checklists and global rating scales; and

- any other role that they may have relating to the OSCE, such as briefing or providing feedback to examinees.

As each examination and the stations within it will change from one examination to the next, even an experienced examiner needs to be briefed. Training is particularly important for new assessors and should be provided with local needs in mind. Preusche et al. (2012) highlighted some key points for examiner training which merit consideration:

- The need for the training programme should be emphasised, with participation of examiners required.

- Separate three-hour workshops focusing on different types of stations, for example history taking, physical examination and procedure stations should be provided one week before the OSCE.

- During the workshop the common examiner errors should be discussed based on what is already known in the literature, for example the problem of 'hawks' and 'doves', and from the findings from examiners in previous years when the OSCE was administered.

- During the workshop, examiners should mark, using a checklist and global rating scale, a video recording of examinees performing at a previous OSCE station or a live station mock-up with a student. The example should be similar to the one for which they will be responsible. Following this they should have the opportunity to discuss their scoring with colleagues and with an experienced examiner.

- Prepare the examiner for situations where something may go wrong in the examination or at the station. For example, the candidate may have taken the incorrect route and arrived late for the station, the patient may be no longer able to take part or a fire alarm signal is sounded.

- Prior to the examination the examiners should be engaged, where possible, with the construction of stations and in the standard setting process by asking them to think about what would be expected at the station of a minimally competent examinee.

As part of the training, the implication of passing or failing a candidate should be fully explored with examiners. Tweed et al. (2013) highlight a concern that, in spite of efforts to improve the quality of assessment data, assessors may lack the confidence to fail a student even when there is adequate evidence to support the decision. Whilst face-to-face training sessions are important, they can be augmented by the use of an online training resource which allows examiners to compare their global ratings of sample students with those of their peers (Gormley et al. 2012b).

There is wide support in the literature for the need for examiner training. Bartman et al. (2013) identified extreme raters in a high-stakes OSCE with a mean of three standard deviations below (hawks) or above (doves) the overall mean. They report that hawks were generally unaware of their extreme marking and were keen to take on board the feedback. There is some evidence that examiners become more 'hawkish' as their experience grows (McManus et al. 2006) and that examiners may be at their most lenient at the start of an OSCE (Hope and Cameron 2015).

A challenging role

The role of an examiner at an OSCE station can be extremely challenging, and studies have pointed to the high mental workload of OSCE examiners (Tavares and Eva 2013; Byrne et al. 2014). Given the importance of the rater's decision, particularly in high-stakes examinations, an understanding of the potential limitations of the rater's observation skills (Holmboe 2004) and of the ability to process the resulting information (Young et al. 2014) is important. Tavares and Eva (2013) suggest the rater's role might need to be simplified. It is important that even after training, we should be mindful of the potential limitations of examiners.

Take-home messages

- Examiners from a range of backgrounds can be used in the OSCE, including junior and senior doctors, other healthcare professionals, simulated and real patients, and students.

- Advance knowledge of the examiner's medical background can impact on examinees and their learning.

- Examiners can have different roles before, during and following the examination; these must be clearly defined and made explicit in written instructions.

- Training and full briefing of the examiner is essential.

  Is there a formal training programme for examiners that equips them to fulfil their roles in the OSCE in your institution?

Implementing an OSCE 10

There are 'good' and 'bad' OSCEs. Advance planning and effective organisation on the day are necessary to deliver a 'good' OSCE.

Plan for a successful OSCE

In previous chapters we have looked at the elements that go to make up an OSCE – the patients (simulated, real or represented by a model or video), the examiners, the venues and the number, length and content of stations. We have looked at what can be assessed in an OSCE, and different OSCE formats have been illustrated. In the case studies in Section D we include examples of how the OSCE can be implemented in different phases of education and in different areas.

In this chapter we describe the steps necessary to successfully deliver an OSCE, the decisions to be taken and the actions required. The delivery of an OSCE requires input from a number of people and the process may appear complicated and demanding. Whilst this is true, if the steps described are followed, a successful OSCE will be the result. We have seen in practice 'good' OSCEs (some astonishingly innovative and beautifully executed) and 'bad' OSCEs where the necessary attention to detail has not been paid and where there was a failure to grasp some of the basic underlying requirements for an OSCE. At an Ottawa Conference we referred to 'The OSCE as a POSCE' (a Potentially Objective Structured Clinical Examination). The OSCE has the potential to serve as a reliable and valid tool to assess clinical competence and to offer the advantages discussed in the early chapters. Its success or failure, however, will depend on the advance preparation and how well it is executed on the day. Bad OSCEs are the result of poor preparation. Validity and reliability are not functions of the OSCE approach *per se* but rather of how it is delivered in practice.

The following recommendations should not be seen as a rigid prescription for the creation of an OSCE but rather as guidelines which can be adapted to meet local needs. In some situations the process can be simplified, but serious consideration first needs to be given before any stages or action points are omitted.

Advance planning for an OSCE

It is impossible to place too much emphasis on the need for advance planning. To allow insufficient time for the preparation of an OSCE is to court disaster. Careful planning is essential if the problems sometimes found associated with the administration of an OSCE are to be avoided and a successful examination is to be delivered (Khan et al. 2013). The decisions and required actions in advance of the OSCE are listed below:

1. **Identify and agree the individuals and committee members responsible** for the OSCE. It is important that the organising committee includes the key stakeholders. For example, if an integrated examination is to be delivered covering a range of disciplines, the major disciplines should be represented. It is essential that one person – the OSCE Lead – is identified as the overall manager and coordinator with responsibility and accountability for the advance planning and for the implementation of the examination on the day. The responsibility may be assigned to a more junior member of staff who is linked to and works with a more experienced individual. In addition to the OSCE Lead who has responsibility for the OSCE, individuals should be designated with specific responsibilities as listed in Table 10.1.

2. **Confirm the purpose of the examination, the areas to be assessed** and how the examination relates to the teaching and learning programme. This should be obvious but can usefully be restated. The examination may be intended to assess the communication skills and other competencies acquired in a 3-month introduction to clinical skills course and to be used for both summative and formative purposes, or it may be a summative final examination as part of the assessment of the student's competence to graduate and practise as a junior doctor under supervision. The aim and purpose of the examination will determine the stations to be included and the skills to be assessed at each station.

Table 10.1 Individuals should be designated with the following OSCE-related responsibilities

- Developing and testing a station once the station brief has been specified
- Serving as a circuit organiser when there is more than one simultaneous circuit
- Identifying and briefing patients and simulated patients (SPs)
- Organising the venue and the resources required
- Serving as an examiner at the stations
- Marking any written responses
- Briefing candidates on the day of the examination
- Timekeeping on the day of the examination
- Shepherding the candidates around the stations
- Looking after patients and SPs on the day of the examination
- Briefing and training examiners

The examination, particularly when part of a postgraduate training programme, may be designed to assess in depth a more narrowly focussed range of skills.

3. **Agree a timeline** for the work to be undertaken in preparing for and delivering the OSCE. Whilst an OSCE may be prepared in days or weeks, for the steps to be undertaken as described below, including the necessary consultation, several months are usually necessary. If a similar examination has been delivered in the past, the timescale may be shortened but sufficient time should still be allocated for the necessary preparation, including the briefing of the examiners.

4. **Decide the number and duration of stations to be included** in the examination and the number of circuits required. This will be influenced by:

   - the number of examinees (Table 6.1 in Chapter 6 may be helpful).

   - the range of learning outcomes or subjects to be assessed (see Chapter 5); and

   - the level of reliability required. The reliability is influenced by the number of stations on which the examinee is assessed (see Chapter 3). More stations may be included in a high-stakes examination.

5. **Arrange a suitable venue or venues** to accommodate the examination. The options are discussed in Chapter 7. They include:

   - a custom designed examination centre, for example in a clinical skills unit.

   - a ward or outpatient hospital accommodation; and

   - areas, such as a large hall or teaching rooms, adapted for the purpose.

Depending on how many candidates are to be examined, more than one circuit at the same venue or circuits at other venues will be required. This is discussed in more detail in Chapter 6. Rooms should be of the appropriate size and specification to meet the station requirements, including personnel and equipment. Lighting should be adequate, and appropriately placed power sockets or extension cables should be provided if necessary. Soundproofing should be taken into account in order that participants at neighbouring stations are not overheard, although this may be less easy if stations have been formed by placing dividers in a large room, as is sometimes the case. If a rest station is located next to the following station, it should not be possible for the 'resting' candidate to overhear the discussions taking place at the adjacent station.

If there is an examinee with a disability, the venue should be checked to ensure that the examinee can be accommodated and that any required resources and personnel can be provided. This is covered further in Chapter 13.

A room should be available where the examinees will assemble and be briefed and a separate rooms where the examiners and simulated patients (SPs) can assemble and relax during breaks.

6. **Prepare an examination grid or blueprint**. The blueprint for the examination provides a summary of what is covered in the examination. It may relate the body systems to the key learning domains to be tested, such as communication skills, physical examination, practical procedures, patient investigations and problem solving. At best an examination can test only a sample of competencies in a specific area. Communication skills can be assessed, for example in the respiratory system (a patient with breathlessness), in the renal system (a patient with haematuria) and in the alimentary system (a patient with abdominal pain), whilst physical examination skills may be assessed in the cardiovascular systems (a patient with a cardiac murmur), the musculoskeletal system (a patient with rheumatoid arthritis), and the endocrine system (a patient with a goitre). An example of a grid is given in Table 1.3 in Chapter 1. Other examples are provided in the case studies.

Where linked stations or double stations are planned as described in Chapter 6, this should be noted on the grid. An example of two linked stations is a station where the candidate is observed taking a history from a patient with breathlessness followed by a station where he/she is asked questions on paper about his/her findings or is asked to write a note about them and perhaps their interpretation. This option is discussed further in Chapter 6.

7. **Prepare a list of stations** and their proposed sequence based on the grid. The list of stations as shown in Table 10.2 should include the station number and the learning outcome to be assessed. Space is left for the name of the examiner and whether a real, SP or manikin is required to be added later.

The list of stations will identify linked and double stations and will note the 'rest' stations to be included. Although there is no strict rule, it is common practice to have a rest station for every 60 minutes of examination time. If the stations are located at a distance as in the layout in Figure 7.2 in Chapter 7, it is helpful to have a rest station separating them.

Table 10.2 Headings for table listing OSCE stations

Station No.	Description of station	Learning outcomes assessed	Examiner	Patient	Other resources

8. **Develop individual stations** based on the grid and list of stations. Responsibilities for this task should be allocated to those with an interest in the area and may be shared. For example, a surgeon and a general practitioner may take joint responsibility for a station on abdominal examination. For each station the following should be prepared:

    *   instructions for the candidate.

    *   instructions for the examiner, including a checklist and/or global rating scale as discussed in Chapter 11.

    *   details of a patient representation (as discussed further in Chapter 8), for example a real patient, SP or manikin, including a brief where an SP is required; and

    *   a list of resources required.

    Examples of the documentation required are given in the case studies in Section D.

9. **Proposals for each station,** including the supporting documentation, should be reviewed and agreed by the OSCE committee with attention paid to:

    *   Does it fulfil the station brief and represent a valid assessment of the outcome(s) to be tested?

    *   Does the content of the station map to the curriculum and education programme?

    *   Can the candidate complete the task required in the time available?

    *   Are the instructions to the candidate, examiner and SPs (where included) clear and unambiguous?

    *   Are all required resources stated and available?

    It is useful to pilot a new station. This can be done in a mock OSCE or in a low-stakes OSCE. If used for the first time in a high-stakes OSCE the result must be closely monitored, and if difficulties arise, the station should be excluded from the final assessment.

    The task required of the candidate at the station, the examiner's checklist or rating scale and the instructions to the SP will vary with the level of the experience of the candidate, with relatively simple requirements of students in the early years of the medical course and more complex and demanding stations for senior students or doctors.

10. **Agree the marking scheme** for each station and for the examination overall. This is discussed in Chapter 11. What standard is expected of the examinee at each station and in the examination overall? Should an examinee be able to compensate for poor performance at one station or in stations covering one domain, such as communication skills with better performance in the rest of the examination?

11. **Appoint examiners** for each station where an examiner is required and ascertain their availability and commitment to the examination. Add the names of the examiners to the list of stations (Table 10.2). (Examiners are not needed at a question station, a data interpretation station, at one part of a linked station or a rest station). It is usual practice in OSCEs to allocate only one examiner for each station – the added value of a second examiner is only minimal. Using any further examiners at additional stations has a greater impact on the reliability of that examination than allocating two examiners to one station. Examiners will be required to mark the candidates' written responses.

    It is essential that the examiner is briefed fully in advance and a formal briefing session should be organised for examiners not familiar with the OSCE process. The training of examiners is discussed further in Chapter 9. It is useful to have one or two examiners in reserve in case the assigned examiner is unable to participate in the OSCE on the day.

12. **Arrange SPs** and fully brief them as discussed in Chapter 8. Add the details to the list of stations. Real patients may be assumed to be available in the hospital at the time of the examination or identified from a bank of available patients with chronic conditions. Decide what, if any, role the SP has as an assessor of the examinee's competence.

13. **Organise resources** as specified on the list of stations, including:

    - beds, chairs and other furniture.

    - equipment, including, for example, ophthalmoscopes, IV infusion sets and inhalers, with spare equipment in case of malfunction, and spare batteries.

    - patient simulators; and

    - timing device and signal that is audible throughout the venue.

14. **Organise catering** for the examiners and patients and provide water for examinees at rest stations.

15. **Prepare packets for each station,** including:

    - the examination timetable.

    - a set of examinee instructions.

- an examiner's scoring sheet for each examinee to be assessed at the station or an equivalent electronic system for recording the marks (see Chapter 11).

- information about the patient or SP; and

- a list of the equipment available.

16. **Finalise the master list of stations** when the initial preparatory work has been completed, with the addition of the names of examiners and information about the patients and other resources required.

17. **Prepare a map of the OSCE circuit** identifying the position of each station at the venue.

18. **Prepare direction arrows and station identification cards** with large numbers to identify stations. Cards and arrows will be mounted on walls or partitions to direct candidates around the circuit. Ideally arrows should also be located on the floor to indicate the route between stations.

19. **Prepare a smaller set of cards with station numbers** for distribution to candidates at the pre-OSCE briefing. Each candidate will be given one card which will indicate the station at which they should start. Coloured cards should be used for the second station in a linked station sequence.

20. **Prepare a list of candidates,** including their allocation to a circuit where the OSCE has more than one circuit.

21. **Inform candidates in advance** with regard to the format of the examination and when and where they are expected to attend.

22. **Set up stations** the day before the examination is scheduled to allow time for troubleshooting. Where the venue is normally used for teaching or clinical work, it may only be possible to set up the stations the evening before the examination.

    An example of helpful guidelines and information that should be provided to the designated person responsible for setting up the OSCE station is given in Case Study 3. It includes the resources and equipment needed and how the furniture in the station should be placed so that the examiner can clearly see the faces of the SP and the examinee.

Implementing the OSCE on the day

The OSCE should proceed smoothly on the day of the examination if the advance planning as described above has been carefully undertaken. The individual with the responsibility for the examination – the OSCE Lead – has an important coordinating role on the day of the examination. This includes managing the overall process and dealing with any problems as they arise. Where there are multiple circuits, a coordinator should be appointed for each circuit, responsible to the OSCE Lead.

The following actions are required on the day of the examination:

1. **The OSCE Lead** should be present at the examination venue at least 1 hour prior to the scheduled start time to check:

    •   the position and numbering of each station.

    •   the direction signs are clear, with arrows on the walls or preferably prominently placed on the floor.

    •   each station is laid out appropriately with chair, bed, etc.; and

    •   any equipment or manikins required are available at the station.

2. **Simulated and real patients** should be present at their station 30 minutes prior to the examination start.

3. **The examiners** should arrive at least 30 minutes prior to the examination for a final briefing. They should be handed their station packet with instructions and examinee scoring sheets, directed to their station and introduced to the patient at the station.

4. **Where an examiner fails to arrive,** the reserve examiner must be briefed about the station and his/her role.

5. **Examinees** should be instructed to assemble 30 minutes prior to the start of the examination. They should have a final briefing by the member of staff to whom this responsibility is delegated:

    •   Examinees should be given a map showing the circuit for the stations.

    •   Where there are linked or double stations, they should be given specific instructions.

    •   They should be instructed to wear a name badge.

    •   They should be briefed on fire alarm arrangements. (During one OSCE in which we participated, students had to be evacuated because of a fire alarm!).

    •   Examinees should be given a card with the number of the station assigned to them for the start of the examination. A coloured card indicates that the candidate will proceed to the station corresponding to the number on the card at the start of the examination but will rest for the first period and not start the examination until the second signal when they will move to the next station. Alternatively, candidates in a linked station may start the OSCE ahead of the other candidates as in Case Study 12. This is usually more difficult to organise.

6. **When all candidates and examiners are present at their stations,** a bell or other sound should signal the start of the examination.

7. **The timekeeper** should repeat the signal at the prescribed time intervals, ensuring it is audible in all the stations. A 1-minute warning signal may be given, but this is usually thought not to be necessary. The advance 1-minute warning may be indicated by a short signal and either one long or two short signals to indicate that the candidate should move to the next station. The end of the examination will be signalled by a longer time signal.

8. **Instructions and information presented at the second of each pair of linked stations** should be covered at the start of the examination for the first time and only uncovered at the time signal marking the end of the first time.

9. **Where candidates are expected to give a written response at a station**, they can be asked to complete this either on a master answer sheet which they carry round with them during the examination or preferably on a station response sheet which is placed through a slot in a box at the station. Alternatively, an electronic response system may be used.

10. **Refreshments** should be made available for the patients and examiners after the examination or during a 30-minute break between two circuits of the examination.

11. **If there is a second group of examinees**, they should assemble before the end of the first circuit of the examination in order to safeguard the integrity of the examination. The group should be briefed during the break between the first and second circuits whilst the patients and examiners are having refreshments.

12. **At the end of the examination, thank all concerned**. You may be dependent on them for their help on a further occasion!

13. **Ensure that simulated or real patients receive their expenses** and any additional remuneration agreed and that their return journey following the examination is facilitated.

14. Where a paper response system is used, **collect score sheets** from the examiners and written responses from the examinees at the end of the

examination. These can be also be collected during the examination and marking commenced immediately.

15. **A debriefing** may be arranged immediately following the examination when the examiners meet with the learners to discuss the examination and the learners' overall performance at each station. This is not always possible, but when organised it can be a powerful learning experience for the examinee's perspective. Feedback to examinees is discussed further in Chapter 12.

16. The OSCE Lead should **keep a record of the examination,** noting at the time of the examination any problems as they arise. This can be useful in planning future OSCEs and also in dealing with any subsequent complaints from candidates. In our experience, student complaints are very unusual. Also noted may be aspects of the examination which work well or where improvements might be made in the future.

Problems during the examination

Occasionally, unexpected problems arise during the OSCE. Probably the most common problem is that a candidate is unable to complete a station either because he/she lost their way in the circuit or because the patient at the station becomes unavailable for a short period. This can be addressed by asking the candidate to return to the station at the end of the examination and informing the examiner and the patient at the station.

Take-home messages

- The success of an OSCE depends on careful and detailed advanced planning and on the organisation on the day. This is summarised in Table 10.3.

- All of the stakeholders should be engaged and briefed, including:

  - OSCE Lead.

  - committee members.

  - venue/circuit organisers.

  - examiners.

  - patients and SPs; and

  - examinees.

- A blueprint should be prepared for the examination together with a list of stations. This should include the specific requirements for each station.

- Stations should be developed and reviewed as specified in the blueprint.

- Stations should preferably be set up the day before the examination.

- On the day of the examination, ensure that everything is in place, the signposts are clear, and the examinees, examiners and patients are briefed.

 Do all of the stakeholders in your programme work as a team to deliver an effective and efficient OSCE?

Table 10.3 Planning for an OSCE

Advance planning for an OSCE

- Set up Organising Committee, designate responsibilities and appoint OSCE Lead
- Review aim of examination and what is to be assessed
- Agree a timeline for development of the examination
- Decide on the number and duration of stations
- Arrange venue(s) for the examination
- Prepare examination grid or blueprint
- Prepare list of stations and update with details of patients and examiners
- Develop individual stations, confirm appropriateness/feasibility of each station and pilot new stations
- Agree standard settings procedure and pass/fail decision process
- Appoint examiners
- Arrange SPs or real patients
- Organise resources required for each station, including manikins
- Prepare documentation for each station
- Prepare map of circuit
- Prepare station identification cards and numbered candidate allocation cards
- Prepare list of candidates
- Brief candidates in advance
- Arrange catering

On the day

- Check venue well before start of the examination
- Check examiners and patients are at stations where required
- Assemble and brief candidates
- Signal start of examination and keep to time with time signals
- Uncover second part of linked station(s) after first time
- Collect examiner score sheets and candidate response sheets
- Organise examinee feedback (if appropriate)
- Arrange refreshments
- Thank all concerned and arrange expenses for patients
- Document any problems that have occurred

Evaluating the examinee's performance | 11

Different approaches can be adopted for assessing performance in an OSCE, making pass/fail decisions and setting standards.

The challenge

Tuckman (1975, p. 180) described the examination in paratrooper training. Trainees have to jump from a plane from a height of 8,000 to 10,000 feet wearing the parachute that they have packed themselves. Any trainee showing up for graduation the next day receives a diploma. Unfortunately, criteria for success in an OSCE are less objectively defined. There are no absolute rules for examiners to use in recording a student's or trainee's performance during the OSCE or coming to a judgement as to whether the examinee has reached the required standard or not.

The extensive work undertaken in preparing for and implementing an OSCE, including the development of the stations and the participation of the examiners and patients, will be wasted unless careful attention (Figure 11.1) is paid to:

- the collection of evidence during the OSCE which truly reflects the performance of an examinee.

- the use of the evidence to inform decisions as to whether the examinee has achieved the required standard; and

- the provision of meaningful feedback to the examinee and curriculum developers. (The provision of feedback is discussed in more detail in Chapter 12.)

The information needed and the decision-making process may be different depending on the purpose of the assessment:

- for pass/fail decisions where standard setting and decisions particularly around the borderline candidate are important.

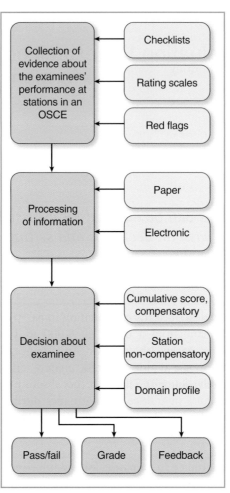

Figure 11.1 Evaluation of examinee in an OSCE.

- for feedback to students and curriculum developers where a detailed evaluation of the student's performance in specific areas is required; and

- to select a specific number of students, for example those most suited to enter medical studies or to be accepted for a postgraduate training programme in a specific field.

Whatever the purpose, it is important to recognise that the overall aim is to increase the validity, fairness and accountability of the assessment.

Collecting the evidence

The OSCE is a performance test. A major advantage of the OSCE is that relevant information is obtained during the examination about the practical and clinical competence of the individual regardless of whether the examinee is a student, a trainee or a practising physician.

Information is collected during the examination by the:

- examiner (who is discussed in more detail in Chapter 9).

- simulated patient (SP) or real patient (who is discussed in Chapter 8); and

- examinees' paper or electronic responses with regard to their findings, their interpretation and the further management of the patient.

Some stations may be captured on video for further analysis later.

Whatever method is adopted to collect the evidence about the student's or trainee's performance, the marking scheme should be part of the development of the station as discussed in Chapter 10. This may be time consuming but is well worth the effort. The items to be included in the scoring sheets for the stations need to be agreed in advance and should be discussed and debated with all the key stakeholders. This process addresses not simply the design of an OSCE station but requires an agreement and clarification of the expected learning outcomes (Box 11.1). Bouhuijs et al. (1987, p. 188) highlighted that in constructing OSCEs, some time is usually spent in overcoming differences of opinion:

> 'Faculty members choose subjects belonging to the domain and construct a preliminary checklist. It's clear that the availability of "standards" is a great help. Subsequently these checklists are screened by a so-called assessment-committee with respect to expected difficulty, content,

---

Box 11.1 Preparation of checklists and rating scales

One of the elements of the OSCE that requires a significant investment of time is the preparation of the rating scales or checklists for each station. In an integrated final qualifying examination in Dundee, medical students were required to take a history from a patient who complained of abdominal pain. In preparing the patient scenario and in constructing the checklist and rating scales to be used at the station, there was an energetic discussion between the professors of surgery and general practice as to what should be expected of the student. This was as much, if not more, about a clarification of the related learning outcomes rather than simply getting an agreement on the items to be included in the checklist. The result of the discussions was an improved specification of the curriculum outcomes as well as the production of the required score sheets for students in the examination.

A similar useful discussion took place between a physician and a chiropodist around a station where the student had to manage the care of the feet for a patient with poorly controlled diabetes.

relevance and adequacy of operation. After screening by the committee and consulting the constructors of the list a definite version is determined.'

The marking scheme or scoring rubric, as it is sometimes termed, is the means by which the examinees' performance is measured during the OSCE. It can include:

- checklists, which record individual elements of the examinee's performance – this is sometimes termed an 'analytic approach'.

- rating scales that provide a more overall judgement of the examinee's performance – a 'holistic approach'.

- red or yellow flags indicating a serious problem with the examinee or bonus points indicating an exceptionally good performance; and

- narrative comments from the examiner.

Checklists

Checklists are widely used in the assessment of the examinee's performance in the OSCE as can be seen from the examples in the case studies in Section D. A checklist is a list of what is expected of the student at the station. It is basically a set of instructions to the examiner relating to the evaluation of an examinee's performance. It is a way of taking the criteria that have been agreed by those responsible for creating the station and externalising and systematising them by writing them down. The criteria for the satisfactory completion of the task as set at each station in the OSCE must be clearly defined in advance and this is reflected in the checklist.

The number of items in a checklist usually ranges from 10 to 30. Stations of longer duration assessing a wider range of competencies, as in the case study by the Medical Council of Canada, tend to have more items (Case Study 7); shorter stations have fewer items.

Each element in the checklist (e.g. 'examine the jugular venous pressure') may require the examiner simply to tick the box if the item is undertaken. Options can be offered to score each item as illustrated in the case studies:

- yes/no.

- yes/partially completed/no.

- performance competent/performance not fully competent/not performed or incompetent.

- yes/yes, with reservations/no.

- clear pass/borderline/fail/clear fail; and

- did not perform/needs improvement/below average/above average/excellent.

Within the one checklist, some items may be scored on a binomial two-point scale, for example in Case Study 8 'offers the family member a tissue', whilst in the same checklist, other items, such as 'gives family members time to talk', may be scored on a five-point scale.

The items on a checklist may represent the critical actions required in relation to the task to be undertaken at the station. A critical action item may be defined as an 'OSCE checklist item whose performance is critical to ensure an optimal patient outcome and avoid medical error' (Payne et al. 2008).

The items in the checklist may be arranged in groups. Individual items in each group may be scored separately as in Case Study 7, or they may be assessed as a group as in Case Study 5 or Case Study 14.

Usually all the items in a checklist carry equal weight, although sometimes as in Case Study 11 the panel of examiners attaches differential weights to the items on the checklist. Research has suggested that weighting checklist items in an OSCE does not have an appreciable impact on the reliability and validity of the examination. However, differential scoring weights are used in some OSCEs. It is obvious to see why – examiners may wish what they perceive as the relative importance of individual items on the checklist to be reflected in the scores for the station. Complex weighting models have been described and, in a recent study, Sandilands et al. (2014) investigated the application of four different weighting models of various complexities. Less complex weighting models were found to yield similar reliability and pass rates to the more complex model, and minimal changes in the candidates' pass/fail status were observed. The general consensus is that the benefit of weighting items is not worth the extra effort.

Advantages of a checklist

As evidenced by the wide use of checklists, this scoring methodology or scoring rubric offers a number of advantages:

- The checklist spells out the performance expected at the station and makes the examination more transparent.

- The checklist appears straightforward and easily and objectively scored, for example 'Did the examinee assess the jugular venous pressure?' or 'Did the examinee ask about the site and radiation of the chest pain?'

- The checklist encourages the examiner to concentrate on the student's performance and to score the student systematically and objectively over the duration of the station.

- Less training and judgement from the examiner is required compared to the completion of rating scales.

- The record of the examinee's specific actions at stations provides useful feedback to students and curriculum developers.

- Schools may collaborate in the production of a checklist. Macluskey et al. (2011) suggested that the development of a checklist for dental student suturing skills could lead to the standardisation of the assessment in different UK-based dental schools.

- As described below, checklists can contribute to the setting of a pass mark for the station.

Disadvantages of a checklist

The checklist also has a number of potential disadvantages:

- It may be perceived as putting examiners into a straitjacket and removing their freedom to assess a student's performance.

- It may be seen as representing a reductionist approach to the task, reducing it to a series of low-level performances. This represents a more general criticism of fragmentation in the OSCE and is discussed in Chapter 16.

- Overall aspects of the student's performance may not be captured in the checklist.

- Students may be prompted to mechanistically rehearse the items on the checklist to the detriment of their overall approach to the patient.

- The checklist is station dependent and has to be developed for each station.

- The same checklist may not capture well the different levels of mastery from novice to master.

Rating scales

A rating scale is a device where the examiner is asked to make a judgement about a student's performance based on an observation of the student's behaviour and performance at the station. It captures an overall judgement by an examiner of the student's competence. A numerical scale may be adopted often accompanied by a verbal description. The rating scales represent a continuum of performance (e.g. from 'poor' to 'excellent'). The number of points on the scale can vary from three to seven or more. An even-numbered scale with, e.g. four or six points on the continuum is sometimes advocated rather than an odd-numbered scale with three or five points on the continuum, as examiners in odd-numbered scales tend to select the middle number. However, this probably does not represent a significant problem. Examples of the continuum as exemplified in the case studies are:

- clear fail/borderline/clear pass.

- clear fail/border fail/border pass/clear pass/excellent.

- clear fail/border fail/border pass/clear pass.

- inferior/poor/borderline/unsatisfactory/borderline satisfactory/good/excellent; and

- 1/2/3/4/5/6/7/8 with the points anchored from 1 ('poor') to 8 ('outstanding').

The examiner's overall rating of the trainee's performance in the cultural skills OSCE in Case Study 6 had a four-point global rating scale:

1. *very little to no sensitivity to differences* – did not establish rapport, did not complete station tasks.

2. *inadequate sensitivity to differences* – rapport was suboptimal, inadequately completed station tasks.

3. *adequate sensitivity to differences* – rapport was good, completed station tasks; and

4. *excellent sensitivity to differences* – rapport was outstanding, completed station tasks with great skill.

Rating scales may be used to assess holistically the examinee's overall performance at a station (a global rating scale), or they may be used to judge specific elements of the overall performance. For example, in Case Study 1, examiners were asked, in addition to a global rating, to rate the student in five areas: accuracy, skilfulness, supportiveness, efficiency and safety on a five-point scale from 'clear fail' to 'excellent', with criteria set for each domain. In the Manchester OSCE described in Case Study 3, 15 skill domains are assessed in the OSCE, with three to five domains assessed at each station.

Advantages of rating scales
Rating scales are widely used in OSCEs alongside checklists because of the advantages they offer:

- They capture general areas of competence, such as organisation, rapport and similar constructs, which may well not be captured in a binary checklist

(Regehr et al. 1999). A rating scale may identify the degree to which the candidate demonstrated an organised approach to the problem and showed a courteous and compassionate attitude toward the patient (Cohen et al. 1991a).

- Rating scales are simpler to construct than checklists and are not station specific.

- Different levels of mastery from novice to master can more easily be identified in a global rating scale.

Disadvantages of global rating scales

A rating scale also has disadvantages:

- The criteria to evaluate the examinee's performance may not be completely explicated or clarified.

- The rating scales are more subjective and are influenced by the personal preferences of the examiner – 'I know a good student when I see one.'

- Some examiners are more severe ('hawks') and others less so ('doves').

- The score is more easily influenced by previously informed opinions of the examinee – the 'halo' or the 'horn' effect.

- Ratings may be affected if the examiner sees several either bad or good students immediately beforehand.

- There may be a tendency towards the average where the examiner plays safe and scores in the middle range.

- The score awarded is less transparent and more difficult to communicate as feedback to a student.

- Because the criteria are less specific, examiners are less accountable for their decisions.

Checklists versus global ratings

Much effort and research has gone into comparing the reliability and value of global rating scales and checklists. Newble and Swanson (1988) suggested that inter-rater reliability improved when detailed behavioural checklists as opposed to rating forms were used. Other studies conclude that global rating scales are more reliable than checklists in terms of interstation reliability (Rothman et al. 1996; Hodges et al. 1998; Regehr et al. 1998; Hodges et al. 1999).

When comparing rating scales and checklists, it should be noted that rating scales are more station independent and assess more general characteristics of the examinee whereas the checklists are more station dependent. One might therefore expect to see greater correlation between scores across stations when global rating scales are used. In contrast, when inter-rater reliability at stations is examined, checklists prove to be more reliable than rating scales (Patricio et al. 2015). There is a strong possibility that checklists and global ratings when used together by the same rater are not independent instruments and that the scores on one scale may influence the scores on the other (Hodges et al. 1997).

Rating scales may be more valuable when assessing the expert level rather than the novice level (Hodges et al. 1999) (Box 11.2), but this may simply mean that we have not yet found the optimum form of checklist to assess an examinee at the level of expert.

The rating scale may give a more holistic overview of the examinee's clinical competence, but the checklist provides a more specific analysis and feedback in relation to the examinee's performance at a station. Waterston et al. (1980) described one of the first OSCEs in paediatrics and reported that the value of checklists compared to a rating scale was that the checklist provided feedback to students (Box 11.3). In some ways the strengths and weaknesses of checklists and rating scales can be

Box 11.2   Global rating scales

Hodges et al. (1999) suggested that global rating scales were more appropriate when assessing experts:

'… we have begun to wonder if checklists might penalize more experienced clinicians who arrive at diagnoses but no longer use a long list of questions in interviews. Indeed, experienced clinicians did not score more points on content checklists even when told this was the way to achieve a high score …'

Box 11.3   Checklists and feedback

Waterston et al. (1980) noted that a common complaint from the student after a clinical examination was that:

'he didn't know what he did wrong … if he is to understand his failings and improve his technique, it is essential for him to learn from the examination and we show students the checklists after each OSCE and discuss individual questions. Any deficiencies in particular aspects of teaching … will quickly become apparent and remedies can then be applied'.

Waterston suggested that feedback that highlighted the student's weaknesses and strengths may not be achievable with assessment based on global rating. Aspects of a student's performance are more amenable to recording using a checklist.

equated to the strengths and weaknesses of multiple-choice questions (MCQs) and essays. The MCQ tests detailed information and understanding in specific areas tested and are more objectively marked, whereas the essay question gives a more holistic assessment of the candidate's ability and tests attributes not tested with an MCQ but is more subjectively scored.

However, comparisons between checklists and rating scales are of more theoretical than practical use. In reality, in almost all situations, it is preferable to use both a checklist and a global rating scale and perhaps also a rating scale in specific learning outcome domains, such as communication skills. All except one of the 15 case studies in Section D used both a checklist and a rating scale. In the original description of the OSCE we described the use of both checklists and rating scales (Harden and Gleeson 1979).

In fact, there may be a fine line between a checklist and a rating scale. Each of the rating scales covering the 15 domains used in the Manchester Medical School OSCE (Case Study 3) has embedded in it a series of items which might have been included in a checklist. Some items included in checklists may almost be viewed as rating scales. An example, in the checklist in Case Study 4 is the item 'systematic and organised history taking'. The item is scored not simply on a 'yes/no' scale but on a five-point scale: 'not done/partially done/inadequately done/adequately done/well done'. The checklist in Case Study 5 has the items arranged in four categories, and a decision is simply required with regard to each category in terms of 'clear pass/pass/borderline/fail/clear fail'.

Narrative comments

Narrative comments by the examiner may also be encouraged but are not essential. They may have something useful to communicate that is not covered in the checklist or rating scales. Kachur et al. (1990) described how examiners in the OSCE were encouraged to add written comments to the traditional scoring forms. This may be valuable in a number of ways:

- The comments can fill gaps where items are missing in the checklist or rating scales. Hopefully, such items would have been picked up in advance when the station was being planned, but this may not always be the case.

- The comments can provide an explanation or further information about the examiner's ratings (e.g. Case Study 7) and can provide feedback to the examinee.

- The examiner can comment on problems or on unexpected issues that arise at the station, for example with regard to the SP's behaviour.

- The comments can provide feedback to the OSCE designers about the construction of the station.

Assessment by the simulated patient

At stations where there is an SP, the SP may also contribute to the assessment of the examinee's performance at the station. As with the examiner, the SP may use a checklist and/or a global rating scale. An example of an SP scoring sheet is given in Case Study 6. In this case, the SP is requested to rate their general satisfaction with the student's performance on a four-point scale and also an assessment of the cultural skills demonstrated by the examinee on a four-point scale.

Vu et al. (1992) suggested that checklists for use by SPs should have 10–20 items for optimal accuracy. They found that there was a loss of accuracy when a checklist item included more than once piece of information. The incorporation of the SP's evaluation of the examinee into the score for the station is discussed later.

Red flags

Consideration should be given as to whether particular attention should be paid to aspects of the examinee's performance which are considered inappropriate but may not be covered by the checklist or rating scales. In the Medical Council of Canada's Qualifying Examination (Medical Council of Canada 2013), the examiner is asked to note whether the candidate demonstrated any lapse in professional behaviour during the examination and if so the reason, for example being disrespectful to the patient or nurse, over-investigation or over-management of the patient or acting in a way that was of ethical and/or legal concern.

In the OSCE described in Case Study 15, examiners can raise a red flag to express serious concerns about the candidate's suitability for practising medicine.

In the UK, the General Medical Council commended the use of a yellow card system at Barts' Medical School in London, where an examiner could flag concerns about a student's performance not covered by the mark sheets. Queen's University, Belfast, developed a serious-concern 'yellow card' reporting system in its OSCEs (Gormley 2011). Issues that arise during the OSCE that warrant a serious-concern report, including unprofessional practice (e.g. being rough with a patient) or unsafe actions that would potentially cause harm to a patient in clinical practice (such as administration of an incorrect or dangerous drug), are recorded.

Linked product or 'post-encounter' stations

As described in Chapter 6, students may be asked at a second linked product or 'post-encounter' station to record electronically or on paper their findings at the previous station, their interpretation of the findings and further action required. They may be in the form of a:

- short constructed response question.

- multiple choice question.

- note to be inserted in the patient's records; and

- discharge or referral letter.

Following the OSCE, the responses are marked by an examiner using either a checklist or rating scale. An alternative is for the examiner to spend the final 1 or 2 minutes at an OSCE station questioning the examinee about the findings or the further action to be taken, as described in Case Study 7.

Deciding about the student's performance

On the basis of the evidence collected about the student's performance at the stations during the OSCE, a decision has to be taken about the student's overall performance. Should the student pass or fail? Does the student have the competence to pass on to the next phase of the curriculum or to graduate and practise as a doctor? Does the trainee have the abilities and competence to practise in the chosen specialty whether in a hospital or in the community? Is the practising physician competent to continue practising? It may be more difficult to make such pass/fail decisions at intermediate points in the course when the milestones are not clearly defined and there is still room and opportunity for the student to acquire the necessary competence in the later years (Pell et al. 2012).

There is considerable variation in how a decision can be reached, and there is no one best method that the examiners can be advised to adopt. Different approaches to arriving at pass/fail decisions have been described along with variations of each approach. One challenge is to take into account the different sources and types of evidence and scoring collected during the OSCE:

- What weight should be attached to the scores in the marking sheets compared to the global ratings?

- What account should be taken of the evaluation of the examinee by the SP?

- How are an assessment of the examinee's performance and technique and an assessment of the findings and their interpretations reconciled when these assessments differ?

- How are red flags or penalty points assigned during the OSCE recognised in the final assessment?

- How should the performance of the examinee at each station contribute to the overall score?

Such judgments need to be discussed and agreed prior to the examination, and the decisions taken should reflect the consensus of the responsible educators. We will explore these issues further.

Pass/fail decisions can be arrived at based on:

- a cumulative score for all of the stations, including process and product stations (compensatory).

- achievement of a pass score at an agreed number of stations (non-compensatory).

- assessment of the required standard in the key domains assessed in the OSCE, for example history taking, physical examination, practical procedures and data interpretation (examinee profile).

- the penalty points or red flags awarded to the student during the OSCE (danger signals); and

- a hybrid methodology combining a number of approaches.

Cumulative score

The OSCE score for the examinee is arrived at by the addition of the marks awarded at each station in the OSCE. These can be adjusted so that each station contributes in the same measure to the final score. In a 20-station OSCE, each station contributes 5% of the final score. Alternatively, the stations can be weighted so that some stations contribute more than others.

In this compensatory method, students can compensate for poor performance at some stations or poor performance relating to certain competencies, such as history taking, by good performance in other stations or other competencies.

An arbitrary mark can be selected as the pass mark. In Case Studies 3, 9 and 14, the mark selected was 57%, 80% and 60%. At the National University of Ireland, Galway, the traditional standard is a 50% pass mark (Kropmans et al. 2012).

Alternatively, the mark required for a pass may be determined by a standard-setting procedure as described below. In this case the pass mark or cut-off score is likely to vary from examination to examination.

Another approach is to equate the performance of the examinee to the performance of other examinees. A test scored in this way is referred to as a *norm-referenced test* because the norm of acceptable performance is set by the group of examinees. A decision is taken as to the number of students who will pass or fail the examination. In most instances this approach is unacceptable. For a better group of students, some students who might otherwise have passed may fail, and for a poorer group of students, some students who may pass might otherwise have failed. However, this approach may be appropriate in special circumstances, such as in the use of an OSCE for selection purposes where places are available only for a limited number of students.

A pass is required in a specified number of stations

A non-compensatory or conjunctive marking scheme based on the student's performance at individual stations has been widely adopted. Here a pass mark is set for each station, and the examinee is required to achieve a pass grade on a set number of stations. This is usually a significant proportion of the stations, for example 80%. In this model, the student is not required to achieve a pass mark in all of the stations, but there is a limit to the extent to which the student(s) can compensate for poor performance. The requirement for a minimum number of stations to be passed prevents excessive compensation and adds fidelity to the requirement for a competent all-around doctor.

The use of conjunctive and competency standards in an OSCE is explored by Friedman Ben-David (2000b). If a conjunctive or non-compensatory standard is rigidly applied, the failure rate may be high, and in a long OSCE, even the better students who may fail a station due to some measurement error will fail the examination (Hambleton 1995). The counterintuitive result is that the more stations included in an OSCE, the less reliable the examination becomes.

Penalty points

A variation of the above approaches is a penalty point methodology adopted at the Hull York Medical School in the UK (Cookson et al. 2011). Pass/fail decisions are made on the basis of penalty points accumulated during the examination. These are awarded to grades below C+:

- C– = 1 penalty point.

- D = 2 penalty points; and

- E = 3 penalty points.

The penalty points are summed over all the stations, and candidates who acquire too many penalty points are at risk of failing the examination. In this way, candidates are allowed to make some errors in the OSCE, but not too many.

A competence profile

Examinees can be assessed in an OSCE based on their performance relating to the key learning outcome domains. Each domain is assessed at a number of stations. A minimum standard is set for each of the domains, and students are expected to achieve this standard for each domain. Poor performance with regard to attitudes and ethics, for example, cannot be compensated by a good performance in other domains (Examinee C in Figure 11.2). Several domains may be assessed at one station.

In the original description of the OSCE by Harden and Gleeson (1979) students' performance was recorded in relation to history taking, physical examination, laboratory investigation and interpretation. The mark for each competence contributed an

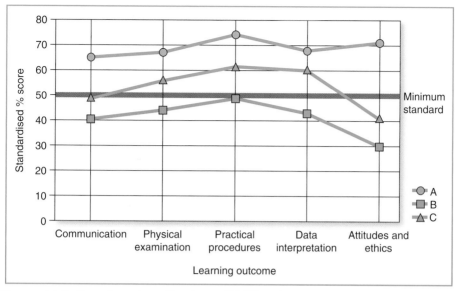

Figure 11.2 Examinees' profiles in an OSCE with marks standardised and a minimum standard set (50%) for each key learning outcome domain.

agreed percentage to the total cumulative score for the examination. With the move to outcome-based education, however, the scores for each learning outcome domain are more properly considered separately as part of an examinee's profile. A key feature of outcome- or competency-based education is that the individual is assessed and has to achieve a required standard in each of the domains.

Hybrid approaches

Variations on the above approaches are frequently adopted and a hybrid approach implemented. Evidence obtained about a student's performance in an OSCE can be combined in different ways. Candidates at Leeds School of Medicine, for example, are required to achieve a specified overall pass score, a minimum number of stations passed, and a minimum number of acceptable SP ratings (Pell et al. 2012).

Kachur et al. (2013) describe how students are assessed in an OSCE at New York University School of Medicine in four competency areas: communication skills, history gathering, physical examination and clinical reasoning. Poor performance in one area cannot be compensated for by good performance in another. Students who fail in the communication skills domain or any other two domains are deemed to have failed the OSCE. Students who received a 'would not recommend to a friend or family' global rating from more than one SP are also reviewed (Box 11.4).

A minimum requirement for SP comments may be required as a proxy for patient satisfaction (Pell et al. 2010). In this case, attention needs to be paid to rigorous training of the SPs. Typically the SP rating should contribute 10–20% of the total station score (Homer and Pell 2009).

In the clinical skills summative OSCE at New York University School of Medicine, students' performance is reported in four competency areas: communication skills, history gathering, physical examination and clinical reasoning:

> '...normative passing cut-off score is set at the lowest decile for each competency. Students in this lowest decile across two or more competencies are identified, and then all students who "fail" communication skills alone (because we have found that this is predictive of failure on the USMLE Step II CS exam) are added to this list. Students' scores that fall close to the threshold (above and below) are further scrutinized to better make pass/fail decisions. Finally, any student who received a "would not recommend to a friend or family" global rating from more than one SP is added to the list because we have found this identifies additional students who go on to struggle with communication issues clinically and on other OSCEs.'

(Kachur et al. 2013, p. 32.)

Process and product

In an OSCE, evidence can be collected as to the examinee's technique, whether it is in history taking, physical examination or undertaking a procedure – their technical skills. Evidence can also be collected as to the candidate's understanding and interpretation of the findings and any further actions necessary. This may be carried out at the second of two linked stations (a product station) or in the final few minutes of the process station. The candidate may be asked to undertake a cardiovascular examination at the process station and at the product station to record the findings and any further action necessary in relation to the patient examined. As shown in Figure 11.3, a candidate may carry out a satisfactory examination and come to the right conclusions or may fail to carry out a satisfactory examination and also fail to come to the right conclusions. Occasionally a candidate may undertake a satisfactory examination, as identified with the checklist and rating scale, but record incorrect findings or recommend inappropriate action relating to the patient. Or the student may come to the correct conclusions, but demonstrate mistakes in their technical performance. Examiners have to determine whether students in these last two categories should be deemed to have achieved a 'pass' score at the station. The decision may vary at different phases of the curriculum. For example, it may be perceived with a more junior student that it is more important to have the correct technique than to come to the right conclusions.

Problems with the examinee's technique may relate to an inappropriate attitude towards the patient. This can be scored as a separate learning outcome. Clinical reasoning may be assessed as a learning outcome at the second linked station and may also be reported and scored as a distinct learning outcome and presented as such in the candidate's profile in the overall assessment.

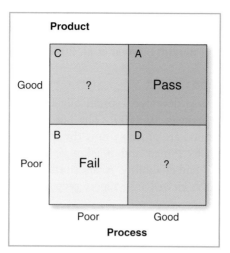

Figure 11.3 An assessment at an OSCE station of the candidate's technique and their findings. A = good technique and correct findings; B = poor technique and poor findings; C = poor technique, but correct findings; D = good technique, but incorrect findings.

Standard setting

The pass mark or cut-off score for an OSCE may be set arbitrarily at 50%, for example, or it may be determined using a formal standard setting process. As described above, evidence is collected during the OSCE about the student's perform-ance and a score is arrived at based on the checklist and rating scales. An educational tool is needed with which examiners can determine the pass or cut-off point on the scoring scale which separates the non-competent from the competent (Friedman Ben-David 2000b). The traditional approach in defining such a cut-off point, for example 50%, does not provide robust and valid evidence for pass/fail decisions. To address this problem, the standard setting process was designed to translate a con-ceptual definition of competence to an operational version called the *passing score* (Norcini 1994). A range of standard setting methods has been employed for written and performance tests (Norcini 2003; Boursicot et al. 2014). The different methods are based on the judgement of a group of subject matter experts following their examination of:

- *The examination material – test-centred models.* The judges set standards by viewing test items and provide judgements as to the 'just adequate' level of performance on these items. The Angoff procedure is the most commonly used test-centred model in the OSCE (Kaufman et al. 2000; Kramer et al. 2003; Boulet et al. 2003). The Medical Council of Canada's Qualifying Examination, as shown in Case Study 7, used an Angoff standard setting procedure but has moved from this to a borderline group method.

- *The examinee's performance – examinee-centred models.* Here to set the standard the examiners make decisions based on the performance of examinees in the test. An example is the borderline group and borderline regression method (Cohen et al. 1991b; Dauphinée et al. 1997; Wilkinson et al. 2001; Kramer et al. 2003; Wood et al. 2006).

Borderline group method

The borderline method was developed specifically for a performance assessment such as the OSCE (Kaufman et al. 2000). The borderline group method and the borderline regression method are probably now the most widely used approaches to standard setting in OSCEs (Smee and Blackmore 2001; Boursicot et al. 2007) because of their efficiency and credibility. A description of other methods, including the Angoff method, can be viewed in a report prepared by McKinley and Norcini (2014).

Advantages of the borderline group method – *The borderline group method offers the examiner a number of advantages:*

- It does not require a complex statistical process, and the cut-off point is easy to calculate. For this reason it can be readily adopted where statistical expertise is not available.

- The approach is based on the actual performance of candidates and examiners find it easier to rate the performance of candidates in practice rather than through a theoretical consideration of a checklist (Boulet et al. 2003).

- It is efficient in the use of examiners' time, as the process happens at the same time as the examination and does not require the time consuming advanced work required with, for example, the Angoff method.

Implementing the borderline group method – *The borderline group method is implemented relatively easily:*

- During the OSCE, the examiners at each station in the OSCE evaluate the examinees' performance at the stations by completing the station-specific checklist and global rating scales as described above. The number of points on the rating scale does not matter as long as the borderline is identified. It may be *'fail, borderline, pass, or excellent'*, or *'fail, borderline fail, borderline pass, pass, or excellent'*.

- The borderline candidates at the station are identified. Their marks on the checklist are noted and added and a mean checklist score for them is calculated and presented as a percentage. If, for example, the mean is 58%, it is assumed that all examinees scoring 58% or more would pass the station and candidates with 57% or less would fail at that station.

- The mean of the pass marks or cut-off scores derived in this way for all of the stations in the examination is calculated. This becomes the cut-off score for the overall examination.

Instead of gathering the examiners' judgements during the OSCE administration, a panel of judges can be used prior to the examination to categorise performance at the examination station as 'clear fail/borderline/pass' (McKinley and Norcini 2014). The borderline examinee is defined as one whose knowledge and skills are not quite adequate, but are not inadequate. The pass mark for the station and for the examination is then calculated as described above.

Problems with the borderline group method – *Whilst it is easy to use, problems have been identified with the borderline group method:*

- Only borderline examinees are used to set the pass mark and in a small-scale OSCE, the number of borderline candidates may be small, with the result that the cut-off score is less reliable.

- Using only the borderline candidates' scores may also introduce a statistical bias (Wood et al. 2006).

To overcome these disadvantages whilst preserving the benefits of the borderline group approach, an adaptation – the borderline regression method – has been introduced and is now widely adopted.

Borderline regression method

The borderline regression method uses a linear regression approach to overcome the problems with the borderline group method (Wood et al. 2006). The checklist scores and global ratings from all the examinees are used. The method regresses all of the examinees checklist scores onto their global rating to produce a linear equation. By inserting into the equation the global rating corresponding to the borderline group, a checklist score can be determined. This becomes the cut-off score for the examination (Figure 11.4).

For the borderline regression method it is necessary to run a linear regression, but this can be carried out easily using a statistical and spreadsheet programme with most statistical packages. This is straightforward and can be done using a Microsoft Excel worksheet.

Having established the cut score for a station, the overall cut score or pass mark for the OSCE is calculated, as for the borderline group method, as the mean of the station scores. Details and an example of how the borderline regression method is implemented in practice can be seen in the report by McKinley and Norcini (2014).

Data processing

When the OSCE was first introduced in the 1970s, the students' performance was recorded on paper checklists and rating scales. Following the examination the score for each station and for the overall examination was calculated using a programmable calculator. The raw score sheets were photocopied and copies given

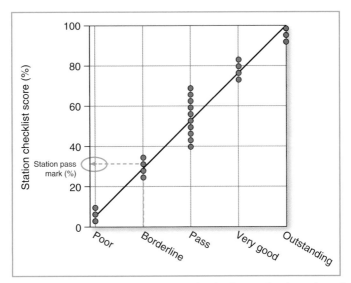

Figure 11.4 The borderline regression method of standard setting. A linear regression is shown of a station checklist against the station global score. A borderline examinee corresponds to a cut score of 35% (Gormley 2011).

to the students following the examination. Handling the data in this way can be time consuming and may introduce errors. With technical developments other more effective and efficient approaches are available. Consideration needs to be given to:

- the method of data collection during the examination.

- the processing of the data and calculation of scores for stations, specified learning domains and the overall examination.

- the preparation of reports for the examination and curriculum committee on the students' performance; and

- the provision of feedback to students.

The advances in technology resulted in the widespread use of optical-marked reader sheets on which the examiner recorded the examinee's performance. This remains the method adopted in many OSCEs.

Electronic tools are now widely used to support the administration of an OSCE, and significant progress has been made since the earlier experience of using personal digital assistants (PDAs) to record data during an OSCE (Treadwell 2006; Van Schoor et al. 2006). With the advent of the tablet computer and Wi-Fi, a number of systems have been developed to mark OSCEs electronically. This eliminates the need for printing and scanning the scoring sheets used in the OSCE. The implementation of real-time electronic marking for clinical examinations was described by Hunkeler and Zimmermann (2014).

At the National University of Ireland, Galway, Kropmans et al. (2012) described an OSCE Management Information System (OMIS) used to streamline the OSCE process and improve quality assurance. OSCE data were captured in real time using a web-based platform. The examiners logged into the system on a computer desktop, laptop or iPad, and opened the dedicated assessment forms for their station. Marking criteria and discriminators were visible whilst hovering over the markers with a mouse or fingertip. The OMIS software included assessment and data analysis tools. Using the system, significant improvements were found in the Galway OSCEs in terms of accuracy, financial feasibility and time costs. A more detailed analysis of student performance was also possible.

Examples of capture and processing systems used for OSCEs:

- *Clinquest* (website: www.clinquest.com) can be used to create individual station or assessment sheets, with candidate responses interpreted by Speedwell's OSCE software Clinquest and Optical Mark Reading (OMR) technology.

- *eOSCE* (website: www.e-osce.ch): The Electronic Registration of Objective Structured Clinical Examination (eOSCE) aims to create a more efficient and entirely digital preparation, execution and analysis process of OSCEs, which is less erroneous and quicker to evaluate.

- The *moscee* (website: www.moscee.com) system was designed to run on mobile devices, such as the Apple iPhone with a web-based interface or any mobile device that had a wireless Internet on a mobile connection.

- *OSCEonline* (website: www.osceonline.com) is a web app plus iPad or Android app combination for online, paperless OSCEs.

- *Qpercom* (website: www.qpercom.com) is an OSCE Management Information System (OMIS) which allows universities to create forms, administer OSCEs and analyse results (Kropmans et al. 2012).

- *OSCE Manager* (website: www.osce-manager.com) is another example of a web-based application developed at the Medical Faculty of the University of Basel.

- *MyKnowledgeMap* (website: www.MyKnowledgeMap.com) is yet another example of a mobile application for marking and reporting on an OSCE.

Without doubt, there will be significant developments in OSCE data processing applications in the years ahead. The above represent examples of what is available at the time of going to press.

A range of approaches to data handling in an OSCE is now in current use, including manual machine-readable forms and electronic capture on tablets. Data capture and processing become increasingly important with demands for more detailed analysis of an examinee's performance in relation to content areas, tasks and learning outcomes across different domains. The need for more detailed feedback both to the learner and to the education developer is also recognised.

Take-home messages

- The collection of information about the examinee's performance during the OSCE, its analysis and the pass/fail decisions taken on the basis of this are of the greatest importance.

- Information about examinee performance during the OSCE should be captured using both checklists and rating scales, as each offers advantages.

- An evaluation of the examinee by the patient or an SP should also be captured.

- Serious points of concern, with regard to the examinee's performance or 'red flags', can be recorded.

- Unless for special purposes, such as selection, an absolute or criterion scoring system should be used rather than a norm referenced system where the candidates' performance is judged relative to their colleagues.

- Decisions about the examinee should be based on his/her total mark across the OSCE stations with a requirement that he/she has to achieve a prescribed standard in a set number of stations and/or a minimum standard on each of the key learning outcome domains.

- A standard-setting procedure should be adopted. Although there is no one 'right' method, the borderline group method or borderline regression method is widely considered to be the most effective and efficient for use in an OSCE.

- Information can be captured electronically during the OSCE and used to produce a detailed analysis of the examinee's performance to allow a pass/fail decision and to provide feedback to examinee and educators.

Consider the approach adopted in your OSCE to capture information during the examination, and make decisions about the evidence on the basis of this information. Compare this with the approaches described in this chapter.

Providing feedback to the learner | 12

The OSCE can be a powerful learning experience, and a variety of approaches may be adopted for the provision of feedback to the learner.

The importance of feedback

Feedback is important. It can be defined as *'specific information about the comparison between a trainee's observed performance and a standard, given with the intent to improve the trainee's performance'* (van de Ridder et al. 2008). Feedback tells the learner that the teacher or trainer cares enough about their work and progress to think about what they have achieved and what they still have to achieve. Failure to provide the learner with appropriate feedback, however, is probably the most common complaint that students have about their teachers and junior doctors have about those responsible for supervising their training programme. The provision of feedback about performance to the learner has been described as one of the four key principles in making learning effective. **F**eedback, together with **A**ctivity, **I**ndividualisation, and **R**elevance make up the **FAIR** principles (Harden and Laidlaw 2012, p. 9).

Providing students with feedback has been demonstrated unequivocally to enhance students' learning (Hattie and Timperley 2007). Indeed, providing feedback may even be the most valuable thing that a teacher can do in facilitating learning. Feedback addresses both cognitive and motivational factors at the same time (Brookhart 2008). If the feedback is done well, students and trainees receive information that helps them understand what they have learned or mastered and what they have yet to learn or master – the cognitive factor. Providing the learner with information in a suitable form helps them recognise their achievements and at the same time understand what they need to do to improve their performance. In this way they can develop a feeling of control over their own learning – the motivational factor. Student self-regulation where students learn to control their own thought processes is receiving more attention in medical education (Butler and Winne 1995; Sandars and Cleary 2011). Feedback is an important part of self-regulation.

Much has been written about feedback and medical education, and some of the published journal articles and resources can be found in the MedEdWorld Update on Feedback (Kennedy 2013).

Feedback and the OSCE

Feedback has an important role to play in the OSCE. Through feedback to the student or trainee, the OSCE can promote learning and not just measure it (Box 12.1). Feedback is basic to formative assessment and should be integrated into the assessment system (van der Ridder et al. 2008). The OSCE offers the teacher or trainer special opportunities to provide powerful feedback to the learner. Feedback often features prominently in descriptions of the OSCE and is highlighted in the case studies in this book. As highlighted in Chapter 4, the OSCE can be used as a formative assessment tool, designed as part of the learning process to provide the learner with information on their strengths and weaknesses – assessment *for* learning and not just assessment *of* learning.

Telling a student or trainee that they have passed or failed an OSCE, that their score was 48% or that they got a 'D' grade is not useful feedback. To be helpful, the feedback to the learner in an OSCE should relate to their performance in individual stations and to their overall performance in relation to outcome domains, such as communication skills, physical examination and practical procedures. A student might be competent in physical examination and practical procedures, but not competent in their communication skills.

Relevant to feedback and the OSCE is:

- the timing – when feedback is given, either during the OSCE or subsequently.

- the mode – individual or group feedback; and

- the amount, nature and specificity of feedback.

Feedback during the OSCE

An important factor in the provision of effective feedback is that it should be timely (Box 12.2). The OSCE can be designed with feedback built into the examination.

Box 12.1

Students at Dundee were asked to complete a questionnaire on the teaching they received. They were asked to list the three most valuable learning experiences they had encountered in the previous term. Would it be the sessions in a new problem-based learning (PBL) course, the learning opportunities in the community or the lectures by a member of staff renowned for his performances before the class? To our surprise, it was none of these. The end-of-term OSCE with the associated feedback was widely acclaimed by the students as their most memorable learning experience.

During the examination, feedback may be given at a station or immediately following a station (Figure 12.1).

Feedback at a procedure station

Time may be scheduled towards the end of a procedure station for the examiner to provide feedback to the examinee. In an OSCE to assess physical examination skills, for example, students were provided with 2 minutes of feedback from the examiner before they proceeded to the next station (Smith et al. 2009). An earlier study from Hodder et al. (1989) to evaluate a 2-minute period of feedback given immediately

---

Box 12.2

In a continuing professional development (CPD) programme developed in Dundee, more than 30,000 General Practitioners throughout the UK were mailed a series of patient management problems. They were invited to make decisions about the patients' further investigation, diagnosis and management. They were able to compare their decisions with those of experts in the field and with those of a group of individuals recognised as 'excellent' General Practitioners. The programme was well received by the doctors and rated as a valuable CPD initiative. Identified as the key feature in its success was the feedback provided and the fact that this was offered immediately through a latent image printing technique. Indeed, the immediacy of the feedback gave the series its name – the 'IF' (Immediate Feedback) programme.

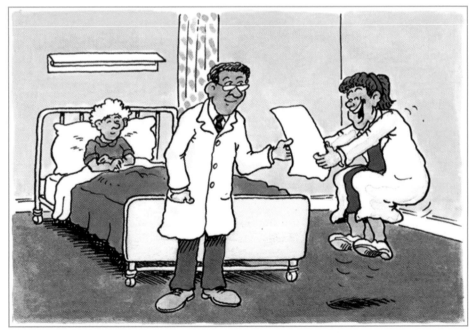

Figure 12.1 The examinee may be given feedback about his/her performance during the OSCE.

after a 4-minute OSCE station compared two groups, one receiving the feedback and the other taking 6 minutes for the station without receiving feedback. Both groups repeated the station. There was a significantly greater increase in the scores of the students receiving feedback.

There are a number of examples in the Case Studies, where a period of feedback is incorporated into the final minutes of the station. In the Manchester Medical School formative OSCE (Case Study 3), a 2-minute period is included at each 10-minute station for feedback provided to the examinee by the examiner and the simulated patient (SP). Similarly, a 2-minute period is incorporated for verbal feedback by the examiner at the end of each station in the Monash University (Malaysia) formative OSCE for second-year undergraduates (Case Study 4). The abdominal ultrasound OSCE for undergraduates (Case Study 14) incorporates 1.5 minutes at the end of each station for feedback, and specific suggestions for improvement are given to the students. A longer period, 5 minutes, is included for feedback to paediatric residents by examiners and SPs after each station in the formative Culture OSCE (Case Study 6). The formative patient safety Orientation to Residency OSCE (Case Study 13) provides immediate feedback from SPs for stations with checklists, as well as exemplars where the examinee completes the station on computer.

Feedback immediately following a procedure station

Rather than the incorporation of feedback into a station, the examinee can be provided with feedback at the following station. A number of strategies can be adopted:

- The examinee uses the time to study their score sheet for the previous station, including the checklist, global ratings and narrative comments from the examiner.

- In addition to looking at their score sheet, the examinee is given the opportunity to watch a video illustrating the performance expected at the previous station.

- Examinees are given their score sheets and remain at the station to observe the next candidate's performance.

- The examinee remains at the station and adopts the role of the SP for the next student. An example of this can be seen in the ultrasound OSCE case study (Case Study 14).

We have had experience of using all of these approaches effectively in an OSCE. In one study (Black et al. 1986), we compared the students' perceptions of feedback provided during the examination through the students' personal score sheets and a video of what was expected of the students, feedback provided during the OSCE through the score sheet plus observation of their peers' performance, and finally

Table 12.1 Students' preference with regard to timing and method of feedback (Black et al. 1986)

| | During examination | | After examination score sheet and expert video |
	Score sheet and observation of peer	Score sheet and expert video	
History taking station	17%	67%	17%
Physical examination station	25%	56%	19%

feedback provided following the examination through the score sheets and a video of the expected performance. As can be seen from Table 12.1, both feedback formats offered during the examination were preferred to the after-examination format. The only difference between the formats where students were given their score sheets with the opportunity to watch a video of good practice at the station was that one was offered during the examination and the other following the examination. This supports the view that, as has been shown with feedback generally, the timing of feedback in an OSCE is important.

Feedback provided during an OSCE can lead to improved competency of the student (Black and Harden 1986). Students who were given feedback performed significantly better both in the history taking and the physical examination stations in a second examination compared with a control group.

A limitation of providing feedback during the examination, however, is that time is short and examinees may find it difficult to absorb all the information provided within the time available. Moreover, allocation of time for feedback lengthens the duration of the examination. However, as a contribution to the students' learning, this may be a good investment. From the examiner's point of view, providing detailed feedback is challenging in an examination where there is a series of short OSCE stations with little time available between candidates (Harrison et al. 2013). Concerns that feedback provided during the examination, if negative, may be stressful and may interfere with the examinee's performance at subsequent stations have not been confirmed in practice. The reason may be that each station is seen by the student as a mini-examination with the feedback associated at the end of it.

Feedback may be provided during the examination by the simulator or manikin. The Laerdal cardiopulmonary resuscitation model does just that, providing oral feedback to the learner as to the number and rate of compressions, with a printed sheet at the end summarising the performance.

Feedback after the OSCE

Feedback may be given to examinees following an OSCE and a number of approaches can be used.

Feedback given as part of a group exercise

This is best conducted immediately following the OSCE, and ideally the examiner responsible for each OSCE station should be present. The examiner can comment on the examinees' performance overall, highlighting what was seen as good practice at the station while at the same time identifying the common mistakes or omissions encountered at the station. The examiner may display the checklist used to rate the examinees' performance and comment on specific items in the checklist. It is helpful also if the standardised patient is present and gives their view of the experience. The examinees may have their personal score sheets returned either at the beginning or at the end of the feedback session. The OSCE Lead can chair the session and comment on general issues arising, such as the rotation through stations.

An example where group feedback is provided is given in Case Studies 3, 6 and 12. In the culture OSCE for paediatric residents, each station is reviewed with the whole group, with copies of the evaluation forms completed at each station made available.

Individual feedback without score sheets

Individual feedback can be given to examinees about their overall performance that highlights areas of weakness. This may not include the examinee's score sheet, as some examiners, as described in Box 12.3, are reluctant to return these to examinees. The Medical Council of Canada's Qualifying Examination Part II (Case Study 7)

Box 12.3

Details of the stations included in an OSCE and the checklists and global rating scales used were treated in a medical school as confidential with the same security allocated to them as to a bank of multiple-choice questions (MCQs). The staff were concerned that if the station details were known, students would simply study for the test. Requests from students to see their own score sheets were refused.

Over time, staff in the school changed, and new staff responsible for the OSCE were more receptive to the requests from students to see their score sheets. It was decided to offer students, upon request, a copy of their personal score sheets which included the examiners' comments. It was argued that this would not have a disadvantageous effect, as the stations and checklists simply reflected the expected course learning outcomes, and indeed, the score sheets could be seen as an additional means of communicating the learning outcomes to the students.

Almost all 'good' students requested to see their score sheets, whereas a significant number of 'borderline' or 'poor' students did not. This identified a problem with the 'poorer' students. They were unwilling to recognise and face up to weaknesses or problems relating to their performance. Steps were taken to arrange individual interviews with them. Overall the policy of making score sheets available to students was seen as a success, and score sheets continued to be issued on request.

offers feedback to candidates on their scores by domain and compares this to the mean for the class.

Individual score sheets

Individual score sheets, including the checklist, global rating and narrative comments from the examiner, are given to the examinees. In Case Study 4, students are provided with their score sheets together with details of the maximum possible score and median and maximum cohort scores within 2 to 4 weeks of the OSCE. Another example of post-OSCE feedback can be seen in the Dundee summative Year 2 OSCE (Case Study 1). Students receive personal, online feedback incorporating interactive graphs and examiners' free text comments to enable them to see their results both by station and by domain. They can compare their performance to a standard and to the class performance.

Following the Dundee Undergraduate BSc in Nursing Year 1 OSCE (Case Study 9), students are given personalised feedback, including their score sheet and examiners' comments by email. A student's personal tutor also receives a copy so that it can be discussed with the student.

Viewing a personal video recording

Students can view a video recording of their performance at one or more stations in the OSCE; this may be viewed alongside a video recording of the expected performance. Participants in the patient safety OSCE (Case Study 13) can watch videos of their performance and use this together with the immediate feedback received to prepare personal learning plans for discussion with their programme directors. It may be challenging to record every examinee's performance at all of the stations unless the OSCE is located in a clinical skills area designed with this facility. However, it is helpful to record at least one history taking and one physical examination station as examples of the examinee's performance in these domains.

Meetings with individual examinees

Staff can meet with students individually to review their performance. This is demanding on staff time and is perhaps best reserved for candidates who are borderline or have performed poorly in the examination across the board or in one particular domain. Examinees who fail the UCL Medical School Final MBBS Examination (Case Study 5) are given individualised feedback about their performance by the Welfare Tutor after the examinations are over.

Feedback and students in difficulty

A problem with feedback to students is that the poorer student or the student in difficulty who would potentially benefit most from receiving information about his/her performance with suggestions for improvement is less interested and less receptive to personal feedback. Shute (2008) likens formative feedback to 'a good murder' in that effective and useful feedback depends on three things: (1) motive – the student needs it, (2) opportunity – the student receives it in time to use it and (3) means – the student is able and willing to use it. The problem with the student in difficulty is that he or she may lack the motivation and willingness to accept and learn from feedback.

In some circumstances the failing student can be persuaded to consider feedback on their performance. Harrison et al. (2013) found that there was a problem getting students in the 'at risk' category to engage with detailed, interactive web-based feedback provided about the OSCE soon after the results were announced. Third-year students were able to compare their own performance with that of the rest of the cohort for each station or for each skill and to see how close their scores were to the pass mark. Whilst students who failed the examination used the feedback, as did those who performed well, the students who scored a minimal pass made the least use of the feedback. Attempts must be made to engage borderline or failing students with feedback and to demonstrate to them the advantages of reflecting and acting on the feedback provided.

White et al. (2009) looked at feedback provided to remediating students. One group was asked to study resources relating to the station they had failed, to view a video of an excellent performance and to reflect on a video of their own performance. Another group was given, in addition, written faculty feedback on their performance at the station. The authors found that both groups improved performance on the station and there was no significant difference between the groups. Perhaps most important was the comparison, on video, of the student's own performance with that of an expert.

Special consideration should be given in the provision of feedback to the needs of the failing student and how they can best be engaged with the process.

Feedback and a variety of approaches

Whilst feedback to students is important, we still have much to learn about how it can best be provided in an OSCE and how students can be encouraged to make the most effective use of it. It is likely that feedback is best given to students using a variety of approaches. However, not all examiners will go to the lengths described in Case Study 3. An audio recording made by the examiner at the time of the OSCE can be used to provide later personalised feedback to the student. Students received feedback from both the examiners and the SPs following the OSCE as a group exercise, when both common mistakes and things that were generally performed well were highlighted, and later individually in the form of the annotated examiner's score sheet.

The amount, nature and specificity of feedback

In many respects, feedback provided as part of an OSCE should follow the same rules and have the same characteristics as those generally associated with good feedback. Particularly important is that the feedback should relate the examinee's

Table 12.2 Students' preference with regard to the medium of feedback (Black and Harden 1986)

Feedback medium	Preference (% students)
Score sheet and video of expected performance	70%
Score sheet alone	24%
Video of expected performance alone	6%

performance to the expected learning outcomes as assessed at the individual stations in the OSCE. The feedback should be specific, positive and clear. Examinees should be provided not only with their overall grade or mark for the OSCE but also with feedback about their performance at each station, in relation to the learning domains assessed in the OSCE, including history taking, communication skills, physical examination, practical procedures, problem solving, and so on.

The score sheet for a station where the examinee has performed poorly should include a narrative comment from the examiner about the performance and how it might have been improved. Examinees should be given a copy of their score sheet, which includes their performance recorded on the checklist, their global ratings and the examiner's narrative comments about their performance. Some examiners and examination boards wish to keep the content of the stations and the checklist and global rating scales confidential and are unwilling for these to be returned to students (See Box 12.3). However, the practice of returning score sheets to examinees is to be recommended. If all of the OSCE stations over a period were known to examinees, this could even be seen as an additional way of communicating the course learning outcomes. We have found that students preferred feedback that included their annotated score sheets (Black and Harden 1986). As shown in Table 12.2, the vast majority of students indicated a preference for receiving both their score sheets and watching a video.

Taylor and Green (2013) looked at the type of feedback received by final-year medical students after stage one of a two-stage OSCE. They found no difference in the improvement in the stage two OSCE scores of the students who received feedback related to the general competencies assessed, such as communication skills, compared with the students whose feedback was based on their performance at each station. Students preferred the station-based feedback, but it was estimated that the cost of providing station-based feedback was twice as much that for the skills-based feedback. As we have argued earlier, despite any additional work and cost, we should aim to provide feedback to students following an OSCE on their performance at each individual station and core tasks at the station as well as on their achievements relating to the broader learning outcome domains.

Feedback and the educational climate

The use of feedback in an OSCE, as with feedback more generally, should be viewed as part of the bigger picture in an educational programme where the educational climate relating to the provision of feedback matters. A positive learning climate and attitude to feedback in the institution is important if feedback is to be maximally effective. Ramani and Krackov (2012) argue that *'the learning climate should promote the concept that the teacher and learner are working together to help the learner enhance the expected learning outcomes'*. They go on to suggest that trust and respect from the teacher helps ensure that the students are more receptive to feedback and that the medical school or training body needs to establish the expectation that regular feedback is part of the learning process. Students should learn to accept and act on feedback with a view to improving their performance. This is important for their practice as doctors later. Consideration needs to be given as to whether the educational climate and culture sufficiently recognise and support the concept of feedback as a key element in the educational programme.

Feedback and summative OSCE

Feedback is an integral part of formative assessment, and much of the discussion in this chapter relates to feedback in formative assessment. The provision of feedback to students in a summative OSCE, an assessment at the end of a course to decide who should pass and who should fail, however, should not be ignored. The standard practice is that students or trainees who are judged from their performance in an examination to have satisfactorily completed a course of study and are competent to pass on to the next phase of the undergraduate curriculum or to graduate and commence their postgraduate training do so without comment on their performance. However, no one is perfect. Should the student be complimented on the areas where they show particular skill and advised on other areas where continuing attention might be beneficial? Should the teacher or trainer taking over the responsibility for the continuing professional development of the individual be made aware of the individual's strengths and weaknesses? These issues are currently under discussion. Blame might even be attached to an institution where a student who is deemed overall to have achieved the competence to graduate and to practise as a healthcare professional later makes a clinical mistake in an area identified as an issue in the final examination, but this is not communicated to the student or those responsible for his/her postgraduate training.

It has been argued in earlier chapters that OSCEs can have both summative and formative functions, and this is illustrated in the case studies. The end-of-term OSCE assessment of students in Dundee had elements of a summative assessment in that it contributed to their end-of-year assessment, as well as elements of a formative assessment in that feedback was given to students. As indicated in Box 12.1, students welcome feedback and perceive it as a powerful learning experience.

Greater consideration needs to be given to feedback not only in formative assessment but also in summative assessment. Friedman Ben-David (2000a) argued that the cultural reform needed in assessment should include formative information within the summative evaluations.

Take-home messages

- Feedback to examinees is important, but even the most experienced teacher or trainer finds it challenging in the clinical context to provide feedback to the student or trainee. The OSCE provides an opportunity to give effective feedback relatively easily.

- The closer in time the feedback is given to the examinee's performance at a station in the OSCE, the more useful it is likely to be. Consideration should be given to providing examinees with feedback during or immediately after the OSCE, and this should include the return of their score sheets with the examiners' comments.

- Feedback should relate to the examinee's performance at individual stations, on core tasks and overall in relation to the learning outcomes, such as communication skills assessed in an OSCE.

- Feedback given by peers can be a valuable learning process for both those receiving and those giving feedback.

- Feedback to students, whilst essential in formative assessments, should also be given in summative assessments.

- A climate where feedback is welcomed should be encouraged in the school. This is particularly important for borderline or 'poor' students.

Is sufficient attention paid in your institution to the provision of feedback in formative and summative assessments, particularly where poor or borderline students are concerned?

The examinee's perspective | 13

Communicating with learners about the OSCE is important. Examinees can prepare for and maximise their performance during an OSCE.

Examinees' attitude to the OSCE

Examinations are a major cause of concern for examinees – there are too many or too few, the assessment is unfair and not related to the learning outcomes for the course, what is asked is trivial and not relevant to the practices of medicine, the examiners are biased and this is reflected in their marking, no feedback is given as to performance in the examination, what is expected of the examinee is not clear and so on. Whilst the OSCE is not exempt from these criticisms, for the most part, the examinees' attitude to the OSCE has been found to be very positive. Favourable comments, such as those reported in Chapter 2, are typical and consistent with the reports in the literature of examinees' attitudes towards the OSCE. Despite some stress and anxiety, a sense of achievement experienced by nursing students was reported following an OSCE (Box 13.1). A humorous view of the OSCE is portrayed in the YouTube video from the students of Griffith School of Medicine (Griffith Med Revue 2012).

In this chapter, we explore the OSCE from the perspective of the student (Figure 13.1). We look at the briefing of students, how they can prepare for an OSCE, the problem of the underperforming student or the student with a disability, and how students can engage with the OSCE process. Although students are not the primary target, we believe that this book can provide them with a useful understanding of the OSCE process and the roles of the examiner and the simulated patient (SP). The case studies in Section D provide helpful examples of the stations and the associated checklists and rating scales used in OSCEs.

Students should consider the OSCE to be a fair assessment of their competence. For this to be the case, the following are important:

- What is assessed in the OSCE should relate closely to the specified learning outcomes for the course and the students' teaching and learning experiences.

Box 13.1

The sense of achievement despite initial anxiety and stress experienced by nurses when exposed to an OSCE for the first time was described by Fidment (2012).

'I thought it was good to have an OSCE, even though when you mentioned it, it scared the heeby jeebies out of me. Afterwards I realised how good it is and now I have remembered more, because it was more of a personal experience, I think it is a good learning tool definitely.'

'I was scared, at the beginning when you find out what you have to deal with at the end, it was scary. But I really enjoyed it, I didn't think I would, but afterwards I felt a real sense of achievement, I was really proud of myself actually.'

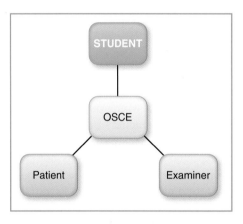

Figure 13.1 The student is a key player in the OSCE.

- Attention is paid to the design of stations, as discussed in Chapter 10, with clear instructions to the student relating to the tasks to be undertaken. It is essential also that what is expected of the student can be completed within the time set for the station.

- Students are briefed adequately in advance of the OSCE and on the day of the examination as to what they can expect with regard to the format of the examination.

- Feedback is provided to students about their performance in the OSCE.

- If the examination is a summative one, students should be given prior practice. Mock OSCEs can be run for this purpose. Such exams have been organised by junior doctors for final year medical students (Bennett and Furmedge 2013). Students who have taken part in a mock OSCE feel less stressed when it comes to taking a real OSCE compared with students who have not. A detailed account of what happens in an OSCE is not a satisfactory substitute for having experienced an OSCE prior to the formal examination.

Briefing of students

Briefing of students is important both prior to the examination and on the morning of the OSCE.

Briefing of students prior to the OSCE

Students should be briefed in advance of the OSCE concerning:

- how the OSCE fits into the overall assessment system and how their marks will be reported.

- the range of competencies to be assessed in the OSCE.

- what students can expect on the day of the OSCE, including the number of stations and the time allocated for each station.

- the types of patient representations used in the OSCE.

- any equipment they are expected to provide, for example a pen, reflex hammer, stethoscope or torch.

- how feedback will be provided to them about their performance in the OSCE; and

- the time and date of the OSCE and where they should assemble.

An online demonstration of the OSCE in action at the UK General Medical Council Assessment Centre is an excellent example of what can be done to brief candidates in advance of the examination (General Medical Council 2014).

Briefing on the day of the examination

Students should be asked to assemble on the day of the OSCE 30 minutes prior to its start. A member of staff should be responsible for briefing the students (Chapter 10). Students should be briefed on:

- the number of stations, their location, and the rotation around the stations; it is useful to have this displayed on a diagram. To avoid any confusion with the rotation, it may be helpful to give students a handout of the rotation which they can consult during the examination. However, with appropriate signposting this should not be necessary.

- the types of stations that students will experience during the examination, including procedure, questions, and rest stations.

- the use of linked and double stations.

THE EXAMINEE'S PERSPECTIVE

- the importance of reading the instructions at each station; and

- the role of the examiners at the stations and whether the student should provide a commentary to the examiner relating to their actions.

Advice to students

The following advice for students may appear redundant, but it is surprising how often the points raised are ignored.

Before the examination

- The OSCE is a performance examination. Prepare for the examination in advance by identifying the areas to be assessed in the OSCE, and think in advance about the tasks you will be expected to undertake at the history taking, physical examination, procedure and data interpretation stations. Think about the different learning outcomes and the core clinical tasks that can be assessed, as described, for example, in Chapter 5.

- Particularly if you have not taken part previously in an OSCE, engage in a mock OSCE. Some institutions offer a formative OSCE a few months before a summative examination to familiarise students with the examination technique; for example, see Case Study 3 and Case Study 14.

- Try out some of the tasks you might face at a station with a colleague or a group of colleagues, taking turns to serve as an SP, an examiner and an examinee.

- Look at examples of OSCE stations. If information is available about stations in previous iterations of the examination you are to take, these should be carefully studied. The case studies in Section D provide examples of stations that might appear in an OSCE at various stages of training. Books are available in many disciplines with examples of OSCE stations (Section F), and a wealth of online material is available.

On the day of the examination

- On the day of the examination, arrive at the correct time and place.

- Be appropriately dressed to take part in a clinical examination with patients (Box 13.2).

- Listen carefully to the briefing provided before the start of the examination, including the time allocated for each station, the time signals to be given and the siting of the stations in the examination area.

- If a map of the station layout is provided, take this with you and look at it as you go around the stations. A member of staff will be available to help should there be a problem in moving from one station to the next.

Box 13.2

The views of students and examiners as to the appropriate appearance of students in an OSCE was studied by Khan (2011). Close agreement was found between students and examiners, with formal rather than casual clothing preferred. Stud piercing of the ear was widely accepted, but nose piercing received a mixed response. Multiple piercing was deemed inappropriate, as were visible tattoos. Length of skirt, makeup and revealing tops were also considerations for females.

- There may be some double stations where twice the amount of time has been allocated for the task you have been set. Recognise this at the start of the station, and plan your use of the time accordingly. Some stations may also be linked so that an activity in one station relates to what is expected at the second station. A linked station may be used if there is a lot of information to read in advance relating to a patient you are to see at the next station.

- Read carefully the instructions provided at each station, and if you are in doubt, ask the examiner for clarification. At some stations the instructions may be quite detailed, and you may be given some useful background to the scenario, as in Case Study 6.

- The instructions may ask you to explain to the examiner what you are doing, as required at Station 1 in Case Study 7, where you are asked also to describe any findings. At other OSCEs, for example Station 7 in Case Study 12, you are told not to ask the examiner any questions during the task.

- Introduce yourself to the patient at a station.

- Show empathy towards the patient, and if an SP, treat them as if they are a real patient. Do not appear rude or inconsiderate towards the patient.

- Ask the patient's consent before carrying out an examination or procedure, and thank the patient on completion of the station.

- Appear confident but not overconfident.

- Most students find that there are one or more stations during the OSCE where they are unhappy with their performance. Do not worry about this, and put a perceived poor performance out of your mind until after the examination. Remember that an advantage of the OSCE is that each station gives you an opportunity for a fresh start.

- The OSCE is likely to include rest stations. At a rest station, do not spend the time rehearsing what you might have done at earlier stations you have completed. Instead, try to relax and think about the stations which you have yet to encounter.

After the examination

- It is likely that you will be given feedback about your performance either during or following the examination. Study this carefully, and if you have any questions, speak to a member of staff. If feedback is not provided about your performance, ask for it. Feedback should be a two-way process in which the learner and the teacher have equal responsibility. With feedback, the OSCE can prove to be a powerful learning experience.

The underperforming student

Teachers have a responsibility to identify students who are underperforming in an OSCE. Particular attention should be paid to the provision of feedback to these students as to their performance in the OSCE. This is discussed further in Chapter 12. It is important to examine the student's performance not only in individual OSCE stations but also across the different learning outcome domains. Does their problem relate to specific tasks they faced in the OSCE or to particular domains, such as communication skills?

The responsibilities of both the teacher and the student do not end with the provision of feedback. Consideration must be given as to any remediation necessary. Appropriate remediation following an OSCE, with support for the student and attention paid to the areas where deficiencies were recognised, is likely to lead to improvement in the student's performance.

As suggested in Chapter 12, it is important that students' performances in OSCEs be profiled over time with long-term support and monitoring for students who not only fail an OSCE but also have several borderline grades (Pell et al. 2012).

The student with a disability

The rotation through a series of stations in an OSCE may be a problem for a student with a disability. The extent to which a medical student's disability should be compensated for in an examination, including an OSCE, is a matter of current debate, and each school has its own policy. While legislation in many countries requires that disabled persons are not placed at a disadvantage in an examination, it is also legislated that adjustments should not compromise professional standards and competence. In the UK, the General Medical Council described what was perceived as reasonable adjustments in an OSCE for a student with a disability, and these are listed in Table 13.1. Box 13.3 describes the length one school went to in order to help dyslexic medical students pass their OSCE.

Student engagement in an OSCE

In line with the greater engagement of students more generally with the curriculum, students can be engaged with the development, implementation and evaluation of an OSCE. This can be a rich learning experience. For example, Heinke et al. (2013)

Table 13.1 Examples of reasonable adjustments for an OSCE as reported by the UK General Medical Council (GMC 2008)

- Sphygmomanometer with a red flipper valve for a blood pressure station
- Amplified stethoscope
- Student permitted to summarise verbally at the end of each station
- Student permitted to use an agreed alternative word or expression
- Student permitted to write down a word if unable to verbalise it
- Extra question reading time
- Paper copies of the instructions for each station
- Extra time at station assessments that do not directly replicate clinical practice
- Physical stations in OSCE to be followed by a rest station or placed at the end of the examination
- A reader
- A 'competent other' who could be instructed by the student in conducting the resuscitation task provided at the station
- Additional practice sessions and support given prior to the OSCE
- Timing of OSCE to earlier rather than later in the day
- Examiners briefed about individual trainee requirements

Box 13.3

The special accommodations made to support students with dyslexia at the University of Ottawa OSCE assessment were described by Renaud and Jalali (2011). The Faculty of Medicine provided an iPod with Kurzweil 3000 software to help students read about the station, and students were allowed 1.5 more time per station to read the instructions at the door of the examination room. At the emergency station, no extra time was allowed. Time and effort were invested by the medical school in working out the process and installing the software. However, the experience demonstrated that providing dyslexic medical students with practical accommodation allows them to participate successfully in an OSCE. The authors also suggested that the innovation should help the students to adapt more successfully to their eventual practice as physicians by using these technologies in their day-to-day activities.

found that students who developed OSCE stations performed better in a summative OSCE. Students can also serve as examiners in an OSCE. Usually this is a mock OSCE or formative assessment, as discussed in Chapter 8. Moineau et al. (2011) used fourth-year medical students as examiners in a formative nine-station OSCE for second-year medical students. Each station included 2 minutes of feedback given by the fourth-year students. Faculty rated the student feedback highly and considered it *'balanced, specific, accurate, appropriate, and given in a professional manner'*. The candidates, student examiners and faculty examiners agreed that using students as examiners was appropriate for formative examinations but not for summative examinations.

Cushing et al. (2011) gave students the opportunity to give and to receive feedback from each other in a formative OSCE. Medical and nursing students took part in a three-station OSCE which was conducted three times, each student taking the role of candidate, examiner and observer. The 'candidate' received immediate feedback from the 'examiner' and the 'observer'. The students found the exercise to be a valuable learning experience.

A feedback OSCE (ICRE 2011) with video recordings of the stations was introduced to help senior residents develop their skills when providing formative feedback to junior residents.

As described in Chapter 17, it is likely that in the future we will see increasing engagement of the student with the development, implementation and evaluation of the OSCE.

Take-home messages

- As with any examination, there can be a measure of stress associated with an OSCE. However, if the OSCE is carefully designed and delivered students generally rate their experience favourably.

- Full briefing of students in advance of the OSCE and on the day of the OSCE is essential with regard to the actions expected of them and how they should behave.

- Students should think in advance how they can best prepare themselves for an OSCE and how they should behave on the day of the examination.

- The OSCE can be a powerful learning experience, and feedback is important.

- Poorly performing students who fail an OSCE or have a borderline performance over a number of OSCEs, should have their progress monitored carefully, and remedial action should be taken to meet their needs.

- Consideration should be given to students with a disability.

- Students can be engaged with the planning, implementation and evaluation of an OSCE. This may include the development of stations and serving as examiners.

 In your institution, are students engaged in the development and implementation of an OSCE as partners in the assessment process?

Evaluating an OSCE | 14

Evaluation and quality control of an OSCE is important, and constant monitoring and improvement are necessary.

The importance of evaluation

The central theme of this chapter is unambiguous. Given the complexity of the process and the different associated elements, the importance of the results and decisions taken with regard to the examinee and the hidden influences of the OSCE on the curriculum and student learning, the evaluation and quality control of the OSCE is essential (Schultz et al. 2008; Pell et al. 2010). Validation of the OSCE is important and should be an ongoing responsibility for those organising the examination, providing guidance for quality improvement (Medical Council of Canada 2011).

Many reports in the literature describe individual teacher's or student's evaluation of an OSCE. Although this is of value, there is a need to go beyond this with a more formal evaluation of an OSCE. The evaluation of the OSCE should be seen as an ongoing process throughout the OSCE cycle and not just as something that happens after the examination has taken place.

Approaches to the evaluation of an OSCE are discussed in this chapter.

The concept of evaluation

First some thoughts on the concept of evaluation. Education evaluation has come a long way over the last half century, and varying definitions exist:

> ' "*Evaluate*," or at least its root word "*value*," finds its origin in the Old
> French value and valoir and the Latin valére, which had the sense of "to be
> worth (something)" and "to work out the value of (something)." Even in
> present everyday usage this has a double meaning, of finding a numerical
> expression for and estimating the worth of, and of course "worth" carries
> several distinct meanings, including personal worthiness, status, how we
> personally estimate someone, judgments of importance, and intrinsic worth.'
> (Mark et al. 2006)

A common functional definition of evaluation involving judgements of values, determinations of merit or worth or significance of something is associated with Scriven's definition (1991): *'Evaluation refers to the process of determining the merit, worth or value of something, or the product of that process.'*

Other definitions of evaluation highlight the purpose of the evaluation (For 'program' read 'OSCE').

> *'Program evaluation is the systematic collection of information about the activities, characteristics, and outcomes of programs to make judgments about the program, improve program effectiveness, and/or inform decisions about future programming.'* (Patton 1997, p. 23)

Such definitions help us think about evaluation in the context of an OSCE, and we will explore this further. How can we determine the merits or worth of using an OSCE? What information should we collect in evaluating an OSCE?

The purpose of evaluation

When consideration is given to evaluation of an OSCE, the purpose of the evaluation should be borne in mind. The reasons for evaluating an OSCE are to ensure that:

- Correct decisions are taken about the learner being assessed. Learners who have the necessary specified competence should pass the examination and those who have not should receive a fail grade.

- Accrediting or other bodies are satisfied that the OSCE as implemented is 'fit for purpose'. In the UK, for example, the General Medical Council needs to be assured in its inspection of schools that the OSCE implemented as part of the final examinations has been appropriately evaluated.

- Appropriate feedback is provided to learners about their performance.

- Appropriate feedback is provided to teachers that impacts the development of the curriculum.

- The results of the evaluation contribute to the further development and improvement of the OSCE. The evaluation may lead to a better understanding of the OSCE as a tool to assess competence and of issues relating to assessment more generally.

Different approaches

The evaluation of an OSCE can be seen from different perspectives. Such philosophical differences are part of the qualitative/quantitative debate that has consumed much of educational research. Differences are a fact of life in contemporary evaluation, and diversity of approaches to evaluate should be encouraged and embraced. The choice of approach to the evaluation of an OSCE will be determined by the question or questions being addressed, but it is almost certain that a range of methods will be required. David Nevo (2006) suggests:

> 'It may well be true that for a complicated activity such as evaluation, the approach needed is one that seeks the best method or set of methods to answer the particular evaluation question at hand, rather than assuming that one method is best for all purposes.'

Psychometrics, such as Cronbach's α (Cronbach and Shavelson 2004), contribute to the assessment of the reliability of an OSCE, whereas other approaches are required where one is concerned with validity and the answer to the question 'Is the examination measuring what should be measured?'

Questions to be addressed

The OSCE should be evaluated both from the perspective of the students' performance in the whole examination and from their performances in the individual stations in the OSCE (Pell et al. 2010). Questions that should be addressed relating to the whole examination include:

- Was the OSCE a valid assessment – was what was assessed in the examination what should be assessed? This question relates to what the examination is used for.

- Was the OSCE reliable? Did it give consistent results? This addresses the question of how the OSCE is used.

- Has the OSCE been cost effective in the use made of the resources, including the venue, the examiners, the patients and the manikins used?

- Were the examiners appropriately trained and briefed for their role in the OSCE?

- Were the instructions for examinees clear, and were the examinees adequately briefed in advance and on the day of the examination?

- Were examinees given appropriate feedback with regard to their performance?

- Was an appropriate standard setting process implemented?

- Does the culture in the school support or prove an obstacle to the use of the OSCE as an assessment tool?

- What, if any, problems were reported during the examination?

- What impact has the OSCE had on the examinees and their learning?

- What impact has the OSCE had on the teachers and on the curriculum planning?

Commenting on the *Assessment Futures* document, an Oxford Brookes University (2014) report noted:

> '...the first question to be asked of assessment should never be: Is it reliable and consistent? Instead, we should ask: Does assessment do what we want it to do in terms of promoting the kinds of learning that are desired for the longer term? If it doesn't do this, then there is no point in moving to other questions.'

In addition to an overall evaluation of the OSCE, the **individual stations** should be evaluated in terms of:

- the validity of the station – what it is measuring.

- whether the task expected of the examinee could be completed in the time allocated.

- the standard expected of the examinee at the station and the number of candidates passing and failing the station.

- the checklists and global rating scales used at the station.

- the role of the examiner.

- the performance of a simulated patient (SP) or manikin; and

- the feedback given to the learner.

Although it may be difficult to video record all of the stations in the examination, doing so for at least one examination and one history taking station can be helpful. This not only provides feedback to learners but also informs the evaluation of the station.

Who should contribute to the evaluation?

It is important that all of the stakeholders contribute to the OSCE evaluation. This will include:

- **Examiners** – Their views should be solicited as to their training and preparation prior to the OSCE and about the station at which they examined the students. This should include the task expected of the candidate; the scoring scheme, including the use of checklists and global rating scales, the SP or other patient representation; the instructions to candidates at the station; the station venue; and feedback to candidates. Overall comments on the OSCE should also be invited.

- **Simulated patients** – The views of SPs should be solicited with regard to the station to which they contributed, both in terms of the organisation of the station and the candidates' performance. Where they are asked to formally rate the candidate, the ratings should be examined and compared with the ratings of the examiners.

- **Candidates** – Comments should be encouraged from candidates on their briefing before the examination, on the day of the examination and at individual stations; on the overall areas tested in the examination and whether they match with the course content and learning outcomes; on the organisation of the OSCE examination and the venue; and on the feedback provided to them about their performance. They should be asked to identify any stations which presented a problem for them, and this should be explored further.

- **The committee and individuals responsible for the organisation of the examination** – Their views should be solicited about the OSCE, including its strengths and weaknesses, and the standard setting procedure, including the pass/fail rate of students. Any problems identified should be explored.

- **External evaluators** – The responsibility for evaluating an OSCE may rest with external assessors not concerned with the implementation of the examination. External assessors, for example, play an important part in quality assurance of the Royal College of Surgeons Intercollegiate OSCE Examination (see Box 14.1).

- **Administrative and support staff** – Comments should be invited from administrative and support staff on the organisation of the examination and the processing of the candidate's score sheets and marks.

- **Clinicians** – At a later stage it may be valuable to compare the students' performance in the OSCE with their performance in subsequent clinical attachments and in medical practice. However, this will not inform immediate decisions about the OSCE.

Validity

Whether the OSCE is a valid examination is the most importation question to ask in the evaluation of an OSCE. If the OSCE is not a valid assessment, the answers to the other questions are irrelevant. Validity in the context of an OSCE is discussed further in Chapter 3.

Box 14.1

The quality assurance of the Royal College of Surgeons Intercollegiate OSCE Examination in the UK is the responsibility of a body of experienced examiners (Joint Committee on Surgical Training 2014). They do not examine candidates but assess the examination. A code of conduct for assessors has been written based on the Nolan principles:

- *Selflessness* – Assessors should act solely in terms of promoting the quality of the examination.
- *Integrity* – Assessors should not place themselves under any obligations to outside individuals or organisations that might seek to influence them.
- *Objectivity* – Assessors should make their judgements on merit.
- *Accountability* – Assessors are accountable to an International Quality Assurance Committee.
- *Openness* – Assessors should be as open as possible about the actions and decisions they take.
- *Honesty* – Assessors have a duty to clear any private interests that may influence their duties.
- *Leadership* – Assessors should promote and support the principles by leadership and example.

Reports from assessors following each diet of the examination comment on any inappropriate examiner behaviour, the standard setting process and scenarios and stations where problems are identified.

The validity of an OSCE is the extent to which the examination actually measures what it purports to measure. Validity is not an entity of the OSCE per se, it is the extent to which the OSCE being evaluated assesses what it purports to test (Schuwirth and van der Vleuten 2011). An OSCE station where the student has to take a history of a patient with an abdominal problem may be a valid test of history taking, but it is not a valid test as to whether the student understands how to obtain informed consent for surgery. A feature of the OSCE is greater authenticity and relating the examination more closely to clinical practice. As in this example, however, authenticity does not always equate with validity.

Content validity

When evaluating an OSCE, content validity is of the greatest importance. This form of validity refers to the appropriateness of what is tested in the OSCE – is it a good sample of what the examinee should be able to do?

Content validity is determined not by a statistical procedure but by a judgement on the part of the examiners. An OSCE that has:

> '...content validity consists of a sufficient number and variety of stations that are representative of the curricular goals and objectives from which the stations were drawn and about which generalizations are to be made.'
> (DaRosa and Kaiser 2001)

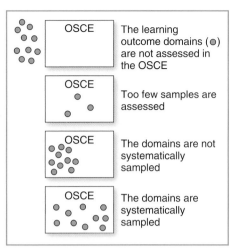

Figure 14.1 Problems with validity in the OSCE. (Modified from Yudkowsky 2009, p. 234.)

For an OSCE to be valued, it must sufficiently and systematically sample the domain to be assessed (Yudkowsky 2009) (Figure 14.1). The development of an OSCE blueprint, as described in Chapter 10, is key to the establishment of the validity for the examination (Newble 1988). The validity of the OSCE should be judged in the context of:

- the disciplines or specialties assessed, for example surgery, medicine and psychiatry.

- the body systems assessed, for example endocrine, cardiovascular and alimentary.

- the learning outcome domains assessed, for example communication skills, physical examination and practical procedures.

- the age of the patient in the stations, for example child, adolescent, adult and elderly; and

- the context for care, for example ambulatory care, hospital practice and family medicine.

Criterion-related validity

In the assessment of the OSCE's validity, it may be of interest to compare the results with other assessments of competence, such as a Mini-Clinical Evaluation Exercise (Mini-CEX), a portfolio or clinical supervisor's ratings. This is referred to as *criterion-related validity*.

Predictive validity

The predictive validity of the OSCE may also be examined, although, by its very nature, this has to be assessed some time later. The question is whether the examinee's score in the OSCE was an accurate estimation of the person's performance at a later stage in the curriculum or following their graduation as a doctor.

Predictive validity can be seen as a type of criterion-related validity where validity relates to how accurately the student's performance in an OSCE estimates their performance on the criteria measured at a later time.

Reliability

The reliability of an OSCE indicates the extent to which the scores in the OSCE are reproducible or dependable. Popham (2009), an assessment guru, has succinctly described three decisively different forms of reliability:

- *Stability reliability* – refers to the consistency of students' scores when a test is administered to the same students on two different occasions.

- *Alternate-form reliability* – describes the consistency of students' performances on two different (hopefully equivalent) versions of the same test.

- *Internal consistency reliability* – describes the consistency with which all the separate items on a test measure whatever they are measuring.

It is often not appreciated that when reliability is described in the context of an OSCE what is usually being described is a measure of internal consistency and of how similar the stations in the OSCE function and their homogeneity. The Cronbach α, as described below, is a unit of internal consistency used to calculate the correlation values amongst the scores for the stations.

It should be noted also that an examination may be reliable but not valid. This was the problem with multiple-choice questions as a test of clinical competence and one of the reasons for the introduction of the OSCE, as described in Chapter 2. In the field of archery, a group of arrows may consistently hit a similar point on the outer edges of the target, as shown in Figure 14.2. This, in terms of an OSCE, is consistent with stations that give reliable but not valid results. What one wants is to hit consistently the centre of the target where one is aiming. It is always desirable to keep the need for validity clearly in mind with, if necessary, a compromise in its favour even if the level of reliability should fall.

Much emphasis has been placed on estimates of an OSCE's reliability, with Cronbach's α being quoted. It should be remembered, however, that this represents only the internal consistency of the stations in an OSCE, and the limitations described above should be noted.

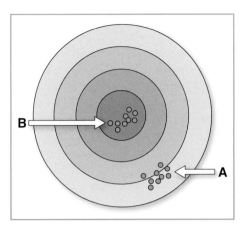

Figure 14.2 A – Arrows consistently hit the same area, but not the centre of the target. This is equivalent to a reliable, but not valid assessment. B – Arrows consistently hit the centre of the target that one is aiming at – a reliable and valid assessment.

Robert Mislevy (2004) has pointed out that *'the internal-consistency reliability indices to aid in evaluating the quality of the evidence, will suit our needs in an assessment situation. Sometimes they won't.'* He goes on to argue that:

> *'...the challenge to test theory specialists is to continually broaden their methodology, in order to extend the toolkit of data-gathering and interpretation methods available to deal with increasingly richer sources of evidence and more complex arguments for making sense of that evidence.'* (Mislevy 2004, p. 239)

Three approaches to the estimates of an OSCE's reliability in current use are:

- classical test theory (CTT).

- generalisability theory (G-theory); and

- item-response theory (IRT).

Classical test theory

The CTT approach is the most widely used and easily understood of the approaches to the assessment of the reliability of the OSCE. In CTT it is assumed that the examinee's score is a function of the true score plus random errors. These errors may relate to many things, including the presentation of the scenario at the station, the checklist, the examiner's scoring or the behaviour of the SP. The true score is a measure of an examinee's true competence in the absence of these errors. De Champlain (2010) has provided a useful primer on CTT.

The statistical procedure most commonly used to estimate reliability is Cronbach's α (Cronbach and Shavelson 2004; Tavakol and Dennick 2011). As pointed out above and by Pell et al. (2010), Cronbach's α is a measure of the *internal consistency of the examination commonly, though not accurately thought of as "reliability"*. The assumption is that in a good assessment, the better student will do well and a poor student less well across the range of stations in an OSCE as determined by their checklist scores at each station. Cronbach's α estimates can range from 0 to 1.0, where 1.0 represents a perfect examination. Reliability as shown by α scores greater than 0.7 or 0.8 is generally thought to be necessary, particularly for a high-stakes OSCE. Schuwirth and van der Vleuten (2011) have illustrated, however, that a test with a high reliability is not always better than a test with a lower reliability.

There is value in generating quality metrics for individual stations as well as for the overall examination. Pell et al. (2010) and Huang et al. (2010) have demonstrated how a measure of the reliability of a station can be estimated if α is calculated with each station deleted in turn. It is also possible to use the correlation between the station score and the total score less the station score.

It is important to recognise, as we have discussed, that Cronbach α is, in some measure, dependent on the homogeneity of the examination. If all stations assess the same learning outcome, one can expect a higher α compared to a situation where stations assess very different competencies. While one might expect the good examinee who is competent in some areas to be competent in other areas, such as obtaining patient consent, this may not necessarily be the case.

Generalisability theory

Generalisability theory is an extension of CTT and uses analysis of variance (ANOVA) to quantify how much measurement error in an OSCE can be attributed to each potential factor, such as raters, SPs, or dates of administration (Lawson 2006; Iramaneerat et al. 2008; Bloch and Norman 2012).

Through the identification of possible sources of error in the OSCE, the use of G-theory can help improve future OSCEs. It is possible to extrapolate what the generalisability or dependability of the OSCE would have been, for example if the number of stations is increased, or which is more efficient – using two examiners per station or having more stations with only one examiner.

Item-response theory

CTT focuses on the test and its errors and ignores issues relating to test difficulty and the candidates' abilities. IRT overcomes this problem. It has many advantages and can provide more precise information about test items and examinees' abilities.

Schuwirth and van der Vleuten (2011), recommend that IRT should only be used if people with sufficient understanding of statistics and the underlying concept are part of the OSCE team. Boulet (2009) suggests that IRT, because of its many advantages, should be applied more broadly in medical education, but also warns that the lack of expertise needed to apply the approach may constrain its use in practice. Donnon et al. (2011) used item analysis to assess the quality of an OSCE checklist.

Further information

A more detailed description of reliability measures is beyond the scope of this book, and further information can be found in guides published by the Association for Medical Education in Europe (AMEE):

- AMEE Guide 57: General overview of the theories used in assessment (Schuwirth and van der Vleuten 2011).

- AMEE Guide 49: How to measure the quality of the OSCE: A review of metrics (Pell et al. 2010).

- AMEE Guide 54: Post-examination analysis of objective tests (Tavakol and Dennick 2011).

- AMEE Guide 66: Post-examination interpretation of objective test data: Monitoring and improving the quality of high-stakes examinations (Tavakol and Dennick 2012); and

- AMEE Guide 68: Generalizability theory for the perplexed: A practical introduction and guide (Bloch and Norman 2012).

See also the books recommended in the bibliography in Section F.

Number of failures

The failure rate in the examination overall and in individual stations in the OSCE should be examined. A higher than anticipated failure rate may be explained if:

- An inappropriate standard has been set for the examination or the station.

- There are technical problems relating to the station, such as ambiguity in the instructions or difficulty with the performance of the SP.

- The examination and the station are not an appropriate assessment of the expected learning outcomes.

- The teaching and the training programme are deficient.

In the presence of a high failure rate the necessary action to be taken will depend on an analysis of the cause.

Circuit equivalence

Examinees may be assessed in an OSCE at one of a number of circuits, sometimes at different locations. It is important to show that the assessment of competence is not affected by the examination circuit to which they have been allocated. If attention is paid to the matching of the patients in different circuits and in the training of the examiners, one would not expect to find an overall difference between the performance of examinees at different circuits. Pell et al. (2010) have described how an estimate can be made as to the extent to which the marks for a student's performance are estimates of competence rather than the particular OSCE environment in a circuit in terms of the location of the OSCE or the attitudes of the assessor – 'hawks' or 'doves'. Provided that careful attention has been paid to the preparation of the assessment, it is likely that any circuit defect will largely be self-cancelling.

Take-home messages

- A rigorous evaluation of an OSCE is important, as key decisions may be taken based on the results. It may be assumed, for example, that the student who passes will be safe to practise in the clinical setting with patients. Quality assessment of the process is important given the impact the OSCE and the evaluation can have on the learner and on the curriculum.

- An overall evaluation of the OSCE as well as an assessment of each station in the examination should be made.

- Validity is key to the evaluation of an OSCE. The question should be asked whether or not the OSCE is assessing what should be assessed.

- The reliability of the OSCE should be assessed using Cronbach's α or some other matrix recognising their limitations.

- The different elements in the OSCE should be evaluated, including the examination blueprint, the role of the examiners and the SPs and the standard setting process.

- All of the stakeholders, including examiners, teachers, examinees and patients, should be engaged with the evaluation.

- An evaluation of the OSCE can lead to a better understanding of the OSCE and to improved future practice.

Are sufficient time, resources and expertise allocated in your institution to the evaluation of the OSCE?

Costs and implementing an OSCE with limited resources | 15

The resources required and the costs incurred can be tailored to the local situation. The OSCE can, but need not, be expensive to administer. Many OSCEs are run at little or no additional cost.

Cost as a cause of concern

The extent of the resources required and the associated costs of developing and implementing an examination are concerns expressed about the use of the OSCE. This, along with other potential limitations to the use of the OSCE, is discussed further in Chapter 16. At many medical schools, cost was said to be a major deterrent to the use of this form of assessment (Reznick et al. 1993b). In this chapter we look at the costs associated with an OSCE in relation to the benefits achieved and how the costs may be reduced and the OSCE implemented in situations where resources are limited.

The cost is frequently not cited in reports on the OSCE. Where it is, these have ranged from $11 to $1,200 (USD) per candidate (Reznick et al. 1993b). A problem in the calculation of OSCE costs is determining what to include in the estimates. As Benbow et al. (1998) noted, '*...the usefulness of estimating the costs is limited by the lack of consensus of what should be included in costing*'. The wide variation in costs reported may be, in part, due to differences in the design of the OSCE implemented, in particular the use made of simulated patients (SPs). Another major factor in the calculation is distinguishing between what is considered a direct cost and what is considered an indirect cost. The direct costs of an OSCE are those additional costs which would not otherwise be charged. The indirect or hidden costs of an OSCE are ones that can be absorbed and considered part of an institution's responsibility.

Estimates of costs

Direct costs vary greatly from institution to institution, depending on the extent to which there is an additional charge made for staff time, accommodation, SPs and resources used in the OSCE. When the OSCE was introduced at the medical school in Dundee, the budget was £0.00 (GBP). This was because there was no charge from the medical school for the examiners' time, the venue, the data handling and other resources. The SPs used in the OSCE donated their time. The fact that there was no need to have additional funding approved facilitated the introduction of the approach. The majority of OSCE developers today, however, may not be in this fortunate position.

In practice, Carpenter (1995) and Kelly and Murphy (2004) respectively estimated such indirect costs as 80% and 70% of a total OSCE budget.

Direct cost per student per station has been estimated as varying from $0.88 (USD) (Feather and Kopelman 1997) to $6.90 (USD) (Cusimano et al. 1994). When all costs were included, the cost per student per station rose to $13.69 (USD) (Gilson et al. 1998) and $12.50 (USD) or $15.68 (USD) if rest stations were excluded (Heard et al. 1998). Reznick et al. (1993b) estimated the cost of administering an OSCE to range from $496 to $870 (CAD) per examinee, depending on the contribution made by the school (Box 15.1). Applying the same approach to costing an OSCE in nursing in Italy, Palese et al. (2012) estimated that the high-end costs, including both direct and indirect costs, were €145 (EUR) per student, whilst the low-end costs were €35 (EUR).

More recently, the costs of implementing a medical OSCE at the University of Ulm, Germany, was estimated at €86 (EUR) per student (Rau et al. 2011). £355 (GBP) per student was estimated by Brown et al. (2015) to be the cost of a final summative OSCE at the University of Aberdeen, UK. The costs attributed to a dental OSCE at the University of Heidelberg were estimated to be €181 (EUR) per student (Eberhard et al. 2011). In postgraduate education, the estimated costs of an American College

---

Box 15.1 Cost estimates for implementing an OSCE, including development and implementation on the day of the examination (Reznick et al. 1993b)

- High-end costs assume that faculty time is compensated.
- Low-end costs assume contributions by the medical school.

Element	High-end cost (CAD)	Low-end cost (CAD)
Examiners	29,100	0
OSCE lead	10,000	0
Support staff	17,700	17,700
SPs	35,500	35,500
Printing and equipment	4,000	1,300
Data processing	4,700	1,600
Catering	3,360	3,360
Total	**104,360**	**59,460**
Total per examinee	**870**	**496**

SP, simulated patient.

of Surgeons' OSCE to assess the clinical skills of surgical residents was estimated to range from $239 to $664 (USD) per resident, depending on the number of residents assessed (Sudan et al. 2014). More than 50% of this was attributed to the cost associated with the use of SPs. An OSCE developed to assess higher medical trainees in rheumatology in the UK was developed and implemented with 12 trainees (Hassell 2002). The cost per trainee was £548 (GBP). This would be reduced significantly if more trainees were assessed in the OSCE or the examination developed was used on multiple occasions.

As pointed out by Reznick et al. (1993b), the costs of a large-scale centralised examination may be significantly higher than an OSCE organised locally in an institution given the added layers of organisation and security required and the travel expenses for examiners.

Cost elements

The costs attributed to an OSCE may relate to the examiners' time, the use of SPs, the venue, the administrative, technical and educational support and other resources required (Figure 15.1).

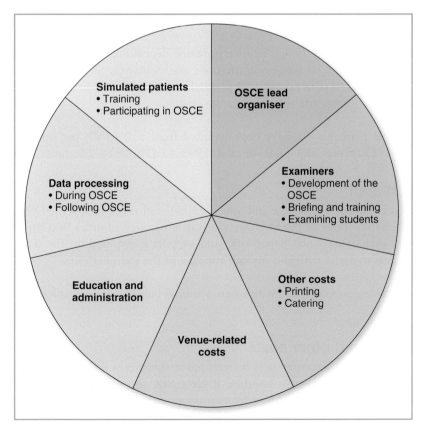

Figure 15.1 Elements contributing to the cost of an OSCE.

Examiner

If physicians are used as examiners and full compensation is paid for their time engaged on OSCE-related activities, the cost can be very high. Reznick et al. (1993b) compensated physicians' time on an academic honorarium basis only at $150 (USD) per half-day. In some situations, because of the cost of using medical examiners, SPs are trained to serve as assessors of the students' competence.

Staff time is required not only on the day of the examination but also for development work on the OSCE blueprint and the OSCE stations and for staff training. Following the examination, input from the examiners is also required in relation to decisions to be taken about the examinee's performance and the award, where appropriate, of a pass/fail grade based on the analysis of the results. In addition, feedback has to be provided to the individual examinees and to the curriculum committee.

OSCE Lead

The OSCE Lead is key to the successful implementation of the OSCE, as described in Chapter 10. This individual, who is usually a member of staff, takes responsibility for the work leading up to the implementation of the examination, for the organisation on the day and for the follow-up after the examination. The responsibility for the OSCE may even be part of the person's job description.

Simulated patients

The costs of SPs for an OSCE will vary greatly, depending on the number of SPs used and the cost per SP. Some examinations use exclusively SPs, whilst others use a mix of SPs and real patients. Trained professional SPs will require to be paid, whilst volunteers may contribute their time at no charge.

Standardised patient costs have been reported from $10 (USD) per hour (Battles et al. 1992; Carpenter 1995; Gilson et al. 1998) to $50 (USD) (Szerlip et al. 1998).

Support staff

Assistance from administrative and other support staff is required if the OSCE is to run successfully. Prior to the examination this is required in order to complete the necessary preparations and paperwork, and support is required on the day of the examination to assist with the smooth running of the examination.

Data processing support and facilities are required before, during and following the examination.

Resources and other costs

Manikins and other resources may be required at stations in the examination. Data processing equipment is also required if electronic marking at stations is to be adopted, including tablets for use by examiners during the examination. Printed materials, including signposts, will also be required.

Other costs that may be incurred relate to catering and travel expenses for SPs and real patients.

Approaches to costing

An alternative approach to costing separately the different elements that go to make up an OSCE, including the examiners, SPs, and so on is to look at the list of tasks and activities undertaken before, during and after the OSCE implementation and assign a cost against each item. These steps are set out in some detail in Chapter 10, but the details will vary from OSCE to OSCE. Direct and indirect costs can be considered for each item, and a total sum for the examination and the component elements can be obtained.

Comparative costs

When comparing the costs of the OSCE with other forms of clinical assessment, some reports have suggested that it is more expensive (Cusimano et al. 1994; Azcuenga et al. 1998) whilst others have suggested that the costs are comparable (Young et al. 1995; Kelly and Murphy 2004). Feather and Kopelman (1997) suggested that the OSCE's cost is 'modest' when compared with overall clinical assessments, and Joorabchi (1991) came to a similar conclusion after comparing the OSCE with a performance-based assessment of clinical skills.

Frye et al. (1989), concerned about the costs of implementing an OSCE at the Bowman Gray School of Medicine, asked the question, 'Is it worth it?' They estimated that conducting the OSCE for 117 medical students required 527 hours of donated faculty time. However, all of the faculty involved in the examination reported that the time they had spent evaluating students in the OSCE was worth it. Walsh et al. (2009, p. 1589) concluded that '...the benefits associated with the OSCE process outweighed the limitations of other forms of evaluative methods and this justified its use'.

When used to assess students for admission to medicine, Eva et al. (2004a) demonstrated that the OSCE required fewer examiner hours than traditional interviews that take place in front of a panel of interviewers. In addition, they found that the OSCE had an impact and that the blueprinting required for the OSCE stations provided a stimulus to prompt the admissions committee collectively to make more explicit the qualities for which they wanted to select candidates.

Given that the OSCE plays a key part in the important task of assessing a student's or graduate's clinical competence, it is not unreasonable to expect that significant resources will be required. The cost of not assessing students' clinical competence and graduating doctors who do not have the necessary skills is higher. Moreover, the costs incurred by an OSCE should not be simply set against the cost of administering a clinical examination. As described in this book, the OSCE can have a major impact on a student's learning and on the curriculum and may be viewed by students as a powerful learning opportunity.

More generally in relation to the financing of education, it can be argued that assessment in healthcare education has probably not been allocated the resources required. The Open University in the UK, which consistently performs in a National Student Survey in the top 10 of UK universities, devotes over half its teaching resources to assessment and feedback (Higher Education Academy 2012). The figures in medical schools will be appreciably lower.

The different purposes the OSCE can fulfil and its impact on teaching have been outlined in earlier chapters. These more than justify the resources required to implement the approach. It has to be recognised, however, that there are financial constraints on the education sector, and in the next section of this chapter we look at how the costs associated with an OSCE can be contained.

Containing the costs or implementing an OSCE with limited resources

Whilst significant costs and resources may be associated with the development and implementation of an OSCE, these need not be a barrier to the use of an OSCE, and it is possible to adopt the approach in resource-limited environments (Poenaru et al. 1997; Vargas et al. 2007). Creative ways can be found to design an OSCE programme with a limited budget (Casey et al. 2009). Palese et al. (2012) also looked at nursing educational strategies for further reducing the costs of an OSCE.

Problems associated with running an OSCE, particularly in a resource-challenged environment, can be related to a lack of experience and technical support and to the availability of and costs attributed to examiners, SPs, a venue for the examination and other required resources.

Lack of experience and expertise

As described by Vargas et al. (2007), a problem in implementing an OSCE may be that the staff in the institution lack experience in developing and administering an OSCE (Box 15.2). This can be tackled in a number of ways:

Box 15.2	Staff training and the adoption of an OSCE in a resource-limited environment (Vargas et al. 2007, p. 197)

'...For OSCEs, specific training in case development, checklist construction, scoring and psychometrics are a few of the topic areas where additional faculty training will certainly be of some benefit. These educational activities can be facilitated in a number of ways, including national and international conferences. Two such conferences were hosted at NUC, bringing interested faculty and international experts together. Providing these educational opportunities was relatively inexpensive and proved to be an effective strategy to maintain faculty support for the assessment program.'

- *Consult published literature or online resources on the subject.* This can provide, as described in Chapter 10, information about the steps and actions required to implement an OSCE and a description of decisions that need to be taken relating to its design, implementation and scoring.

- *Visit other centres.* Talk with colleagues about the lessons they have learned in running an OSCE, and listen to any advice they offer. If possible, take part in an OSCE as an examiner or an observer. Obtaining experience of an OSCE in this way proved to be a valuable element in the spread of the OSCE approach in schools in South Africa (Lazarus and Harden 1985). Travel grants may be available to support such visits to other centres.

- *Attend conferences, workshops or courses where the OSCE is on the programme.* These experiences not only provide useful information on planning and delivering an OSCE, but make it possible to network with others working in the area. At the annual conference of the Association for Medical Education in Europe (AMEE), there are sessions on the OSCE and an assessment course in conjunction with the conference that features the OSCE in the wider context of assessment.

- *Invite a consultant to visit the school.* The consultant selected should be someone who has personal experience and expertise in the organisation of an OSCE.

- *Obtain examples of documentation relating to OSCEs.* Examples of instructions for students, examiners and SPs and examples of OSCE stations are helpful. Some examples are available in Section D, and a search online will provide further useful examples.

Other steps to be taken

From the experience gained at the National University of Cuio in Argentina (Vargas et al. 2007) and elsewhere, there are a number of additional important steps that can be taken to support and facilitate the OSCE implementation in a school where there has been little, if any, previous experience of the approach.

- *Create a culture* within the school, led by the dean, where implementing the OSCE is seen as something worth doing. The use of the OSCE can reassure accrediting bodies and the local population that the graduates from the school have the necessary competence. It can also make a valuable contribution to curriculum development.

- *Involve and engage the faculty and students* in the reasons for introducing an OSCE and in the plans for the development of the OSCE. Obtain their commitment to supporting the OSCE implementation.

- See the development of the OSCE and of stations in the OSCE as part of *curriculum development*. The OSCE blueprint should focus on the core learning outcomes for the education programme, and these may need to be further developed.

- When the OSCE has been developed, initiate a *pilot examination* where the OSCE is used first for formative purposes and then for summative purposes.

Technical support

Technical support is valuable to develop a system of recording scores during the OSCE to review the scores and make pass/fail decisions following the OSCE, as described in Chapter 11. Educational advice on standard setting and the provision of feedback to the examiners can be useful. Technical expertise in these areas is useful but is not strictly necessary. Where resources are limited, a more sophisticated analysis of the results may not be possible, and basic standard setting procedures can be carried out using available computer packages. In the early years of the introduction of the OSCE, paper-based systems were relied upon and worked perfectly adequately. However, there are now greater expectations as to what can be done with data processing, standard setting and the provision of feedback in an OSCE.

Design of the OSCE

Costs can be contained to some extent by limiting the number of stations, the duration of stations and the length of the examination. It is advisable, however, not to go lower than 10×5-minute stations. As described below, the stations should be designed to make best use of the available resources, including examiners and patients.

Sequential OSCEs have been suggested as an approach to reducing costs (Cookson et al. 2011). Students whose performance is judged entirely satisfactory after a small number of stations are not examined further, and it is suggested that this may result in a significant cost saving. At the Hull York Medical School, UK, the savings were estimated at approximately £30,000 (GBP). The sequential approach concentrates resources where they are most needed – to make decisions with regard to borderline candidates. The adoption of a sequential design does, however, require significant additional organisational and judgmental activities.

Examiners

The availability of examiners may be limited, and if fees are paid to examiners, the overall costs can be high. This need not be a problem.

- Examiners and the employing authority can accept that their input to the OSCE is part of their responsibilities and commitment to the school, and no additional charge is levied.

- An advantage of the OSCE, as discussed in Chapter 9, is that examiners can be recruited with a range of backgrounds and seniority. Examiners can come from different healthcare professions. In the final medical examination in

Dundee, for example, nurses, pharmacists and health education officers were used in addition to doctors.

- In some situations, SPs have been used as sole examiners at a station, but in many contexts this is not acceptable. Following a trial, it was decided in a Canadian pharmacy OSCE that SPs should not be used to replace pharmacist assessors (Austin et al. 2003).

- Senior students can also serve as examiners in formative assessments.

- Potential examiners should be involved early and actively engaged with the OSCE process.

- Contributions to the examination and its preparation should be recognised by the dean, and certain privileges or an honorary title should be given to non-faculty members. Consideration should be given to awarding a certificate recognising the input of all who assisted.

- Maximum use should be made of examiners during the OSCE. They should be used only at stations where to assess a student's competence it is necessary to observe performance. Questions about the student's findings and the interpretation of data can be assessed at a linked station where it is not necessary for an examiner to be present.

Simulated patients

When costs have been calculated for an OSCE, a significant sum is usually allocated to expenses relating to SPs. This sum can be kept to a minimum.

- Real patients may be used rather than SPs at many stations, and in some instances this is even preferable.

- SPs can be enrolled from a range of sources, often at no cost. These may include the local community, past patients, or, as described at the National University of Cuio in Argentina, a local theatre group. Many SPs enrolled in this way are willing to donate their time at no charge. Members of staff can be used if other sources are not available (Box 15.3 and 15.4).

Box 15.3 Staff used as simulated patients

At the University of Sharjah College of Medicine in the United Arab Emirates, clinical faculty are used as simulated patients (FSPs) (Abdelkhalek et al. 2009, p. 323). An evaluation of the programme found that:

'... Students were able to think of the FSP as a real patient and faculty generally felt they were able to assess the students' reasoning processes, communication skills and history taking.'

Experience has shown that the recruitment of unpaid volunteers is not a difficult task (Cusimano et al. 1994; Sloan et al. 2001; Kelly and Murphy 2004). The use of pregnant women as volunteers was documented by Grand'Maison et al. (1985). Joorabchi (1991) reported on the *'gratifying willingness of parents and older children to get involved'*. Hodges and Lofchy (1997) found that *'there were more volunteers than needed'* and *'faculty from other teaching sites expressed interest to participate...'*. Battles et al. (1992) and Grand'Maison et al. (1985) noted that SPs helped recruit other SPs and SPs 'suggested friends or relatives'.

- SPs, once recruited and trained, should be encouraged to make themselves available on a number of occasions, and a bank of SPs should be established.

- Only one SP should be allocated to any one station in an OSCE circuit. Sometimes two SPs have been allocated to one station to perform for alternate students, but this is not necessary.

- Scenarios designed for a station may be less ambitious where volunteers rather than professional SPs are used. Some training of patients recruited is required.

OSCE venue

Whilst many OSCEs are implemented in custom-designed facilities, others make use of space adapted temporarily for the purpose as described in Chapter 7. Almost any location can be adapted and improvised as a location for an OSCE. The organisers need only be flexible and imaginative in their approach.

Other resources

Existing resources (e.g. ophthalmoscopes) can be used to provide the required equipment for stations in an OSCE. Simulators available within the institution may be used, or low-cost simulations may be developed for use in the examination, such as plaster pads or locally obtained pig legs used to test suturing skills. We have participated in an OSCE where at the end of the examination the legs were given as a reward to the examiner for cooking and consumption when they returned home!

Catering costs in the OSCE can be kept to a minimum. For example, Young et al. (1995) proposed to reduce costs for meals and coffee breaks by using supermarket food and not catered food.

Conclusions

We have seen OSCEs delivered successfully on many occasions where resources are seriously limited. The attitudes of staff and lack of leadership rather than lack of resources may be more serious barriers.

Myron Dueck (2014), in his book *Grading Smarter Not Harder*, talks about assessment strategies that motivate children and help them learn. Costs and lack of resources should not prevent us from adopting an OSCE. We simply need to be smarter and find more innovative ways of designing an OSCE and making use of the resources we have available.

Putting resources into an OSCE should be seen as an investment into:

- an assessment system that helps to guarantee the quality of the product.

- a high-quality educational programme based on feedback to the learners and curriculum developers.

- motivation of the learners to develop their clinical competence; and

- a competency- or outcome-based approach to education.

Take-home messages

- Costs attributed to an OSCE vary greatly, depending on the design of the OSCE and the extent to which additional direct costs have to be covered or can be built into the educational programme budget for the institution.

- Strategies relating to the use of examiners and SPs that can significantly reduce the costs incurred in an OSCE are available.

- The costs and lack of resources should not prevent us from developing and implementing an OSCE. We simply need to be innovative and find ways to make use of the resources we have available.

  In your institution consider how the benefits from the OSCE outweigh the costs.

15

Limitations of the OSCE 16

The OSCE has an important role to play in the examiner's toolkit alongside other assessment approaches. If recognised, the limitations of the OSCE can be addressed.

The examiner's toolkit

The OSCE offers many advantages as a tool to assess a learner's clinical competence, and these are described in Chapters 2–4 in this book. However, it is not a panacea or a magic bullet that addresses all assessment needs. Just as the tradesman or carpenter has a range of tools in his toolkit, each with a specific function, the examiner also has a range of tools that can be employed in the assessment of a learner's competence to practise medicine. Schuwirth and van der Vleuten (2011) emphasised that '...*a programme of assessment is needed incorporating a plethora of methods, each with its own strengths and weaknesses, much like the diagnostic armamentarium of a clinician.*' If the tools in the toolkit are to be used effectively, one needs to appreciate the principles underpinning each tool, along with not only its advantages and potential uses but also its limitations. We discussed the principles underpinning the OSCE and its uses in earlier chapters. In this chapter we explore the potential limitations of the OSCE.

Limitations of the OSCE

The powerful advantages of using an OSCE to make a valid assessment of the clinical performance of medical students, residents and fellows were noted by Merrick and McCoy (2001). Whilst commending the use of the OSCE they also suggested:

> 'It is cumbersome and expensive to set up, and it requires a great deal of personnel for its implementation. The expense involved in obtaining the examination site, the use of models or simulated patients, and the time of the examiners, can often be intimidating factors for those considering using an OSCE format for evaluating students, residents, and fellows.'

Some limitations, such as the learning outcomes that can be assessed in an OSCE, are intrinsic to and determined by the method itself, whilst others are related to the context in which the OSCE is administered and how it is implemented in practice.

Problems related to an OSCE may be particularly noticeable in a traditional medical school where the climate does not support a rigorous assessment of clinical skills and where minimum attention is paid to faculty development (Troncon 2004). When the culture is changed, a dramatic effect can be seen on the acceptance of the OSCE and the resources invested in its organisation. The announcement by the authorities in Taiwan that the OSCE would be a pre-requisite for the Step 2 Medical Licensure Examination resulted in an increase in the use of the examination and changes in the format of the OSCE, with the number of stations increased and the station duration decreased (Lin et al. 2013). The spaces and resources allocated to the OSCE were also expanded.

We discuss below the common perceived limitations of the use of the OSCE as a tool to assess the learner's clinical competence. These are summarised in Table 16.1.

Not a holistic approach

A feature of the OSCE is that examinees rotate around a number of stations, with only a limited period spent at any one station and with a focussed task, for example an aspect of history taking and/or physical examination. Concern has been expressed that this results in fragmentation or compartmentalisation of medicine, with examinees not assessed on their overall approach to the care of the patient. The result is

Table 16.1 Perceived limitations of an OSCE and possible responses

Limitations	Response
The OSCE does not assess a holistic approach to a patient.	Use the OSCE alongside other tools, such as portfolios and work-based assessment instruments.
The OSCE assesses only a limited sample of competencies.	Use a blueprint to sample across the outcome domains, the body systems and the core tasks.
The OSCE is resource intensive.	With organisation, the resources required can be contained. The cost–benefit ratio is favourable.
The role of the examiner is prescribed.	Within the set framework, the examiner can also use his/her judgement.
Only minimum competence is tested in the OSCE.	The scoring system can also reflect excellence. More advanced stations can be included.
Some learning outcomes are difficult to assess in the OSCE.	Performance in an OSCE can be triangulated with ratings from other assessments.
Students' behaviours are influenced by the context.	Design the OSCE to be as close to real practice as possible.
The OSCE is stressful.	Students should be briefed and prepared.

that medical practice may be viewed simply as a series of tasks represented on a station checklist. There is a need for a more integrated, holistic assessment which incorporates more complex thought processes appropriate for a patient-centred approach to medicine. However, such an assessment can be seen as in addition to an OSCE. As has been pointed out by Friedman Ben-David (2000a) and Mitchell et al. (2009), there is a need to assess in an OSCE the discrete skills appropriate to the expected level of performance and clinical experience at the specific stage of the learner.

Epstein (2007) has argued, *'The use of multiple methods of assessment can overcome many of the limitations of individual assessment formats.'* Friedman Ben-David (2001a) has described how the OSCE should be used alongside other assessment methods, including work-based assessment and the use of portfolios where the candidates produce evidence that they have achieved the required standard in relation to the expected learning outcomes. At the Hull York Medical School in the UK, the clinical examination consists both of a 12-station OSCE and a modified Objective Structured Long Examination Record (OSLER) (Gleeson, 1997). In the OSLER, students are asked to take a history and carry out a physical examination and are given thinking time to prepare a problem and management plan. Following this they discuss their conclusions with an examiner. They are also observed as they give a short explanation to the patient (Cookson et al. 2011).

The OSCE may be modified, as described in Case Study 4 from Monash University Malaysia, so that the learner is assessed on the same simulated patient (SP) but by different examiners. Whilst this does address the issue of a more holistic approach, it has the disadvantage that it limits the number of patients on whom the student is assessed. In an attempt to balance the advantages of the traditional OSCE with a sense of patient continuum, an OSCE was developed in Canada at McMaster University and the University of Toronto, with each of four OSCE stations subdivided into three sequential 10-minute sections that separately assessed physical examination, management and communication skills (Hatala et al. 2011). The stations were designed such that the answers at each section of a station did not influence the performance in a later section. The same examiner rated the candidate's performance across all three sections in a station. It was suggested, however, that the risk of a halo effect would be reduced if different examiners assessed the learner in each of the sections.

In the more traditional OSCE, rather than short 5-minute stations, the time allocated to a station may be extended to 30 minutes. However, the result of this is that fewer tasks are sampled with a reduction in the reliability of the examination. The use of 'linked' and 'double' stations, as described in Chapter 6, can be used to increase the length of a station from 5 to 10 minutes or from 10 to 20 minutes.

The need to assess a holistic approach to the patient should be recognised, and this can be achieved by including other instruments in the examiner's toolkit in addition to the OSCE or by modifying the design of the OSCE.

A limited sample

In any examination, only a sample of the competencies expected of the learner is assessed. This is true with regard to the OSCE as it is with other approaches to assessment. The need to sample as wide a range of competencies as possible is one of the reasons why we have advocated in Chapter 6 the use of an OSCE with more stations that are shorter in length rather than an OSCE with fewer but longer stations. It is not possible in any clinical examination to assess the complete repertoire of a learner's competencies. A more systematic record of the learner's experiences, including procedures undertaken, can be documented as part of the portfolio.

In the OSCE, whilst not all competencies can be assessed in all systems, the competencies assessed can be a systematic sample through the preparation of an examination blueprint, as discussed in Chapters 1 and 10. This ensures that the different domains, disciplines, body systems, core tasks and clinical settings are addressed.

Resource intensive

Essential to the success of an OSCE, as discussed in Chapter 10, is careful advance planning and organisation on the day, involving all the stakeholders. A blueprint for the examination has to be agreed, stations have to be developed and tested, examiners organised and briefed appropriately, SPs enrolled and trained, a venue organised and resources, including manikins and any required equipment, assembled. As noted by Merrick and McCoy (2001), for many this may appear a daunting if not overwhelming task requiring a considerable amount of time and teamwork. If all the contributions to the examination are costed, the examination may be expensive to run.

In a consideration of the work involved and associated costs, however, three things should be taken into account. Firstly, one can expect that any comprehensive, rigorous clinical examination that samples a range of competencies and on the basis of which important decisions are made about the learners' progression and later their competence to graduate and practise medicine will be demanding in the time and resource required. Secondly, whilst accepting that significant resources are required to organise an OSCE, it is possible, as shown in Chapter 15, to do so with more limited resources. How this can be achieved is illustrated, although not all solutions may be applicable in every situation. Thirdly, when looking at the cost–benefit equation for an OSCE, it is important to recognise on the benefit side that the contributions to the educational programme made by an OSCE go well beyond the assessment of a learner's competence. As we have described in earlier chapters, the OSCE has an important role to play as part of the learning process with the provision of feedback to learners (see Chapter 12). It also helps clarify, for both students and staff, the expected exit learning outcomes and the progression to these at each stage of the curriculum. The additional, sometimes hidden, benefits of an OSCE and their impact on the educational programme have been documented (Turner and Dankoski 2008):

Box 16.1

The benefits of introducing an OSCE in the second year at the University of Florida, USA, were reported by Duerson et al. (2000). In the 20-station OSCE, first-, second-, and third-year students served as SPs. Teachers were given feedback as to the performance of the students in the group for which they were responsible compared with the class mean. Data on the class performance were reported to the curriculum committee. Students also received report cards of their performance. The OSCE with feedback to staff resulted in an improvement in the teaching and the teachers' enthusiasm for teaching physical examination. Over a 9-year period, students' performance improved, and significantly fewer students failed stations. Students' confidence in their clinical skills improved, and anxiety about upcoming clinical rotations decreased.

- improvements in student overall performance (Duerson et al. 2000) (Box 16.1).

- increased student confidence in their clinical skills (Duerson et al. 2000).

- improved levels and greater enthusiasm for clinical teaching (Duerson et al. 2000).

- clarification of expected learning outcomes and curriculum content.

- more time spent by students on work-based activities (Newble and Jaeger 1983); and

- reinforcement of the patient-centred nature of medical practice reminding students that they are practitioners and not mere masters of medical knowledge (Barrows 1993).

In summary, if the OSCE resource requirements seem to be a cause for concern, it should be noted that:

- With thought and organisation, the requirements can be kept to a minimum.

- There are many benefits to be gained from implementing an OSCE.

- No cheaper method is available to meet the same needs.

A prescribed role for the examiner

The role of the examiner is prescribed in the OSCE, and this can be seen as both an advantage and a disadvantage. The fact that the examiner has to work within a predetermined framework and is not allowed to engage in dialogue with the candidate outside the framework contributes to a fairer and more reliable examination. However, the repetitive task of observing and completing a checklist for 20 or more candidates over a 2-hour period may be seen as tiring and boring. The OSCE procedure may also be seen as removing the autonomy of examiners and as undervaluing their judgement. However, the score sheet at stations can include a global rating scale as well as a checklist, and it can also offer examiners the opportunity to flag excellence or specific merit when they see it or to identify poor or dangerous practice.

The task of providing narrative feedback on each candidate's score sheet and meeting the group following the examination to discuss the experience at the station with the provision of good and bad examples makes the role of the examiner more attractive and not simply a gruelling, boring exercise.

Examiners may find their role more acceptable if, as described in Chapter 9, they understand the reasons for the OSCE and are more generally involved with the examination process and the principles underpinning the OSCE are discussed in advance. Evidence suggests that despite the repetitive nature of the task, examiners, if appropriately trained, maintain the same standards from the start to the finish of the examination and that they have a favourable attitude towards the OSCE process.

A test of minimum competence

Concern has also been expressed that the OSCE may be seen only as a test of minimum competence and that clinical excellence is ignored. Certainly for the pre-licensure examinations, stations are usually selected to reflect common conditions and core tasks that are faced by a doctor, with rarer problems excluded. Indeed, the purpose of an OSCE is usually to establish whether the learner has the appropriate minimum level of competence to pass on to the next stage of the course, to graduate or to enter specialist practice. Examinations can be created in specific areas, for example the Culture OSCE (Case Study 6), the Ultrasound OSCE (Case Study 12) and the Patient Safety OSCE (Case Study 13), to assess competence in greater depth.

Whilst usually the OSCE is not developed with the main aim of distinguishing the 'excellent' candidate from the 'average' candidate, the excellent candidate may be recognised from their achievement of a higher score in the checklists and global ratings scales across the different stations in the OSCE. The stations may be constructed such that bonus points are awarded by the examiner for an exceptionally good performance at a station relating to the overall task or to one part of it. It is possible also to administer a second OSCE with more advanced stations to further test high-achieving candidates.

Some learning outcomes are difficult to assess

Much attention has been paid in the OSCE to the assessment of communication skills, history taking, physical examination and data interpretation, as illustrated in the case studies in Section D.

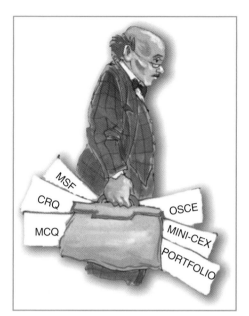

Figure 16.1 **The examiner's toolkit**

Whilst the assessment of other learning outcomes, such as attitudes, professionalism, teamwork, interprofessional practice and health promotion, may not at first sight appear to lend themselves to assessment in the context of an OSCE, increased experience, as described in Chapter 5, has been gained with assessing these learning outcomes. A survey of the literature on the OSCE (see Chapter 5) showed that all the 12 learning outcome domains described in the *Scottish Doctor* were reported as having been assessed in practice in at least one OSCE. What is important to recognise in the assessment of areas such as professionalism, is the need for triangulation as part of the assessment process, and the use of an OSCE alongside other methods to assess students in areas such as attitudes and professionalism (Petrusa et al. 1990; Friedman Ben-David 2000a; Epstein 2007). A cocktail of methods is required as part of a programme of assessment with an OSCE as a component (van der Vleuten et al. 2012) (Figure 16.1).

Student behaviour is influenced by the context of the examination

It has to be recognised that examinees are aware that their behaviours are being observed at the stations in an OSCE, and this may influence how they behave. Mitchell et al. (2009) noted: *'The examination context itself may encourage the individual to behave in a socially desirable manner, which may not truly reflect the way the individual would perform in a real-world situation.'* O'Sullivan et al. (2012) suggested that *'unless assessment is carefully constructed, we risk students learning to fake professional behaviours in order to pass'.*

There is a difference between competence and performance. Competence is assessed by what an individual demonstrates in an OSCE that they are able to do, and performance is what they do in practice when unobserved. Performance has been assessed using incognito SPs to assess the actual performance of practising doctors, with the participating doctors not knowing when they will receive a visit (Rethans et al. 2007).

Whilst students in an OSCE will be aware that they are being observed by an examiner, the more authentic the examination and the closer it relates to real practice, the more likely the assessment will relate to the student's performance in practice. This is an argument for including real patients in an OSCE as well as SPs.

The OSCE is stressful and tiring for students

Stress may be a feature of an OSCE as with any examination. Whilst some studies have identified this as a problem, on the whole, students have responded favourably to an OSCE, and stress does not appear to influence their performance adversely. Concern has also been expressed that an examination duration of 2 hours or more may be excessively tiring for students. Again, there is no evidence that this does interfere with their performance. Indeed, it could be argued that assessment of a student's performance over a period is a better reflection of their later work as a practising doctor.

Failure to integrate with the curriculum

Concern has been expressed by some workers that there is poor integration of what is assessed in the OSCE, the curriculum learning outcomes and what is taught and that in practice there is a lack of opportunity for students to improve their skills following an OSCE (Mavis et al. 1996). However, these are not intrinsic limitations of an OSCE but, rather, limitations of its implementation in practice.

Take-home messages

- The OSCE has an important role to play in the assessment of the learner's competence. However, its limitations should be recognised.

- The OSCE is not a panacea and should be used as part of a cocktail of tools alongside other assessment approaches, such as portfolios and work-based assessment tools.

- Whilst it is valuable to assess the learner's competence in discrete tasks in an OSCE, there is a need also to assess the learner's overall performance with patients.

- The assessment of learning outcomes, such as attitudes and professionalism, require a cocktail of assessment tools, with triangulation of the results from different sources of evidence. The OSCE can contribute useful information.

- The OSCE may be seen as demanding to organise and expensive to run in terms of resources and time. This is not surprising given the important goals of the examination. However, the OSCE can be administered where resources are limited. Use of the OSCE can be associated also with hidden benefits.

- Behaviours of students in an OSCE may not reflect their later behaviours in clinical practice. The closer the OSCE approach is to clinical practice, the more valuable the assessment will be to assess students' competence.

- If the full benefits of the OSCE are to be obtained, the assessment should be closely integrated with the curriculum, recognising 'assessment *for* learning' and 'assessment *as* learning', as well as 'assessment *of* learning'.

Does the OSCE as used in your institution contribute alongside other methods to an overall assessment of a student's competence?

Conclusions and looking to the future | 17

The OSCE will continue to evolve and have a major role to play in response to changes in medical education.

Assessment and the future of the OSCE

In this final chapter we look to the future of assessment in medical education and the role of the OSCE. The vision we present is based on what we know about the OSCE as outlined in this book and on our own experience since we first introduced the OSCE in 1975. It also builds on discussions on the future of assessment more generally and on influential documents on developments in assessment (Boud et al. 2010; Higher Education Academy 2012; Gordon Commission on the Future of Assessment in Education 2013). Boud et al. (2010) highlighted that assessment needs to be rethought and produced seven propositions for assessment reform in higher education (Box 17.1).

Making summative and formative assessments of a student is a key role for the teacher or trainer (Harden and Crosby 2000). Whilst assessment systems can help students learn, inappropriate examinations can have a negative impact on a student's motivation for learning. As noted by Boud et al. (2010):

> 'Assessment is a central feature of teaching and the curriculum. It powerfully frames how students learn and what students achieve. It is one of the most significant influences on students' experiences of higher education and all that they gain from it. The reason for an explicit focus on improving assessment practice is the huge impact it has on the quality of learning.'

In the next decade we are likely to see increasing recognition of the importance of assessment. Almost certainly, the role of the teacher as an assessor will change as a result of the challenges facing medical education, a demand for greater accountability and new expectations about standards (Frenk et al. 2010). Assessment will have a key role to play in the significant changes in medical education that will take place in response to advances in medicine, changes in healthcare delivery systems, developments in education technology and changing public and patient expectations (Figure 17.1).

SECTION C

Box 17.1 Seven propositions for assessment reform in higher education (Boud and Associates 2010)

1. Assessment is used to engage students in learning that is productive.
2. Feedback is used to actively improve student learning.
3. Students and teachers become responsible partners in learning and assessment.
4. Students are inducted into the assessment practices and culture of higher education.
5. Assessment for learning is placed at the centre of subject and programme design.
6. Assessment for learning is a focus for staff and institutional development.
7. Assessment provides inclusive and trustworthy representation of student achievement.

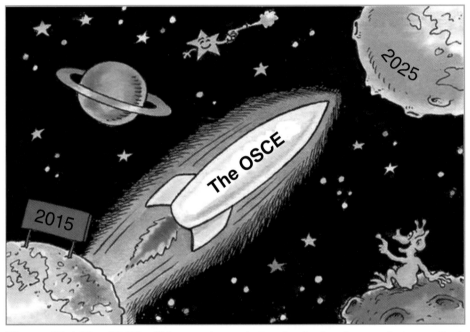

Figure 17.1 The OSCE will have a key role to play in developments in medical education over the next decade.

The future developments in assessment and in the OSCE as an assessment tool have implications for all stakeholders, including policymakers at international and local levels, deans and administrators, teachers and trainers, education researchers and support staff, students and patients. Developments in the OSCE will reflect work undertaken to improve how the OSCE is used, for example through more efficient computer-based recording of the examiner's scores and their analyses. We will also see new thinking about the OSCE and what is assessed in an OSCE, how the OSCE is administered and the role of the OSCE in the curriculum.

17

Promising developments relating to the OSCE which are likely to be pursued over the next decade are noted below. Whilst the themes discussed are addressed in the specific context of the OSCE, many are also relevant to assessment more generally.

The OSCE as an integral part of the curriculum

Traditionally, assessment is often considered separate from the teaching and learning programme, with the assessment decisions and planning executed frequently after the decisions about the curriculum and teaching and learning programme have been completed. However, things are changing, and we will see greater integration of assessment with the curriculum – good assessment is, in fact, good teaching. There will be a move from a psychometric view of assessment to one of assessment as an integral part of educational design and curriculum planning (van der Vleuten et al. 2012).

Key to this integration of assessment and the curriculum is the adoption of an outcome-based or competency-based approach to education. It has been suggested that outcome-based education has been the most significant development in medical education over the past decade (Harden and Laidlaw 2012). Outcome-based education is not simply the determination and communication of the expected learning outcomes or competencies. It is an approach where the learning outcomes, the teaching and learning programme and, importantly, the assessment are closely interlinked, with each supporting the others and the learning outcomes of the curriculum and the assessment fully aligned. As learning outcomes framed in performance terms become increasingly adopted as a currency in education, increasing attention will be paid to the OSCE as a performance assessment tool to assess students' achievement of the outcomes.

The linkage of learning outcomes and the OSCE is implicit every time a student is certified in an OSCE as having the skills necessary to practise medicine or a doctor as having the expertise necessary for a special aspect of medical practice. Related to this is the acceptance of the concept of a greater accountability to the profession and the public.

The importance of assessment to curriculum planning is also emphasised in the powerful concept of 'assessment-led innovation'. If we wish to change the curriculum or the teaching and learning programme, a good starting point is the assessment. We found in Dundee, for example, that the students' attitude to otolaryngology was changed more by the introduction of an ENT station in an OSCE rather than by changes in the ENT curriculum, including problem-based learning. Assessment can be seen as a change agent in medical education. Whilst undoubtedly we will continue to see piecemeal innovations to assessment and the curriculum, perhaps the most significant progress over the next decade will involve a more radical rethink of assessment practice and how the OSCE (and other assessment tools) can be linked to the curriculum as part of an overall educational programme. In the years ahead we will see the continuing development of the OSCE as part of a broader curriculum development alongside changes in curriculum content and new approaches to teaching and learning.

Assessment *for* learning and assessment *as* learning

Consistent with the view of the OSCE as an integral part of the curriculum will be an increasing appreciation of the effect the OSCE can have on the quality and the amount of learning that takes place. The last decade has seen a move away from thinking of the OSCE exclusively as a summative assessment to its role in formative as well as summative assessment. In the next decade we will see greater use made of the OSCE for combined formative and summative assessment purposes and there will be a growing appreciation of how summative assessment can be used to provide learners with feedback that will be helpful in their ongoing development.

The move to formative assessment has been described as a move from 'assessment *of* learning', where the emphasis is on the assessment of what the student has learned and on the student's or doctor's proficiency in a specific area, to 'assessment *for* learning', where the emphasis is on how the assessment can support learning (Earl 2005). Earl makes an unambiguous call to shift the balance away from 'assessment *of* learning' to 'assessment *for* learning'. There is evidence, as seen, for example, in the case studies in Section D, that this move to the use of the OSCE to support learning is already happening in medicine. The OSCE can be viewed as diagnostic, with feedback given to the learner and further appropriate learning designed to meet the individual's needs. The Gordon Commission noted that:

> *'...the future of assessment in education will likely be found in the emerging interest in and capacity for assessment to serve, inform, and improve teaching and learning processes and outcomes. Shall we call that assessment **for** education in addition to the assessment **of** education?'*
> *(Gordon Commission on the Future of Assessment in Education 2013, p. ii)*

We will also see a move to 'assessment *as* learning'. This spotlights the purpose of the OSCE itself as a learning experience. Participation in an OSCE offers, as illustrated in Chapter 12, Box 12.1, a powerful opportunity for learning. The learner reflects on his/her own learning and on the ability to self-assess and to use feedback to improve. Although, to our knowledge, the study has not as yet been done in relation to an OSCE, we expect that if the improvement in competence in a student was to be measured after a 2-hour OSCE and compared with the improvement after 2 hours of study, the former would be significantly greater.

Crisp (2012) used the term 'integrative assessment' to distinguish tasks designed to facilitate and test current learning as in formative and summative assessments from those assessment tasks primarily designed to encourage self-assessment and enhance future learning. We will see in the future greater attention paid to the use of the OSCE as a learning tool to address the acquisition of generic competencies, such as self-regulation and self-assessment, and to prepare the learner with the skills required for his/her continuing education.

Assessment of different competencies

The skills and competencies required of a doctor will change as we move through the twenty-first century. This will be reflected in what is assessed in an OSCE and the context in which the examination will take place. There will be a more complex assessment of competencies extending beyond the basics of history taking, physical examination and practical procedures, and the importance of outcomes, such as professionalism, patient safety and error avoidance, will be recognised. In terms of what is assessed in an OSCE, more attention will be paid to collaboration between the different stakeholders in healthcare, with an emphasis on interprofessional practice. Some of these outcomes are currently being assessed in an OSCE, as described in Chapter 4. In the years ahead we will see the OSCE being used to assess these more prominently and in addition to assessing other areas we can now only dream about.

The OSCE as a progress test

We will see greater recognition given to capturing evidence of student learning at multiple points in time. We need to go beyond obtaining an assessment of a learner's competence at one fixed point in time with a single examination to examining how learners progress in their competence as assessed over a series of tests. Pell et al. (2010) have demonstrated the importance of recognising students who are borderline in a number of OSCEs and found that they will not improve unless they have continued long-term support.

Multiple-choice question papers have been used as a progress test to assess students' knowledge and understanding of different subjects in the curriculum as they pass through the different stages of the course (Freeman et al. 2010; Norman et al. 2010). There is evidence that the OSCE can be used for this purpose (Pugh et al. 2014). We will see in the years ahead the OSCE being developed as a progress test designed to assess students' clinical competence in each year of the curriculum.

Adaptive and sequential testing

In the traditional OSCE, all learners pass through the same set of OSCE stations. Although the logistics are formidable, we may see developed OSCEs where the examinee's performance in earlier stations will determine the later stations on which he/she is examined. Where an examinee is found to be borderline in one area, he/she may be examined on the same domains at a further station or series of stations. The number of stations and duration of the examination will vary from learner to learner.

The development of adaptive testing will be considered where the candidates differ in terms of language, cultural experience or a disability. Alternative versions of stations may be provided to assess the learner's competence whilst taking into account any differences.

A more practical variation of this adaptive testing model that will be developed further is what has been described as a 'sequential test', where all students take a shorter screening OSCE, with an additional sequential test for candidates who fail to meet the screening standard (Pell et al. 2013). This is discussed in Chapter 6. Sequential testing has the potential advantage of increasing the reliability of the examination for borderline candidates and at the same time has financial benefits.

Student engagement and the OSCE

An increased emphasis on student engagement with the curriculum and the medical school has been recognised by the ASPIRE initiative (www.aspire-to-excellence.org). This engagement applies to the role of the student in assessment as well as in peer teaching and curriculum planning and evaluation. We are likely to see greater involvement by students in an OSCE, in relation to:

- a student voice on assessment as well as curriculum committees.

- peer teaching, with more senior students organising a mock OSCE for junior students.

- peer assessment, with students alongside examiners assessing their peers' performance in an OSCE.

- self-assessment, with students assessing their own competence in addition to an examiner's assessment.

- evaluation of an OSCE with an important role to play in the further development of the OSCE; and

- students serving as simulated patients (SPs) in the examination (an example is given in Case Study 14).

We are likely to see stronger partnerships being developed between students and faculty in these and other areas, with students playing a more active part in the OSCE process in addition to their role as examinees. A reduction in cost may result if students work with faculty in the delivery of the OSCE.

The ability to assess one's own competence is a necessary graduate attribute. We know that students (and doctors) are notoriously poor at self-assessment. This does not mean that it should be ignored. Indeed, the opposite is the case. Professionals and practitioners should be *'enquirers into their own competence'*. This ability should be developed in the learner from undergraduate education through postgraduate and continuing education. Self-assessment behaviour of students can be encouraged in relation to an OSCE (Han and Park 2011), and the OSCE needs to be designed with this as one of its goals.

Effective use of technology

The use of technology will be important in the further development of the OSCE through, for example:

- the use of virtual reality and more sophisticated simulators, designed, for example, to test competencies not otherwise assessed in an OSCE.

- more automated capturing of examiners' scores and the subsequent analysis of a candidate's performance overall and in different domains.

- a more detailed evaluation of the performance of individual stations in an examination.

- more powerful feedback to learners with regard to their performance in the examination.

- the development of learner analytics with the provision of a rich source of information about the learner over time and across different assessment tools; and

- online assessment where the candidate or examiner is at a distance – particularly important where there are distributed learning programmes.

Greater collaboration

There are major advantages in medical schools having responsibility for the planning and delivery of OSCEs in their institutions, with the examinations integrated into the curriculum. There are also benefits from greater collaborations locally, nationally and internationally. Collaborations will involve:

- interprofessional co-operation involving different healthcare professions; this may be at a local level.

- the continuum from undergraduate education to postgraduate and continuing education reflecting the expected learning outcomes across the continuum.

- the recording of a learner's progress across the different phases; and

- sharing of OSCE blueprints, individual stations and examiners among institutions.

Areas for discussion

In the continuing development of the OSCE there will be many aspects relating to the OSCE that will continue to be topics for discussion and debate. These include:

- the allowance that should be made in an OSCE for candidates with a disability.

- the optimum approach to scoring a candidate's performance at a station and to setting a required standard.

- the best combination of approaches to patient representation in an OSCE involving real patients, SPs and manikins.

- the place of health professionals or SPs as examiners.

- the tools to be included in the examiner's toolkit alongside an OSCE to provide an overall assessment of a candidate's competence.

- a final summative OSCE organised at a national or international level or a final summative OSCE with the local medical school responsible.

- the provision in a summative OSCE of feedback to a candidate and to teachers/trainers; and

- the use of online or web-based OSCEs.

Conclusions

Michael Peckham (1998) writing in *Clinical Futures* reported, '*Franz Vranitsky, a former Austrian chancellor, is said to have commented that "anyone with visions needs to see a doctor"*' (p. 208). Attempts to predict the future are notoriously wildly inaccurate. We believe, however, in the short to medium term the OSCE will develop along the lines described above. If it is to remain fit for purpose, the OSCE (along with other assessment practices) needs to keep pace with the changes we will see in education in the healthcare professions. The challenge for the OSCE is to conform to the proven basic principles underpinning the approach whilst applying the OSCE in new ways to meet the challenges ahead. The OSCE will continue to evolve to reflect the trend to more authentic and performance-based assessment.

It is likely that new tools to assess clinical competence will emerge in the years ahead and that these will be used alongside the OSCE as part of a mixed economy. To assess the competencies expected in a twenty-first century doctor, rather than

> **Box 17.2** A vision for the OSCE over the next decade
>
> - The OSCE being an integral part of the curriculum
> - Assessment *for* learning and assessment *as* learning
> - Assessment of different competencies
> - The OSCE as a progress test
> - Adaptive and sequential testing with the OSCE
> - Student engagement and the OSCE
> - Appropriate use of technology in the OSCE
> - Greater collaboration

looking at reliability and psychometrics in the context of one test, we will look at triangulation of evidence regarding a learner's competence across a number of assessment instruments of which the OSCE will be one.

To some extent, a vision for the future of assessment, as set out in Box 17.2, is less about the techniques or assessment methods themselves and more about a new frame to think about assessment, where assessment is more closely linked with the curriculum and the teaching and learning programme. The ongoing development of the OSCE will require continued input from curriculum planners and teachers and those with special expertise in the area of assessment, as well as the allocation of resources dedicated for the purpose.

When thinking about the future of the OSCE, we should ask ourselves one final question: Is our enduring legacy to be one that shows we have cared enough about our learners to assess them fairly in the competencies necessary for medical practice in the years ahead and have provided them with feedback to improve their learning and become better doctors?

Take-home messages

When thinking about the further development of the OSCE, consider:

- its closer alignment with the curriculum and the concept of assessment *for* learning and assessment *as* learning as well as assessment *of* learning.

- what is assessed in the OSCE will respond to changes in the practice of medicine and in healthcare education.

- the adoption of the OSCE as a progress test.

- the use of adaptive and sequential testing.

- greater student engagement in the OSCE.

- increasing use of technology; and

- greater collaboration in the development and administration of OSCEs among all the stakeholders and among different institutions locally, nationally and internationally.

Consider whether you wish to have a role in and contribute to the further development of the OSCE.

Case Studies

Undergraduate medicine

Other healthcare professions

Nursing

Dentistry

Veterinary medicine

Case Study

Dundee Medical School – Year 2 OSCE

1

Dundee Medical School – Year 2 OSCE	
Title	Dundee ASSESS Domain Grading
Author	Rob Jarvis
School/institution	Medical School, University of Dundee, UK
Professional background	Medicine
Course including level	Systems in Practice, second-year undergraduate students
Description	This OSCE is designed to assess consultation, examination and procedural skills of students finishing the second year of study. Blueprinting was by system, core clinical problem, key task of the consultation and the GMC (General Medical Council) *Tomorrow's Doctors* 2009 outcomes.
	The Dundee ASSESS (accuracy, skilfulness, supportiveness, efficiency/structure, and safety) domain grading system is designed to improve feedback to both students and examiners to improve performance and calibration. The domain approach rewards a more realistic approach to clinical encounters and relies on guided expert opinion on performance.
Role of examination	Summative and formative. Students were required to pass the examination before proceeding to the next year of the programme.
Venue	Clinical Skills Centre and a simulation suite
Number of students	176 students
Number of stations, duration of stations and length of exam	Two eight-station OSCEs, each station 8 minutes (including 1 minute reading time); total exam time of 128 minutes split over 2 days.
Number of circuits and timing	Each of the 2 days consisted of runs of eight stations across four venues (32 students). Six runs occurred through each day. There was a staggered start such that venues 1 and 2 started at 8.30 a.m., venues 3 and 4 started on run 2 at 9.45 a.m. to allow examiners with early morning commitments to partake.
Examiners	Clinicians from NHS Tayside and university clinical teachers.

Continued

SECTION D

Patients	Simulated patients, simulators and relevant clinical information (investigation results or brief section from the clinical records).
Criteria for pass/fail decision	The standard for pass was set by the borderline group method. The test statistic was the sum of the domains across all stations.
Feedback provided	Students were given personal feedback online with interactive graphs so that they could explore their results by station and by domain. They were able to compare their performance to a standard and to the class performance. Free text comments were inputted by examiners during the exam and made available for the students with their graphical feedback.
Experience gained with exam	2 years
Publications describing exam	Currently being written up for publication

CASE STUDIES

List of stations and basic blueprint

Station number	Key task/interaction	Context	Primary system	Primary core clinical problem	History	Exam.	Procedure	Explain
1	Consultation – skin lump	GP	Derm.	Skin lump	Diagnostic	**Skin lump**		Diagnosis and mgt.
2	Examination of hip	Medical ward	MSS	Trauma		**Hip**		
3	Explain condition and mgt. of septic arthritis	GP	MSS	Joint pain/ swelling				**Diagnosis and mgt.**
4	Review history – RhA	Rh clinic	MSS	Long-term conditions	**Review**			DMARD in pregnancy
5	Diagnostic hx – acromegaly	GP	Endo.	Headache	**Diagnostic**			
6	Examination of thyroid	OPD	Endo.	Lump in neck	Review	**Thyroid**		
7	Acute care – hypo collapse	Community	Endo.	Collapse	Acute			
8	Plot growth chart and reassure mum	Paeds OPD	C+F	Growth and development	Brief diag.	**ABCDE**	**Growth chart**	Neonatal feeding
9	Nasal symptoms	ENT clinic	ENT	Blocked nose	**Diagnostic**			
10	Review of eye, explain mgt.	Eye clinic	Ophth.	Red/painful eye	Review			**Diagnosis**
11	Diagnostic – uraemic itch	Medical admissions	Ren./ Derm.	Itching	**Diagnostic**			
12	Simple UTI – Hx, urinalysis and explanation	GP	Ren.	Urinary symptoms	Brief diag.		**Urinalysis**	Diagnosis and mgt.

Continued

List of stations and basic blueprint—cont'd

Station number	Key task/interaction	Context	Primary system	Primary core clinical problem	History	Exam.	Procedure	Explain
13	Rectal exam	GP	Ren./urol.	Urinary symptoms	Brief diag.	**Rectal**		Examination finding
14	Sub-acute chest pain	Chest pain clinic	CVS	Chest pain	**Diagnostic**			
15	Perform and record PEFR	GP	Resp.	Noisy breathing (wheeze/stridor)			**PEFR**	
16	Abdo. and general exam.	General medicine ward	GI	Abdominal pain		**General and abdo.**		

Notes

Simulated patients (SPs) used for all stations except Station 7 where simulator/manikin was used. Station 6: no goitre present. Examiner asked to examine SP before start of OSCE to know what the student should find.

Text in bold indicates major element to be examined.

Full blueprint includes mapping across outcomes from *Tomorrow's Doctors* (GMC, 2009).

ABCDE, airway, breathing, circulation, disability, exposure; C+F, child and family; DMARD, disease-modifying anti-rheumatic drugs.

Station 2 Examination of the hip
Instructions for candidates

Context: You are a medical student seeing a patient on a medical ward.

Task: The doctor you are attached to has asked you to examine this gentleman's hip.

Essential background: The patient is Mr Joseph Redpath (d.o.b. 3/6/1932). He fell as he was getting up from his bed and has since complained of pain from his left hip. Please explain to the examiner what you are doing as you examine this patient's hip. Treat the examiner as if they were the doctor you are attached to.

Station 2 Instructions for examiner

Examiners score the student on iPads. There is a free text comment box available for feedback to the student.

You are expected to grade each candidate in five domains: **accuracy**, **skilfulness**, **supportiveness**, **efficiency/structure** and **safety** (ASSESS).

ASSESS grading for each domain:

Poor				Good
1	2	3	4	5

Separately, you are expected to identify a global score for each candidate considering their overall performance:

Clear fail	Borderline fail	Borderline pass	Clear pass	Excellent

Please use the following descriptors as a guide of what we are looking for from the students. There may be aspects of the student's performance which are not included here that you wish to take account of in your grading.

Accuracy

Major element: carries out examination

Good students will carry out all steps in the examination: please see the attached checklist. *(The checklist used to teach the students would normally be appended.)*

Minor element: gathers information

Good students may ask the patient about his fall, past problems, reason for being in hospital whilst they examine him.
Good students will explain to the examiner what they are doing as they proceed.

Skilfulness

Major element: examination

All students should carry out this examination in a skilled manner. A good student will appear as though they have done this many times before. They will move from one part of the procedure to the next deftly.

Continued

Minor element: communication

All students should interact with the patient and direction and history taking should be integrated with the examination.

All students should be able to explain what they are doing in the examination clearly. A good student will explain this in terms which both the examiner and patient can understand.

A good student may ask the patient questions and they will gather this in a skilled way – open questions, listening and avoiding jargon.

Supportiveness

All students should display care and concern.

All students should attend to the patient's comfort.

Good students will put the patient at ease through the procedure either by explaining what they are doing or through other means.

Good students will alleviate any concerns expressed by a patient and engender trust.

Efficiency and structure

All students should clarify the tasks of the consultation at the start with the patient.

All students should complete the tasks in the time allocated.

All students should allocate appropriate time to each element of the consultation.

Good students will have a well-structured consultation with the student taking an appropriate level of control.

Good students will reach a conclusion and enable next steps to be discussed.

Safety

All students should identify self and role, and ensure the patient's identity is clear.

All students should work within the boundaries of their professional level.

All students should display good hygiene practice.

No student should cause harm or unnecessary discomfort.

Good students will ensure the patient is clear regarding the findings of the examination and on appropriate management or follow-up.

Station 2 Appendix Hip examination checklist

Look

Gait – antalgic or Trendelenburg?

Trendelenburg test

Asymmetry

Leg length discrepancy – measure if necessary to determine whether real or apparent

Feel

Greater trochanter

Groin

(Pubis – please do not expect students to do this with a simulated patient)

General tenderness

Station 2 Hip examination checklist—cont'd

Move – passive and active

Flexion

Abduction

Adduction

Internal and external rotation

Extension

Thomas test for a fixed flexion deformity

Station 2 Instructions for the simulated patient

You are Joseph Redpath d.o.b. 3/6/32. You are currently a patient on one of the medical wards. You have been here for the last 2 weeks since getting a chest infection. Your chest is much better, but you have to stay here until adequate help can be organised for you at home. You are very keen to get home. You live by yourself. You have no family in Dundee – your daughter is in Glasgow. You are finishing off some antibiotics, but otherwise you are not on any tablets. You have never injured yourself before.

• You fell over whilst getting out of bed this morning.

• You were able to stand with help from the nurses straight after, but your left hip has been painful since.

• You did not injure anything else.

• When they examine you please state that you have pain in your left groin and the outer aspect of your thigh, over the hip bone (please ask the examiner if you are unsure where to indicate).

• When they move your left hip please indicate that it is generally uncomfortable but you are able to move.

• You are able to stand and walk if asked. Be a little cautious when weight bearing on your left leg.

• If they do not ask if you are sore please grimace and complain of pain when they examine you.

Station 2 Resources required

1. Simulated patient dressed as an inpatient

2. Examination couch

3. Chairs

2

Case Study

King Saud bin Abdulaziz University for Health Sciences
Cardiovascular System Block Phase 2 OSCE

King Saud bin Abdulaziz University for Health Sciences Cardiovascular System Block Phase 2 OSCE	
Title	KSAUHS Cardiovascular System Block Phase 2
Author	Tarig Awad Mohamed, Bashir Hamad, Ali I AlHaqwi and Mohi M.A. Magzoub
School/institution	College of Medicine, King Saud bin Abdulaziz University for Health Sciences, Ministry of National Guard Health Affairs, Riyadh, Kingdom of Saudi Arabia
Professional background	Medicine
Course including level	Cardiovascular System Block (CVS), undergraduate education, Phase 2 curriculum: Pre-clerkship, organ-system phase. (OSCE is also used in the clerkship period.)
Short description	The OSCE is used in the college for the assessment of student performance in history taking and communication skills including counselling, consent etc., physical examination and procedural skills.
Role of examination	Summative contributing to end of block exam
Venue	OSCE Area Skills Lab
Number of students	100 students
Number of stations, duration of stations and length of exam	Timing is 7 minutes per station. Ten stations (seven active and three rest stations). Duration of the exam is 70 minutes. Students whose turn is yet to come are kept under observation in a separate hall without their electronic devices.
Number of circuits and timing	Students divided into five groups of 20. Two parallel circuits of 10 students each. Time for both circuits is 70 minutes and to complete the exam for all 100 students takes 350 minutes.
Examiners	Members of medical college staff
Patients	Simulated patients and manikin
Criteria for pass/fail decision	Criterion referenced, decided by faculty beforehand
Experience gained with exam	10 years

King Saud bin Abdulaziz University for Health Sciences Cardiovascular System Block Phase 2 OSCE—cont'd

Costs or resources required	Both the examiners and simulated patients are financially compensated. Refreshments are provided for all including students.
Publications describing exam	Al Rumayyan et al. (2012)

List of stations

Station	Type of station	Title	Patient representation	Examiner
1A	Communication skills	History of presenting illness (PI) for shortness of breath (SOB) as the chief complaint	Simulated patient (good English)	Yes
2A	Clinical diagnostic skills	Precordial examination	Simulated patient	Yes
3A	Rest station			
4A	Procedure skills	Cardiopulmonary resuscitation (CPR)	Manikin	Yes
5A	Communication skills	History taking for chest pain as a presenting complaint	Simulated patient (good English)	Yes
6A	Rest station			
7A	Procedure skills	Blood pressure examination	Simulated patient	Yes
8A	Procedure skills	Doing and interpreting a 12-lead ECG	Simulated patient	Yes
9A	Rest station			
10A	Communication skills	Medication history in post-myocardial infarction patient	Examiner acting as simulated patient	Yes

Note

Only 'A' stations are used in the College of Medicine and students are examined and marked in the same station. In the College of Allied Health Sciences, 'A' and 'B' stations are used where, for example, the student is asked to answer multiple-choice questions relating to the 'A' station.

Station 5A   History taking for chest pain as the presenting complaint
Candidate instructions

Time allowed: 7 minutes

This gentleman presents to your clinic with a feeling of chest pain which makes him worried about having heart disease.

Task: You are asked to obtain a relevant history that can clearly address the patient's concern

Station 5A   Examiner instructions

Station title: History taking for chest pain as a presenting complaint

Time allowed: 7 minutes

Objective: This station tests the student's ability to distinguish cardiac from non-cardiac chest pain.

Instructions for examiner

- Greet the student and give him/her the written instructions.
- Ensure the student's name and number is on the marking sheet.
- Observe the interaction between the student and the simulated patient and complete the marking sheet according to the marking schedule (circle the mark given).
- Total the student marks.
- Sign the marking sheet.
- Please do not interact with the student or simulated patient during and after completion of the task.

Station 5A   Marking schedule

Student name: _____   **Number:** _____

Item	Performed completely	Performed but not fully completed	Not performed
Greets patient, makes him comfortable and **introduces** himself/herself	2	1	0
Explains the purpose of the interview/asks patient's **permission**	2	1	0
Asks about history of present (chest pain) illness:			
• Onset and duration of present illness	2	1	0
• Character of pain	2	1	0

Station 5A   Marking schedule—cont'd

Item	Performed completely	Performed but not fully completed	Not performed
• Site and radiation	2	1	0
• Severity and duration of episodes	2	1	0
• Aggravating and relieving factors	2	1	0
• Any associated symptoms (SOB, palpitations…)	2	1	0
Asks about past cardiac history:			
• Cardiac events or admissions	2	1	0
Asks about past medical history and other coronary risk factors:			
• Diabetes mellitus	2	1	0
• Systemic hypertension	2	1	0
• Family history of coronary artery disease	2	1	0
• History of tobacco smoking	2	1	0
• Occupation and diet	2	1	0
Student's reply to patient's query of the possible cause of chest pain as non-cardiac or musculoskeletal pain	2	1	0
Thanks the patient at the end of session	2	1	0
Overall approach	2	1	0
TOTAL MARKS:	/34		

Name of examiner: _____   Signature: _____

Badge number: _____

Station 5A   Simulated patient instructions

Station title: History taking for chest pain as a presenting complaint

Time allowed: 7 minutes

Objective: This station tests the student's ability to distinguish cardiac from non-cardiac chest pain.

Continued

Station 5A Simulated patient instructions—cont'd

Scenario

- You are a 25-year-old unmarried male shopkeeper.
- You have two brothers and two sisters.
- Your father is 59 years old and your mother is 52 years old.
- Both parents, brothers and sisters are healthy and did not suffer any heart problems.
- You do not have diabetes or high blood pressure.
- You do not know about your cholesterol level.
- You do not smoke or drink. You take a main meal at lunch time and light meals for breakfast and dinner, not more than one soft drink a day and two spoons of sugar per cup of tea or coffee.
- You are complaining of chest pain which started 3 days ago and continued until now.
- The pain is sharp, moderate in severity (5/10), over the junction of the rib with sternum, which can be localised by one finger. The pain is easily triggered by pressure and not felt anywhere else in the body.
- Chest pain is not related to physical activity, but increased by deep breathing and arm movement.
- You have no difficulty in breathing (except the pain), no dizziness, no palpitations or loss of consciousness, no cough or leg swelling.
- During the session you **ASK the student: please tell me is this pain due to a heart attack or not, and if it is not from the heart, what could be the cause?**

Station 5A Requirement list

1. Chair and table for the examiner
2. Couch
3. Simulated patient

Case Study

Manchester Medical School MBChB –
Phase 2 Formative OSCE

3

Manchester Medical School MBChB – Phase 2 Formative OSCE	
Title	Manchester Medical School MBChB – Phase 2 Formative OSCE
Authors	Alison Quinn, Clare McGovern, Emyr Wyn Benbow and Kamran Khan
School/institution	School of Medicine, University of Manchester, UK
Professional background	Medicine
Course including level	Phase 2 – Clinical years Third-year undergraduate students
Short description	This OSCE is designed for third-year medical students as an introduction to the forthcoming clinical years' summative OSCEs. The examination takes place in the third year of the MBChB programme 6 months after the commencement of formal clinical experience. This OSCE assesses either Heart, Lungs & Blood (HLB) or Nutrition, Metabolism & Excretion (NME) modules depending on the students' placements in the preceding 6 months. Each student has to appear in an eight-station OSCE assessing their respective module.
Role of examination	This examination is purely formative. It was originally designed to give the students who were transferring from other medical schools, at the beginning of year 3, an insight into the nature of the OSCE examination in Manchester, so that they were not at a disadvantage at the summative sitting. However, being the first purely clinical OSCE it enables all students to gain appropriate feedback to refine their examination technique, leaving all students on an equal footing.
Venue	The examination is run over four main sites, in purpose built facilities at the education centres of the four main teaching hospitals. No student is examined at their usual place of study, to avoid examiner bias because of familiarity.
Number of students	470 students with a 50/50 split between HLB and NME modules. Therefore, approximately 235 students are examined in each examination.

Continued

229

Number of stations, duration of stations and length of exam	Eight stations, each 10 minutes long with 1 minute to read the instructions for the station, 7 minutes to complete the task and 2 minutes for feedback at the end of the station. The total time is 80 minutes.
Number of circuits and timing	There are seven or eight circuits run at each of the four locations. Each location runs two parallel circuits at any one time, enabling twice as many students to be examined. There is a strict quarantine in place during the examination period.
Examiners	Members of staff from local hospitals and primary care. All examiners have completed a central examiner training course; regular updates are also provided, to be undertaken every 3 years. Examiners also attend a standardised briefing on the morning of the examination. All stations are marked real time by the examiners present.
Patients	Real patients, simulated patients and student volunteers are used depending upon what is appropriate for each individual station. Part task trainers and simulators are also used and investigation results are available as appropriate.
Criteria for pass/fail decision	The examination is marked using a global rating scoring system, which is based upon performance in 15 skill subsets. For each OSCE question, between three and five of these marking domains are selected, as detailed in the marking guidance for that individual question. As this is a formative examination, there is no pass or fail. Any candidate scoring below 57% would be required to meet with their hospital dean in order to form an action plan in preparation for the summative examination.
Feedback provided	There are 2 minutes incorporated into each station for the examiner to give verbal feedback. Feedback may be given by the simulated patient also. The examiner will also document their feedback on the mark sheet; this is scanned and the written feedback given to the student at a later date. The year group as a whole is also given feedback on common mistakes and things that were commonly performed well. Feedback is also collected from the examiners, post-examination, as to how each individual station performed and areas of improvement for the conduct of the examination. Students also have the ability to feedback on the examination itself.
Experience gained with exam	14 years

List of stations

No.	Question type	Time in mins	Patient/volunteer	Examiner
1	History – Abdominal pain	7	SP, F (25–35)	Observed, scored and verbal feedback, including SP verbal feedback
2	Examination – Examine abdomen	7	Real patient with abdominal signs	Observed, scored and verbal feedback
3	Explanation – Explain renal stones	7	SP, M (45–55)	Observed, scored and verbal feedback, including SP verbal feedback
4	Examination – Thyroid	7	Healthy volunteer, F	Observed, scored and verbal feedback
5	Practical – Venepuncture	7	Healthy volunteer, M or F Part task trainer	Observed, scored and verbal feedback
6	Explanation – Diverticulosis	7	SP, F (50–60)	Observed, scored and verbal feedback, including SP verbal feedback
7	Practical – Venous cannulation	7	Healthy volunteer, M or F Part task trainer	Observed, scored and verbal feedback
8	Prescribing	7	SP, M (50–60)	Observed, scored and verbal feedback, including SP verbal feedback

SP, simulated patient

Example of blueprint for year 3 OSCE NME

	Obtaining history in order to make a diagnosis (1 station)	Clinical examination (2 stations)	Explanation and planning, including data interpretation (2 stations)	Procedural skills (2 stations)	Prescribing (1 station)
Nutrition	Abdominal pain		Diverticulosis		
Metabolism		Thyroid			
Excretion			Renal stones		
Any		Abdominal examination on patient		Cannulation Venous blood sampling	Medication history and write prescription chart

Question

Prescribing – Medication history and write prescription chart

SP age and sex

M (50–60)

Resources and equipment needed

The instructions to the candidate should be clearly visible inside the station.

Paper and pens with clipboard for students to make notes.

BNF

Student prescription chart with patient name, date of birth and hospital number filled in already. A sticker may be used for this and placed on the relevant sections of the chart. The students should not be given blank prescription charts. This information should be completed already on both pages of the chart.

Patient details – These should be on the chart and on a hospital wristband on the patient. The patient may be fully dressed, there is no need for a hospital gown or nightclothes.

James Murrat

DOB 02/01/1955

Hospital number 24689

Setting up the station

The examiner's chair should be positioned so that he/she can observe faces of both candidate and simulated patient.

A desk or table for the student to use whilst writing the chart. It should NOT form a barrier between the candidate and the patient.

This station is set on the surgical ward.

This is James Murrat.

He is being admitted for elective surgery to ward A9 under the care of consultant surgeon Mr Patel.

Your consultant has asked you to take a medication history and prescribe his usual medications on his prescription chart.

Examiner's role

Please let the candidate start immediately when they enter the station. The instructions to the candidate should be clearly displayed inside the station as well as outside. You do not need to read the instructions to the candidate but you may do so at the start if you think this will help a hesitant candidate to get started.

If the candidate is making very slow progress with the allocated task, you may remind them that they will need to speed up if they are to complete the station.

When the candidate has finished the station they should remain within the station area until the bell rings for the end of the station.

What are the objectives of the station and what is expected of the candidate?

Focused medication history taking and writing a prescription chart.

Clinical information relevant to the station

The student should concentrate on taking a focused medication history and writing the chart.

They may spend a short amount of time discussing the medical problem for which the medication is prescribed. You may advise them to move onto writing the chart if they have obtained the relevant information and they are running short of time so that they can gain the marks for this. They should not spend a lot of time discussing the surgical problem or surgery – you should remind them that this is not part of the task.

The student should cover

Medication history:

- Prescribed medications – Medication, dose, frequency, time of day taken.
- Patient knowledge around the medication – The indication for the medication.
- Adherence to prescribed medication.
- Non-prescribed medication – Over the counter, herbal/homeopathic, bought through the Internet, etc.
- Allergies/intolerances including the type of reaction experienced.

Prescription chart:

- Patient name, date of birth, hospital number – This should already be filled in. This is often the case when a chart is presented for completion. The student must check the patient's identity to ensure that they are completing the correct chart.
- Consultant, ward, date when chart was written and allergies.
- Prescribed medicine – Correct section of the chart, approved name, dose (checked in BNF), route, start date, time of dose, indication, signature and name.

1: Overall conduct of the consultation

- Candidate introduces self, states role and checks the patient's identity (name and DOB)
- Explains the purpose of consultation
- Keeps the patient's confidentiality, safety and dignity foremost
- Seeks consent
- Maintains a courteous and caring demeanour
- Listens attentively and acts with empathy, honesty and sensitivity
- Demonstrates a fluent, coherent and confident approach
- Considers patient's preferences and makes no attempt to force or coerce patient
- Manages time and closes appropriately, thanking the patient
- Dresses appropriately

2: History taking skills

- Uses a structured, fluent and focused approach
- Uses a combination of open questions and closed questions
- Responds to information given by patient, rather than appearing to follow a set formula of questions
- Obtains key and relevant information and shows the ability to use the information
- Elicits and acknowledges the patient's ideas, concerns and expectations
- Discovers the impact of the problem on the patient's life
- Repeats, reflects, summarises and clarifies
- Avoids premature or false reassurance

7: Prescribing – Writing a prescription

- Correctly enters or checks patient's details, location and consultant
- Correctly enters or checks known allergies
- Selects appropriate medications to prescribe as per clinical scenario
- Prescribes accurately (dose, route, frequency, date and sign)
- Prescribes legibly
- Avoids any serious drug errors
- Documents additional instructions as appropriate

13: Non-verbal communication

- Establishes a rapport early and maintains it
- Maintains positive and open body language and eye contact
- Maintains a calm and composed demeanour
- Responds to cues and follows up appropriately
- Uses or offers appropriate and understandable visual methods for conveying information, e.g. diagrams if applicable
- Uses appropriate seating position

Publication describing this format of station design: Khan et al. (2013)

234

4411318877

MANCHESTER
1824

The University of Manchester

FACULTY OF MEDICAL AND HUMAN SCIENCES
MANCHESTER MEDICAL SCHOOL
YEAR 3 OSCE RE-SIT – TUESDAY 5 AUGUST 2014

D1808	PRESCRIBING

STUDENT NAME: STUDENT ID NO:

EXAM SITE   CYCLE   BASE

EXAMINER SURNAME   EXAMINER PIN

PLEASE READ THE INSTRUCTIONS IN THE SCRIPT BEFORE YOU BEGIN MARKING
DO NOT MAKE MARKS ON THIS FORM OUTSIDE THE DESIGNATED BOXES

COMPONENT OF SKILL (PLACE A 'X' IN ONE BOX ON EACH LINE)

Overall conduct of consultation

Uses no elements	Uses few elements	Uses half elements	Uses most elements	Uses all elements
☐	☐	☐	☐	☐

History taking skills

Uses no elements	Uses few elements	Uses half elements	Uses most elements	Uses all elements
☐	☐	☐	☐	☐

Prescribing – writing a prescription

Uses no elements	Uses few elements	Uses half elements	Uses most elements	Uses all elements
☐	☐	☐	☐	☐

Non verbal communication

Uses no elements	Uses few elements	Uses half elements	Uses most elements	Uses all elements
☐	☐	☐	☐	☐

PLEASE ASSESS THE CANDIDATE'S PERFORMANCE BY PLACING A 'X' IN THE APPROPRIATE BOX BELOW

1 ☐	2 ☐	3 ☐	4 ☐	5 ☐	6 ☐	7 ☐
Unsatisfactory	Borderline (fail)		Satisfactory	Good		Excellent

THE FOLLOWING SECTION MUST BE COMPLETED FOR ALL STUDENTS

Please give concise, constructive comments on how the student can improve their performance

- _____
- _____
- _____
- _____
- _____

PLEASE ENSURE THAT YOUR COMMENTS STAY WITHIN THE BOX

SECTION D

Who are you?

- James Murrat

- Date of birth 02/01/1955 (this is important as it is already entered onto the prescription chart and the patient ID band which you will need to wear).

- You are a software designer and work for a company in Manchester designing accounting software. It is an office-based job.

- You live in a flat with your partner near the city centre.

- You have no children but have plenty of family support, i.e. nearby parents (elderly) and sister if needed.

- You do not smoke.

- You drink alcohol after work with your friends. This would be three to four glasses of wine a week on average.

- You are relaxed and easy to talk to.

- The student may ask you what your weight is for the drug chart, if asked please tell them your weight in kilograms.

History

Past medical history – You do not have any other medical problems apart from those described here and you have never been admitted to hospital before.

Medication – See below.

Medical problems in the family – Your parents and sister are alive and well. No other medical problems in the family.

Details of current health problems

Surgical problem – Inguinal (groin) hernia, which is the reason for admission

- The student is not required to ask about this and the examiner will steer them back on track if necessary but the following is included for your information.

- You have an inguinal (groin) hernia which is the reason you have been admitted to hospital today.

- You are due to have surgery to repair this under general anaesthesia tomorrow afternoon.

- The hernia is in your right groin. There is a visible bulge at the bottom of your abdomen near the top of your leg which you can see and which increases in size if you cough or strain. It does ache from time to time but had never caused you a serious problem.

- Two weeks ago you came to surgical outpatients to see your consultant and he advised you to have the inguinal hernia repaired. You understand that there is a weakness in your abdominal wall here which the surgeon will repair and strengthen by making a cut a few inches long in the lower part of your abdomen above the top of your leg.

- The surgeon explained the procedure to you, you have no further questions.

3

Gastro-oesophageal reflux – For which you take your regular medication

- The student may ask you about this as it relates to your medication.
- If the student asks if you take any medication tell them that you take an antacid tablet.

If asked specifically

- Your medication is a capsule – Omeprazole 20 mg (milligrams) which you take once a day in the morning at about 7–8 a.m. before breakfast.

Background to this

- You started getting a burning sensation (heart burn) in the mid-lower part of your chest about 6 months ago. It happened after meals and was quite uncomfortable.
- Your GP referred you for an endoscopy where a camera was passed down your throat, through your oesophagus (gullet) and into your stomach whilst you were sedated.
- You were told that you had a small hiatus hernia inside where a small part of your stomach pushes up into your chest through your diaphragm. This allows stomach acid to pass up into your oesophagus (this is acid reflux or gastro-oesophageal reflux) and causes the burning sensation in the chest known as heart burn.
- You were started on medication to supress stomach acid production and you have lost a bit of weight as your doctor recommended. You were told that no other treatment was required for this.
- This is a capsule – Omeprazole 20 mg (milligrams) which you take once a day in the morning at about 7–8 a.m. before breakfast. It works very well and relieves your symptoms completely.
- You understand the reason for your medication – To reduce acid production by your stomach and therefore prevent the burning sensation from the acid reflux.
- You very rarely forget to take a dose (maybe once every 3 weeks or so at the most).
- You don't find it difficult to take and don't believe that this has caused any side effects.
- You did try to stop taking it a month or so ago and the burning sensation returned after about a week so you started again.
- You are not sure if you are supposed to take this medication forever (don't ask the student if this is the case). You intend to go back to your GP to review this in a month or so.
- You have never had the following (which may be related to these symptoms):
  - Weight loss
  - Anaemia
  - Difficulty swallowing.

Continued

Allergies/sensitivites

- You are allergic to erythromycin. You were given this a couple of times in your early teens. You think that it was for tonsillitis but you can't remember the exact reason. The first time you took it you got a mild red rash on your chest and abdomen. The second time you got a severe red blotchy rash all over and your lips and face swelled up. The reaction subsided quickly without any special treatment when you stopped taking the medicine. You were told by your GP that this was definitely an allergy and not to take erythromycin again.

Others

- You do not take any 'over the counter medication' (bought directly from a pharmacy or any other shop without prescription).
- You do not usually take any pain killers, although in the past you have occasionally taken paracetamol and ibuprofen (Brufen) without any problems.
- You do not take any herbal homeopathic or alternative medicines.
- You have never bought any medicines over the Internet or from any other alternative source.

Details of your concerns/perceptions

Feelings and concerns. (These are minimal in this station as a significant task for the student in this station is completing the prescription chart accurately.)

- You are keen that your medicine is documented on the chart as you think it is important that your acid reflux does not start happening again around the time of your operation. You don't want to be bothered by it whilst you are recovering
- You have no concerns regarding the surgery, the anaesthetic or pain after surgery as all your questions about these have already been covered by the consultant surgeon, Mr Patel, in surgical outpatients.

What you should say and what you should not say

- Tell the student readily that you take an antacid tablet.
- Give the other information if asked specifically.
- If the candidate uses medical jargon, ask them what they mean.

What you should ask

- You may express your concern – That you want to continue your medication whilst in hospital to avoid any symptoms but do not delay the student excessively with this as they need to move on to writing the drug chart.

Specific standardisation issues

- As this is an exam, it is important to perform the same role time after time, and for simulated patients to perform the same role on different sites. All aspects of the script have been inserted for good reasons. Please do not divert from the script.
- Please ensure that they are given the relevant information readily when they ask for it so that they can complete the task in time.

The simulated patient should receive the entire script including the student and examiner instructions and the marking domains.

Case Study

Monash University Malaysia Formative OSCE

4

Monash University Malaysia Formative OSCE

Title	Monash University Malaysia Formative OSCE
Author	Wee Ming Lau
School/institution	Jeffrey Cheah School of Medicine and Health Sciences, Monash University Malaysia, Malaysia
Professional background	Medicine
Course including level	Monash MBBS Programme
	Second-year undergraduate students
Short description	This OSCE format adopts a four-linked station approach. Station 1 is always (constant) on history taking from a simulated patient. Stations 2 and 3 may be on performing a physical examination (e.g. respiratory system), conducting a procedure (e.g. taking blood pressure) or providing explanation (e.g. use of the combined oral contraceptive pills in family planning). Station 4 is always (constant) an integration station where students are required to summarise their findings from the previous three stations to their respective examiners. In Station 4 students need to generate a problem list (medical and non-medical issues that their patient is facing), red flags (possible pathological causes for the patient's presenting complaints) and yellow flags (possible psychological causes for the patient's presenting complaints), and demonstrate appropriate clinical reasoning to further discuss the case with their respective examiners.
Role of examination	Formative. This is held at the end of the first semester and provides a learning and feedback opportunity for students. They are assessed on their knowledge, communication and hands on skills, and their ablity to integrate key information related to the patient. They are provided with immediate verbal feedback and written results (scoresheets) 2–4 weeks later. Students are advised to reflect upon their performance, take appropriate steps and seek academic support, if needed.
Venue	Learning suites on campus
Number of students	120 students

Continued

Number of stations, duration of stations and length of exam	Four linked stations each with an 8-minute task. The reading time for the first 3 stations is 2 minutes; with 3 minutes for the final station. The total exam time for each student is 49 minutes (inclusive of the examiners' verbal feedback time of 8 minutes. Each examiner provides an immediate 2-minute verbal feedback to the student at the completion of each station).
Number of circuits and timing	Five circuits on two half days. There are 60 students in each session. There are five circuits as 12 students are allocated to each circuit. The remaining 60 students will be examined in a similar manner the following day. Similar stations are used on both days.
Examiners	Members of staff, who are clinicians. Each student will have a different examiner for each of the four stations. The examiner moves from room to room, and examines a different station each time. Therefore, all examiners are trained in all four stations.
Patients	Simulated patients (SP) only. Each student will have the same SP throughout the exam. The student and SP stay in the same room throughout the 49 minutes. The SP moves with the student as they progress from Station 1 to 2 to 3. The SP leaves the room at the end of Station 3 as they are not involved in Station 4.
Criteria for pass/ fail decision	The pass mark in each OSCE station is based on the average of the global rating of the borderline (BL) score of the cohort. For example, in the cohort, the average of the BL scores of five students (12,13, 11, 10, 14) is 12; then students who score above the borderline pass the station and those below fail the station. This is done for each of the OSCE stations, i.e. the four different stations will have individual BL scores. The total BL score/pass score for the OSCE is the sum of BL scores for the individual stations.
Feedback provided	Each student will be given a 2-minute verbal feedback by the examiner, immediately at the completion of the task/s at each station. Each student will receive their respective score sheet from the Curriculum Office within 2–4 weeks of the activity. The score sheet provides details of the candidate's score, maximum possible score, cohort median and cohort maximum scores. Each student will also be provided with written feedback on the patient's perspectives from the SP at the completion of the circuit.
Experience gained with exam	7 years with the OSCE
Publications describing exam	None to date.

Formative OSCE for second-year medical undergraduates
List of four stations that student A will undertake

Station	Learning outcomes assessed	Patient representation	Examiner
1 Reading time = 2 min Task time = 8 min Feedback time = 2 min	History taking in a patient with chest pain: • Take a focused medical history of the cardiovascular system. (Chest pain is the presenting complaint for this set of integrated stations.)	Simulated patient (same)	Observed and scored by examiner 1
2 Reading time = 2 min Task time = 8 min Feedback time = 2 min	Examination of the respiratory system (RS): • Perform a competent and thorough physical exaimation of the respiratory system. Note, instead of proceeding to examine the CVS as in the traditional format (since the presenting complaint was due to a CVS problem), here, the student is instructed to examine a different system such as the RS to ensure adequate sampling of the scope of materials taught. The SP will have a RS problem in their history, such as a 'chronic smoker', so that examination of RS is relevant.	Simulated patient (same)	Observed and scored by examiner 2
3 Reading time = 2 min Task time = 8 min Feedback time = 2 min	Examination of the thyroid gland: • Perform a competent and thorough physical exaimation of the thyroid gland to assess the thyroid status. Note, explanation is as above. Here, the patient may have presented with palpitations associated with the chest pain but may also have a family history of thyroid disease and therefore asked for examination and assessment of the thyroid status.	Simulated patient (same)	Observed and scored by examiner 3
4 Reading time = 3 min Task time = 8 min Feedback time = 2 min	Integrated station: • Summarise the findings from Stations 1–3 with an appropriate level of detail. • Apply the knowledge from themes I, II, III and IV to discuss the issues pertinent to the patient. **Note:** Theme I (personal and professional development); theme II (population, society, health and illness); theme III (scientific basis of clinical practice); and theme IV (clinical skills).	Not required	Observed and scored by examiner 4

Note

The same simulated patient is used across the first three stations. However, different examiners are used across each of the four stations to maintain station reliability (Hay et al., 2012).

Station 1 History of chest pain

Examiner's scoresheet – These are marked on softcopy using Qualtrix generated forms.

The following data are entered: Campus, name of examiner, gender of SP, name and (identification) number of the student.

Key points in history

Items	Not done	Partially done	Inadequately done	Adequately done	Well done
Task 1 – Preliminaries					
Patient's name, age, occupation					
Consent, explanation of purpose, confidentiality					
Task 2 – Presenting complaint					
Use of opening question					
When, duration, frequency, circumstances					
Where, radiation					
Quality (description) and quantity (scale of 0–10)					
Alleviating and aggravating factors					
Associated factors					
Belief, impact, concern, expectation					
Systems review (relevant)					
Task 3 – Other histories					
Past history (details)					
Family history (details)					
Drug history (details)					
Smoking, alcohol (details)					
Social history (details)					
Task 4 – History taking skills					
End interview and thank patient					
Systematic, organised, patient-centred history taking					
Use of appropriate non-verbal communication					

Station 1 History of chest pain—cont'd

Global rating

Clear fail   *Borderline*   *Clear pass*

Notes

1. Examiners are required to select the global rating which best describes the student's overall competence. This assessment will be used to determine the pass mark for this station.

2. Depending on the information sought, not all five options may be used for each item.

3. Examiners are trained to allocate marks according to how well the student performs (e.g. asking appropriate questions and seeking details where required) and not just on what the student did.

4. Examiners are not to intervene or ask students any questions unless specifically instructed to do so in the examiner's instructions.

Station objectives

This station tests the student's ability to:

Take a focused medical history

Establish rapport to enable the patient to feel understood, valued and supported

Demonstrate communication skills necessary to end a medical interview

Station set-up requirements

The following are placed in each examining room, depending on what is being tested at the station:

Tables and chairs

Stationery for the student and examiners

Hand sanitiser

Stethoscope

Couch, pillow, blanket, bedsheet, screens, stopwatch, box of tissues, waste bin

Tendon hammer, bottle of water, disposable cups

Desktop computer and/or iPad for examiners

Students attendance list for examiner

Backup scoresheets (in case the Internet fails unexpectedly)

Printed copies of candidate's instructions for all the four stations

Simulated patient requirements

Age range

Gender

Ethic origin

Dressing

Body build

Language (must be proficient in English)

Expectations required of the SP in each of the three tasks

Station 1 Student instructions

You are a second-year medical student on your urban GP placement. Peter has come in to see his GP today. Please take a complete medical history from Peter.
You will not be asked any questions by the examiner.

Station 1 Simulated patient instructions

Background: Your name is Peter Ng. You are a 45-year-old gardener and have come to see the GP today. You experienced sudden onset of chest pain while clearing weeds at your workplace this morning. It felt like a sharp pain but disappeared after 5 minutes of rest. The pain resumed when you restarted your work. You never had this before but you were concerned as your best friend had a similar pain recently and was later diagnosed to have a heat attack. You have hypertension and take perindopril 4 mg daily. You are overweight due to excessive indulgence and smoke 20 cigarettes a day, but do not consume any alcohol. You have a family history of hypertension (father) and thyroid problems (mother and sister). You are keen to get this problem sorted out as this job will help pay off your outstanding mortgages incurred from your car and house.

Note: Simulated patients are provided with 2 to 3 pages of detailed information on the role play. They are seen on a minimum of two sessions by the OSCE coordinator who provides face-to-face training sessions on the role play.

Case Study

UCL Medical School Final Examinations – Short Station OSCE

5

UCL Medical School Final Examinations – Short Station OSCE	
Title	UCL Medical School Final Examinations – Short Station OSCEs
Author	Kazuya Iwata, Daniel S. Furmedge, Alison Sturrock and Deborah Gill
School/institution	University College London Medical School, UK
Professional background	Medicine
Course including level	MBBS – Final-year medical students
Short description	The short station OSCE (SSO) is a component of the final medical school examination that students need to pass in order to receive their medical degree (MBBS). It consists of approximately 18 stations covering short clinical cases and tasks such as practical procedures and history taking to assess the students' preparedness for medical practice as junior doctors (interns). There is a particular focus on common situations that junior doctors are likely to face in their first year of practice.
Role of examination	Summative. In order to graduate from medical school, students are required to pass this examination, along with two single best answer papers on clinical problems and a separate (4 × 30 minute station) long-station OSCE which tests their clinical method.
Venue	Clinical skills centre (side rooms; dividers used to make teaching rooms into individual stations)
Number of students	400 students
Number of stations, duration of stations and length of exam	Eighteen stations of 5 minutes duration, although one or two double stations of 10 minutes are also included per examination circuit. Double stations require the station to appear in the circuit twice. One student is an 'early starter' to commence the double station. Total exam time of 100 minutes.
Number of circuits and timing	A circuit of 18 students running in parallel at three different sites, held up to four times a day over 2 days.

Continued

245

Examiners	Members of clinical staff from medical school and teaching hospitals.
Patients	Simulated patients, plastic models, real patients, multimedia (video recordings), investigation results such as blood tests.
Criteria for pass/fail decision	The pass mark is calculated using the borderline regression method of standard setting, which involves collating the mean checklist scores and global judgement scores for each station. These are then statistically regressed and the point where the line of best fit crosses the midpoint of borderline passes and borderline fails becomes the pass mark for that station. The overall pass mark for the SSO is the sum of individual station pass marks. The final SSO score then contributes to the overall final MBBS examination score.
Feedback provided	Students who fail the final MBBS examination as a whole are given individual feedback about their performance by the Welfare Tutor after the examinations. These students are usually given another opportunity to resit the examination at a later date.
Experience gained with exam	10 years
Publications describing exam	Iwata et al. (2014)

List of stations

Station	Learning outcomes and competencies assessed	Patient representation	Examiner
1	Discussion of ECG with colleague (5 minutes)	ECG tracing and simulated colleague	Observed and scored by examiner
2	Prescription of an antibiotic (5 minutes)	Brief synopsis of patient's condition	Proctored and scored by examiner*
3	Examination of a hernia (5 minutes)	Real patient	Observed and scored by examiner
4	Interpreting abnormal blood results (5 minutes)	Blood results with simple history	Proctored and scored by examiner*
5	History taking in a patient with breathlessness (5 minutes)	Simulated patient	Observed and scored by examiner
6	Handing over a patient to a colleague – linked to previous station (5 minutes)	Notes made in previous station and simulated colleague	Observed and scored by examiner
7	Examination of the cardiovascular system (5 minutes)	Real patient	Observed and scored by examiner

Station	Learning outcomes and competencies assessed	Patient representation	Examiner
8	Male catherisation (5 minutes)	Plastic model with simulated patient	Observed and scored by examiner
9	Assessment of abnormal gait and associated knowledge (5 minutes)	Video of a real patient	Proctored and scored by examiner*
10	Assessment of an acutely unwell patient (5 minutes)	Simulated patient	Observed and scored by examiner
11	Discussion of a radiological investigation request (5 minutes)	Patient history and simulated colleague	Observed and scored by examiner
12	Performing cannulation and aseptic technique (5 minutes)	Plastic model with simulated patient	Observed and scored by examiner
13	Prioritisation of ward jobs (5 minutes)	Description of patients on paper	Proctored and scored by examiner*
14	Communication skills: Breaking bad news (5 minutes)	Simulated patient	Observed and scored by examiner
15	Discharge prescription (5 minutes)	Brief synopsis of a patient's condition	Proctored and scored by examiner*
16a (double)	Integrated station on explaining medical condition and treatment to a relative (10 minutes)	Simulated relative	Observed and scored by examiner
16b (double)	Integrated station on explaining medical condition and treatment to a relative (10 minutes)	Simulated relative	Observed and scored by examiner
17	History taking in a patient with headaches (5 minutes)	Simulated patient	Observed and scored by examiner
18	Cranial nerve examination (5 minutes)	Simulated patient	Observed and scored by examiner

Notes

*Can be scored later if lack of examiners or other emergencies arise.

Two identical 10-minute stations 16a and 16b are needed in order that students do not have to wait for the previous candidate to finish since all the other stations are 5 minutes.

CASE STUDIES

Station 16: Double station on explaining medical condition and treatment plan with a relative

Station 16   Instructions to student

You are a foundation year doctor on the respiratory team.

Golda Phillips is a 73-year-old woman with severe chronic obstructive pulmonary disease (COPD) requiring long-term oxygen. Over the last 6 months, she has become increasingly frail with reduced appetite and has been saying she is 'fed up' with using oxygen all the time. She has not attended her GP appointments since she had an acute chest infection 3 weeks ago.

Two hours ago, she was brought to the Emergency Department by her daughter as she was confused and disoriented. Her temperature is 38.6°C, BP 120/80 mmHg, and oxygen saturation 78% on air. She has been started on controlled oxygen therapy (28%), nebulised bronchodilators, antibiotics and intravenous fluids. The card provided shows the results of her initial investigations.

Mrs Phillips's daughter, Karen Baldwin, wants to speak to someone about her mother's condition. Your consultant is busy and has asked you to see her. Please respond appropriately to her questions.

Station 16   Examiner's checklist

This is an OSCE station for final-year students who are about to become junior doctors. The standard of a pass is that of a standard acceptable for a junior doctor on their first day.

Candidates are being assessed on both their clinical knowledge of chronic obstructive pulmonary disease (COPD) and related causes of confusion, and their knowledge and explanation of the law around withholding/withdrawing life-prolonging treatment and deliberately ending life. They should demonstrate knowledge of the following:

- The patient's condition is consistent with an acute confusional state.
- There is evidence of infection, which is exacerbating the COPD.
- Management includes taking blood cultures and starting broad spectrum i.v. antibiotics.
- The patient's ABG results are indicative of type 2 respiratory failure and deterioration despite controlled oxygen therapy and non-invasive ventilation. BiPAP is indicated.
- The patient might not survive, even with maximum treatment.
- Without treatment, the patient's prognosis will be very poor – hours to days rather than weeks.
- Treatment that is futile or not in the non-competent patient's best interests can be withheld even if it is life-sustaining.
- It is illegal for doctors to administer drugs with the intention of ending life.
- Doctors are legally bound to consider the opinions of those close to the patient when deciding on a patient's best interests.

	Clear pass	Pass	Borderline	Fail	Clear fail
Demonstrates clinical knowledge • Causes of condition • Management of condition • Prognosis					
Demonstrates knowledge of legal and professional guidance • Treatment can be withheld if futile or if not in best interests • Illegal to administer drugs with intention of ending life • Role of those close to the patient in best interests decision					
Demonstrates professional behaviour/communication skills • Introduces self (name and role) • Establishes and maintains rapport • Gives information in clear, jargon-free way • Treats actor with sensitivity and respect					
Ends consultation appropriately • Clarifies concerns/queries have been addressed • Agrees on appropriate plan • Offers further support					

Global judgement

☐ **Clear pass**   ☐ **Borderline pass**
☐ **Borderline fail**   ☐ **Clear fail**

Notes

The examiner completes the checklist manually on a machine-read form.

A global rating for each series of bullet points is given to allow flexibility since the station assesses both clinical and ethical/professional skills.

SECTION D

You are Karen Baldwin, daughter of Golda Phillips. Your mother has had lung disease for 15 years and has been on long-term oxygen therapy. Normally she tolerates this well and has hardly ever complained about it. However, during the last couple of months she has been saying she is fed up with having to use oxygen all the time. Over the last 6 months, you have also noticed that her appetite has been steadily decreasing and that she is becoming increasingly frail.

Two weeks ago she got a lung infection and this really upset her, so much so that she stopped attending her regular appointments with the GP and told you that she'd 'had enough' and 'wanted to die'. She has not written anything down about refusing BiPaP (breathing machine) or any other treatment (an advance decision) and, to the best of your knowledge, has not told anyone else about wanting to die.

You love your mother and have always been fully involved in her medical care and you do not want to see her suffer. You are not upset or angry with the doctor (the candidate), you just want to do what's best for your mum. You want to understand what's happening to your mum and what her chances are of living and regaining some quality of life. Given what she's recently told you, about wanting to die and her loss of appetite and increasing fragility, you want to consider whether it would be best to not treat her and let her die.

Please ask the questions below using the wording in the script as much as possible and try to avoid becoming sidetracked into other areas. The candidate should start by introducing him/herself (name, role) and offer to answer your questions. Say to the candidate:

- Thank you for agreeing to see me, doctor. I know you're busy, but I'm so worried about my mother. Can you tell me why she's confused? It's so unlike her.
- What can you do to make the confusion better?
- If BiPaP not mentioned by student: Does she need to go onto a machine – I think it's called a BiPaP machine? (If BiPap is mentioned: How will you put her onto this machine?)
- What do you think her chances of survival with treatment are?
- If my mother doesn't have treatment, what is likely to happen to her?
- My mother's suffered a lot in the last few months. Last week she told me she'd had enough and wanted to die. Do you have to treat her?
- Given my mother's suffering, can't you just give her something that will help her to die quickly and peacefully?
- Do I have any say about whether my mother has treatment or not?
- Please end the consultation by saying: Thanks for explaining all of that. What will happen now?

Station 16   Resources required

- Blank paper and pens for students to make notes
- Laminated card with clinical information
  - Her blood tests on admission
    - White cell count: 16.6 × 109/L (4–11)
    - CRP: 268 mg/L (<10)
  - Her ABG on air
    - pH: 7.33 (7.35–7.45)
    - PaO_2: 5.2 kPa (11–15)
    - $PaCO_2$: 7.5 kPa (4.6–6.4)
  - Repeat ABG (on 28% oxygen)
    - pH: 7.30 (7.35–7.45)
    - PaO_2: 6 kPa (11–15)
    - $PaCO_2$: 8.5 kPa (4.6–6.4)

Case Study

Culture OSCE for Pediatric Residents

6

Culture OSCE for Pediatric Residents	
Title	Culture OSCE for Pediatric Residents
Authors	Elizabeth K. Kachur, Lisa Altshuler, Ingrid Walker-Descartes, Lita Aeder and the Maimonides Pediatrics OSCE Committee
School/institution	Maimonides Medical Center, Department of Pediatrics, New York, USA
Professional background	Medicine
Course, including level	Pediatric Residency Program (Postgraduate) Year 2
Description	This OSCE is designed to assess and improve residents' cultural competence which is vital for the practice of medicine. Culture is defined broadly to include ethnic, language, racial, religious and sexual orientation differences. Second-year residents were chosen because at this level they already have a significant amount of cross-cultural clinical experience, but there is still room for acquiring and implementing new skills. Station development has been challenging since it is important to bring complicated cultural underpinnings to life without stereotyping. The OSCE rounds are preceded by a 90–120 minute workshop to prime learners and a 45 minute debriefing to help learners contextualise the OSCE concepts in their day-to-day practice.
Role of examination	Formative
Venue	First 13 years were in the clinic exam rooms and after that the hospital simulation centre was used
Number of students examined in each OSCE	20–30 residents, depending on size of the yearly cohort
Number of circuits and timing	2 days, two–three staggered circuits per day organised to allow concurrent orientations and debriefings with multiple small groups of residents
Number of stations, duration of station, and length of examination	5–6 stations, 2 minutes to read scenario, 10 minutes for the faculty-observed encounter, 5 minutes for feedback from faculty and simulated patients (SP)

Examiners	Interprofessional group of healthcare providers (including physicians, psychologists, genetic counsellors, child life specialists and chief residents)
Patients	SPs, parents and residents
Criteria for pass/fail decision	Residents with low scores in three or more stations will have to undergo some remediation as determined by the programme director and OSCE committee
Feedback provided	5 minutes of feedback by observing faculty and simulated patient after each encounter, post-OSCE debriefing for the whole group with a review of each station, copies of the evaluation forms completed at each station and additional reading materials keyed into the station topics
Experience gained with the examination	Yearly since 1999
Costs or resources required	Direct costs: SPs, food/refreshments, props Indirect costs: Faculty time and loss of revenue from clinic space
Publications or further information available describing the examination	Altshuler and Kachur (2001); Altshuler et al. (2003); Kachur and Altshuler (2004); Aeder et al. (2007); Aeder et al. (2012)

Sample culture OSCE timetable

Approximate time	Activity
8.00–9.45	**Resident workshop** (all residents that day, breakfast)
9.00–10.00	**SP and faculty assembly and practice** (breakfast)
9.45–10.00	**AM group goes to sim centre** (take positions at respective first station)
10.00–11.42	**AM group completes OSCE** (five residents)
11.45–12.00	**PM group assembly and orientation**
11.45–12.00	**AM group returns to department**
11.45–12.10	**SP and faculty lunch** (at sim centre)
12.00–12.10	**PM group goes to sim centre** (take positions at first station)
12.00–12.45	**AM group debriefing** (and lunch)
12.10–1.52	**PM group completes OSCE** (five residents)
1.55–2.10	**PM group returns to department**
2.10–2.55	**PM group debriefing** (and lunch)

Notes

AM, morning; PM, afternoon.

List of Maimonides culture OSCE stations (5–6 stations selected each year from the pool)

Title & cultural group	Learning outcomes assessed	Patient representation	Examiner
1. Life threatening illness (Nigerian)	Explore parental beliefs about illness (cancer) and the need to inform adolescent child of condition, develop joint plan	Simulated parent	Scored by SP & observing examiner
2. Informed consent (Jehovah's Witness)	Obtain informed consent from the mother of a 12-year-old girl who needs surgery; negotiate alternatives to blood transfusions with a Jehovah's Witness	Simulated parent	Scored by SP & observing examiner
3. Pelvic exam (Iranian Muslim)	Discuss the need for a pelvic exam with a sexually active adolescent whose culture/ religion severely punishes sexual activity prior to marriage. (While parents 'wait outside')	Simulated patient	Scored by SP & observing examiner
4. Down syndrome (Sephardic Orthodox Jew)	Explore parental beliefs/ concerns about raising a child with Down syndrome in family and community; negotiate a plan for child placement with opposing parents	Simulated parental couple	Scored by SPs & observing examiner
5. Suspected child abuse (Orthodox Jew)	Discuss the need for making a report of suspected child abuse and explore its community ramifications on the marriageability of older siblings	Simulated parental couple	Scored by SPs & observing examiner
6. Cough/cold (Chinese)	Explore the use of alternative medicines which might be harmful; negotiate a mutually acceptable plan about their use	Simulated mother	Scored by SP & observing examiner
7. Preparation for surgery (Roman Catholic)	Develop a rapport with a teenage patient and their parent who request that the physician holds hands with them and prays for the success of the operation	Simulated patient & mother	Scored by SPs & observing examiner
8. Photo ID/ alternative medicines (Caribbean, Asian, Latino, Middle Eastern)	Identify pictures of alternative treatments as distinct from child abuse and recognise herbal remedies commonly used by specific cultural groups	Paper & pencil task	Observing examiner

List of Maimonides culture OSCE stations (5–6 stations selected each year from the pool)—cont'd

Title & cultural group	Learning outcomes assessed	Patient representation	Examiner
9. Lost in translation (Bengali)	Address differences in parental levels of concern when the father is the only interpreter available	Simulated parental couple	Scored by SPs & observing examiner
10. Autopsy consent (Pakistani)	Explore cultural and religious beliefs about autopsy with parents of recently deceased child	Simulated parental couple	Scored by SPs & observing examiner
11. Seizure disorder (African American)	Communicate a change in medication to a mistrusting African-American mother who has had negative experiences with the healthcare system	Simulated parent	Scored by SP & observing examiner
12. Paediasure please (Pakistani/ various)	Recognise and address unprofessional behaviour (i.e. stereotypes and racist comments) with a colleague	Video featuring inappropriate encounter; simulated resident	Scored by standardised resident & observing examiner
13. Sexually transmitted infection (Hispanic)	Recognise and address different sexual preferences in a teenager; provide non-judgemental advice	Simulated patient	Scored by SP & observing examiner
14. lifestyle changes (Mexican)	Address weight gain issues in a recent immigrant (identified through a school fitness report); counsel the parent as appropriate	Simulated mother	Scored by SP & observing examiner
15. HEADSS Up (Homosexual, Roman Catholic)	Recognise and address sexual identity conflict in a teenager (adapted from case 13, above)	Simulated patient	Scored by SP & observing examiner

Note

List of stations as of October 2014.

Station 1   Life threatening illness
Station objectives

This station is designed to test residents' ability to:

- Discuss with mother the need to speak openly with adolescents about their medical condition

- Explore mother's beliefs about the illness and about informing her son of his condition

- Jointly with mother develop a plan for handling the situation

SECTION D

Patient information	Parent:	Mrs Odeji
	Patient: Age: Health status: Cultural background:	Aeyi 17 Newly diagnosed leukaemia Recently immigrated from Nigeria
Reason for visit	Meet with mother to discuss how to communicate with Aeyi about his illness	
Your role	Paediatric Resident on inpatient unit	
Situation	• Aeyi is a 17-year-old boy, recently diagnosed with acute lymphoblastic leukaemia (ALL). He has been treated in the hospital for the past week.	
	• During the medical workup, his parents asked that staff not discuss the diagnosis with their son so as not to upset him. So far you have complied with their wishes.	
	• Parents have recently been informed of the diagnosis and you have spent time with them discussing specifics of the illness, including a etiology, prognosis and treatment options. They continue to resist your suggestion that this information be shared with their son.	
	• Aeyi has been told that he may have a problem with his blood and that the medicine is to help his blood become stronger. He has begun to ask questions about his situation, tests and treatment, and has hinted that he thinks something 'terrible' is wrong with him.	
	• Hospital staff (nursing, child life, etc.) have voiced increasing concerns about how to respond to his questions and comments.	
	• You believe that this boy has a right to be informed of his condition, and that not knowing may contribute to emotional difficulties as he copes with the illness and treatment.	
	• Your attending has asked that you speak with the mother about the need for more honesty with this adolescent.	
Your tasks	1. Explore with mother the concern of parents about sharing medical information with their son.	
	2. Begin to develop a plan to deal with Aeyi's concerns and needs.	

Note

The 'attending' is the supervising physician.

The scenario Your name is Mrs Odeji. You and your family moved from Nigeria a year ago, and it has been a big adjustment for everyone. You have four children, and Aeyi is your oldest and your only son. All your children have been in good health generally, until recently when Aeyi became ill. He had been tired and run down for a few months, but you did not think this was due to any serious illness.

Aeyi was admitted to the hospital for a workup of his symptoms. The diagnosis was made 5 days ago. The doctors have been very helpful in explaining Aeyi's illness and the necessary treatments, but it has felt quite overwhelming to take in all that was discussed. You are still struggling to make sense of this and feel quite frightened. All the people you knew with cancer died quickly (these were people you knew when you were in your country) and you cannot bear to think about that possibility for your son. You feel quite helpless to change the situation and feel that the only thing you can do is to pray for your son.

You have asked the doctors not to discuss with Aeyi the nature of his illness. You fear that if your son is told that he has leukaemia, he will feel as helpless as you do and will give up his will to live. In addition, you wish to shield your son from pain and worry.

You are frightened about how Aeyi might react if he finds out what is really wrong with him. You consider it essential to his recovery that Aeyi remain optimistic. You believe strongly that it is your duty to assume the burden of Aeyi's illness, taking care of him and making all decisions about what is in his best interest. This is what you have done in all other matters pertaining to your children.

Your current life situation and past history The family, including parents, Aeyi, and his three younger sisters, ages 14, 8 and 4, moved from Nigeria about 1 year ago. This was at the urging of Mrs Odeji's brother who has been in this country for several years and who owns a business. Mr Odeji now works for his brother-in-law and Mrs Odeji stays at home to care for the house and the children.

Aeyi has been a good son who has helped out with his younger sisters. He is obedient and respectful of his elders and, as is customary for adolescents from your country, has relied on his parents to make important decisions for him.

It has been difficult leaving your life in Nigeria and, although you have some family connections here, you continue to feel isolated and uncertain about how to handle life in such a different environment. You miss the relationship with your elders and the advice and guidance they gave you. In many ways, it has been easier for your children to adjust to this new life and accept these new 'American' ways.

The medical encounter You are respectful and polite towards the doctor, but are still convinced that it is inappropriate for Aeyi to hear the details of his illness, and particularly to hear the words 'cancer' or 'leukaemia.' In a soft-spoken way, you attempt to express your wishes about this issue to the doctor.

Continued

Timing	**Beginning:**	You are quiet and subdued, and very respectful of the doctor. You nod as the doctor speaks, and often look down rather than directly at him or her.
		Do not discuss your fears and emotional reactions without being asked. Begin by focusing on what you feel is best for Aeyi (i.e. for his well-being the diagnosis should not be shared with him).
	Two-minute warning:	Begin to acknowledge that there may be different ways of dealing with adolescents who are ill. Begin to consider the possibility of talking more openly with your son. Close with agreeing that you would discuss it with your husband.

Station 1 Life threatening illness
Observer evaluation form

Resident name: _____

Faculty observer: _____

Resident ID: _____

	Not done	Minimally done	Done adequately	Done well	Notes
General communication skills					
1. Allows patient/parent(s) to express self (does not interrupt, expresses interest in hearing more, asks how parent feels)					
2. Communicates in non-judgemental fashion (no leading questions, is respectful/courteous, no patronising/arrogant comments)					
3. Makes empathic and supportive statements (expresses concern, acknowledges emotional content and/or coping efforts)					
4. Uses language appropriate to parent's understanding (avoids jargon or slang, explains unfamiliar medical terms)					

Continued

CASE STUDIES

Station 1 Life threatening illness
Observer evaluation form—cont'd

	Not done	Minimally done	Done adequately	Done well	Notes
5. Uses non-verbal behaviour that is facilitative and culturally appropriate (appropriate distance, tone of voice, attentive posture, gestures and verbal message match)					
6. Proceeds in organised fashion (clear beginning, middle and end; moved through encounter in efficient manner)					
Exploration of cultural beliefs and practices (station specific)					
7. Elicits parents' perception of problem/model of illness (telling truth will lead to depression and poor outcome, cancer = death)					
8. Elicits parents' perspective on dealing with the situation (don't tell patient about cancer so that he can remain optimistic)					
9. Acknowledges parents' perspective respectfully (acknowledges parents' concern for child's welfare)					
Management of differences (station specific)					
10. States medical opinion/obligations clearly (open discussion will lead to improved outcomes)					

CASE STUDIES

	Not done	Minimally done	Done adequately	Done well	Notes
11. Provides rationale for preferred option(s) (secrecy can't be maintained as this diminishes trust)					
12. Concludes with plan that includes patient's/parents' perspective (no immediate action necessary; discuss issue further)					

Overall cultural skills demonstrated

1	2	3	4	
Very little to no sensitivity to differences, did not establish rapport, did not complete station tasks	Inadequate sensitivity to differences, rapport was suboptimal, inadequately completed station tasks	Adequate sensitivity to differences, rapport was good, completed station tasks	Excellent sensitivity to differences, rapport was outstanding, completed station tasks with great skill	

Strengths: _____

Area(s) needing improvement: _____

Station 1 Life threatening illness
Standardised patient evaluation form

Resident name: _____   Resident ID: _____

SP initials: _____

Satisfaction with doctor

1	2	3	4
Not satisfied, would not come back to this doctor or refer any friends to this doctor	Only slightly satisfied, but would prefer not to have more to do with doctor	Satisfied with interaction, would be willing to continue working with doctor	Very satisfied, strongly pleased with interaction and would certainly continue with doctor

Overall cultural skills demonstrated

1	2	3	4
Very little to no sensitivity to differences	Inadequate sensitivity to differences	Adequate sensitivity to differences	Excellent sensitivity to differences

Strengths:_____
_____
_____

Area(s) needing improvement: _____
_____
_____

Case Study

Medical Council of Canada's Qualifying Examination Part II

7

Medical Council of Canada's Qualifying Examination Part II	
Title	Medical Council of Canada's Qualifying Examination Part II
Authors	Sydney Smee and Members and Consultants, MCC OSCE Test Committee, Medical Council of Canada
School/institution	Medical Council of Canada, Ontario, Canada
Professional background	Medicine
Course including level	Successful completion of 12 months postgraduate training – all specialties
Short description	An OSCE to assess the core clinical skills of history taking, physical examination, communication and patient management, which are common to all physicians. Implemented nationally in 1993. Basic format is a series of short patient encounters combined with a series of paired stations comprised of patient encounters linked to written tasks related to the first component. Patient problems are drawn from five disciplines (medicine, surgery, obstetrics–gynaecology, psychiatry, paediatrics), and sample across age groups, gender and body systems. Stations assess one or a combination of clinical tasks according to sampling criteria. The OSCE is administered twice per year.
	As an important disclaimer, all station content is strictly confidential. Further, the blueprint, test form specifications, scoring criteria and station formats are all being revised for a proposed 2018 implementation. While this case is representative of the format, scoring approaches and content for this OSCE currently, it is not representative of its future. The anticipated shift is towards more complex patient presentations with a stronger focus on physician communication and management skills.
Role of examination	Summative; a prerequisite for licensure and therefore for practice in Canada
Venue	Administered in hospital outpatient clinics at university-based sites
Number of students	2012: 3,547 candidates
	2013: 4,240 candidates

Continued

Number of stations, duration of stations and length of exam	1993–97: 20 stations, e.g. ten 10-minute stations, 10 paired stations with two 5-minute components; testing time of 4 hours. 1997–98: Sequenced administration – 10 station screening portion (comprised of both station formats) with 60% of candidates continuing on to complete 10 more stations; testing time of 2 hours or 4 hours. 1998: 14 stations; both station formats equally; testing time of 2.8 hours. 2003–12: 12 stations plus two pilot stations; seven 10-minute stations and five paired stations; testing time of 2.8 hours. 2013–15: 12 stations; eight 10-minute stations and four 15-minute simulated office orals for family medicine candidates and eight 10-minute stations and four paired stations for all other specialties. Testing time is 2.3 hours or 2.4 hours. 2016: To be determined.
Number of circuits and timing	1993–12: Increasing number of sites until all 17 universities were running the examination. Each site ran from one to six circuits, administered twice a day. Two to three tracks were the most common layout. 2013–15: Test form is administered at 18 sites, across 2 days, with two to eight circuits per site, and three administrations per day.
Examiners	Community and faculty physicians
Patients	Simulated patients
Criteria for pass/fail decision	1992–93: modified Angoff; 1994–2012: borderline group; 2013–14: Hofstee; 2014–15: panel-based borderline group
Feedback provided	Standing, total score and pass score, graphical representation of scores by domain relative to the mean and a supplementary report with limited information regarding stations and their link to the objectives of the Medical Council of Canada (www.mcc.ca)
Experience gained with exam	23 years
Publications describing exam	Reznick et al. (1992); Reznick et al. (1993a,b); Reznick et al. (1996); Dauphinée et al. (1997); Rothman et al. (1997); Smee et al. (2000); Smee et al. (2003)

Sample list of stations (14-station version)

	Clinical problem	Primary domain
1	Older man presents with chest pain	Management
2	Adult child regarding elderly parent's medications	Management
3	Man brought to ER with hypotension/shock (nurse present)	Management

Sample list of stations (14-station version)—cont'd

	Clinical problem	Primary domain
4	Older woman with post-op delirium	History
5	Teenage woman brought to ER after suicide attempt	History
6	Woman refusing treatment for cancer	Communication
7	Parent regarding 7-year-old child with behaviour problem	History
8a	Parent regarding seizure in infant	History
8b	Short written answer related to station 8a	Written – scored later
9a	Young woman presents with lumps in her neck	Physical examination
9b	Extended match questions related to station 9a	Written – scored later
10a	Woman presents with vaginal bleeding	History
10b	Extended match questions related to station 10a	Written – scored later
11a	Older woman presents with altered sensation in hands	Physical examination
11b	Short written answer related to station 8a	Written – scored later
12a	Young man presents with chest pain and shortness of breath	Physical examination
12b	Short written answer related to station 8a	Written – scored later
13a	Woman presents with abdominal pain	Physical examination
13b	Extended match questions related to station 13a	Written – scored later
14a	Man presents with hoarseness	History
14b	Short written answer related to station 8a	Written – scored later

Notes

All stations were based on an encounter with a standardised patient. At Station 3 a nurse was present. Physician observers were present at Stations 1–7 and 8-14 'a' stations only.

Station 1 Instructions to candidates
Older man presents with chest pain

Raymond McKenzie, 55 years old, has been brought to the *Emergency Department* by ambulance because of chest pain which has now resolved with oxygen in the ambulance. The **initial** ECG was normal and the vital signs are as follows:
BP: 130/85 mm Hg
Pulse: 70/minute, regular
Resp.: 20/minute

In the next 9 minutes, assess and manage this patient. An Emergency Department nurse is present in the room. Direct the nurse to order any tests or perform any procedures you believe are appropriate for this patient.

As you proceed with the physical examination, **explain to the examiner** what you are doing and **describe any findings**.

In the last minute, you will be asked a question about this patient.

Station 1 Examiner checklist

	Done satisfactorily
1. Orders initial management	
• oxygen	☐
• intravenous line	☐
• blood pressure monitoring	☐
2. Elicits history of presenting problem	
• information about the pain	
• nature	☐
• radiation	☐
• severity	☐
• gastrointestinal complaints	☐
• previous episodes	☐
• precipitating	☐
• associated complaints	☐
• coronary artery disease risk factors	
• smoking	☐
• diabetes	☐
• hypertension	☐
• hypercholesterolaemia (no knowledge)	☐
• family history (brother had angioplasty at age 55)	☐
• drug allergies	☐
• medications	☐
• specifically asks about Viagra, Cialis or Levitra	☐
• risk factors for thrombolysis	☐
3. Conducts physical examination	
• auscultates chest	☐
• auscultates heart	☐
• assesses jugular venous pressure	☐
• abdominal examination	☐
4. ECG requested *prior* to change in status. [Nurse reports findings]	☐
5. ECG requested *after* change in status. [Nurse provides ECG.] [Candidate asked to interpret]	☐
• correct interpretation	☐
• any other answer	☐
6. Orders further appropriate initial investigations	
• cardiac enzymes	☐
• other blood work	☐
• specifically orders INR or PT/PTT	☐

CASE STUDIES

Done satisfactorily

7. **Management of patient's pain**

- nitroglycerin ☐
- morphine or other narcotic ☐
- clopidrogel ☐
- IV or PO beta blockers ☐
- IV heparin/low molecular weight heparin ☐
- arrange admission/consult Internal Medicine/Cardiology ☐

8. **Orders aspirin (ASA)** ☐

Oral question – from examiner

Q1. **The patient refuses to be admitted to hospital. You have explained, at great length, the risk of severe complications or death. He seems to understand the risk well. You consider him to be capable. What action will you take? [Check only ONE item]**

A1 Explore reasons with patient; respect his final decision ☐

A2 With permission, enlist family or friend to discuss; respect his decision ☐

A3 No further discussion; document discussion in chart ☐

A4 No further discussion; have patient sign release ☐

A5 Try to convince the patient further by repeating risks and benefits ☐

A6 Involuntary admission to hospital ☐

A7 Restrain the patient ☐

A8 Consultation with a psychologist/psychiatrist ☐

A9 No action required ☐

A10 No answer or other answer given ☐

Notes

Some explanatory content to guide examiners has been removed.

Oral question from examiner asked in last minute of station. Candidates do not see options.

Station 1 Global rating completed by the examiner

Did the candidate respond satisfactorily to this patient's needs and problem(s)?

- ☐ Borderline Unsatisfactory
- ☐ Poor
- ☐ Inferior

- ☐ Borderline Satisfactory
- ☐ Good
- ☐ Excellent

If **unsatisfactory**, please specify why:
- ☐ Inadequate medical knowledge and/or provided misinformation
- ☐ Could not focus in on this patient's problem
- ☐ Demonstrated poor communication and/or interpersonal skills
- ☐ Actions taken may harm this patient
- ☐ Actions taken may be imminently dangerous to this patient

Other: _____

Station 1 Professionalism question completed by examiner

Did this candidate demonstrate a lapse in professional behaviour? ☐ Yes ☐ No

If yes, please specify the reason:

- ☐ Disrespectful to others (e.g. to patient, nurse)
- ☐ Over-investigated/over-managed the patient
- ☐ Actions raised ethical and/or legal concern

Briefly describe the behaviour for any of the above reasons or any other observed lapse:

_____

Station 1 Information for simulated patients

Starting position: Lying on a stretcher/exam table, head raised. BP cuff on arm. The patient holds his hand over lower sternum.

Opening statement: 'I had this terrible chest pain'. (He holds his hand over his lower sternum.)

Patient behaviour, affect and mannerisms:

At beginning of encounter:

1. Perspiration on forehead and nostril area. BP cuff is already on the patient's arm.

2. He is in mild pain, but appears frightened. Initially he is mildly distressed (anxious), mildly short of breath (20/minute) and coherent.

3. He tends to minimise the pain, but is clearly feeling unwell and worried. He seeks to be reassured and, when encouraged, answers questions fully.

4. He holds his hand over the end of his breast bone when asked where the pain is. He does not move a lot because he is afraid the pain might return.

At 4 minutes into the encounter:

The severe pain returns. He becomes very frightened, presses his hand to his sternum and speaks in very short, broken sentences.

History of present problem:

Raymond Mckenzie, 55 years old, was brought to the A&E because of severe chest pain (10/10). The pain is almost gone now (1/10). The chest pain started fairly suddenly about 2 hours ago. A co-worker was concerned with how he looked and called the ambulance.

- The very severe pain eased to 1/10 in the ambulance after oxygen was administered. The pain is in the pit of his stomach and lower chest. He describes it as a burning feeling, like indigestion. He also has an ache in the inside of both upper arms that runs to about his elbows. He is nauseated and slightly short of breath.
- Raymond has never had this severe pain before. He does get occasional mild heartburn after meals but nothing like this. He takes no medication. He smokes 2 packs of cigarettes per day and has been smoking for 30 years. He only drinks alcohol when he is socialising (once or twice a week).
- His father died at age 50 from a stroke. His mother, who is 80, has Alzheimer's disease and lives in a nursing home. The mother is on some heart pills but he doesn't think she has ever had a heart attack. Raymond's 58-year-old brother had a 'balloon in his heart' to prevent heart attacks 3 years ago. The brother had angina for several years before that.

Simulation information

Chest pain and shortness of breath:

Initially the simulated patient (SP) is breathing quietly, is mildly short of breath and occasionally belches.

Arm pain:

The SP demonstrates pain in both arms *only* when asked, by rubbing his biceps area. The pain in the arms is only elicited on specific questioning.

After 4 minutes into the encounter:

The pain radically intensifies to 10/10. The patient becomes very apprehensive and breathes at 26–28/minute. He says: 'Oh my, the pain is back!', while simulating pain and fear.

To simulate the shortness of breath and nausea, he should break up his sentences by taking a breath in the middle. As the rapid breathing is hard to maintain, the SPs will need to vary it from 26 to 28/minute down to 18 to 20, and up again to maintain the sense of being short of breath without hyperventilating.

This only needs to be maintained until/if the pain is relieved.

Note

Responses to different pain and nausea medications and other interventions are specified and provided to trainers for coaching SPs and nurses. This information includes responses to overdoses.

CASE STUDIES

Station 1 Instructions to nurse

As the candidate enters the room, the nurse should be just finishing taking the patient's blood pressure. She gives the *first* ECG to the candidate and says: 'This patient has just arrived and just had an electrocardiogram; how do you want to manage him?' As the candidate asks for different things, the nurse will carry out the task as per the nurse's chart and instructions.

If candidates order a cardiac monitor before 4 minutes, the nurse will report the vitals given at the beginning of the station: pulse 70/minute.

If candidates order an external or internal pacemaker, the nurse reports that 'it's being asked for and it is on its way'.

Two main responsibilities: Respond to the candidates and facilitate SP simulation:

1. **Respond to the candidates** *upon request only* and as specified in the nurse's chart. The candidates' approach may be logical or disorganised, not necessarily reflecting the order of information on the nurse's chart. The nurse must respect the candidates' decisions and not attempt to influence them in any way.

2. **Facilitate the SP's simulation**. The patient's condition may vary according to the candidate's decisions. The nurse must help the SP to change his affect or behaviour appropriately. The SP and the nurse need, therefore, to agree on specific signals for each action outlined in the script.

Station 1 Nurse's chart and instructions

Candidate	Nurse's response
Candidate enters the room	**Give the ECG # R and make opening statement**
Orders aspirin	Simulate giving aspirin. (Nothing changes for SP)
Asks to confirm initial **vital signs**	**Report only if asked. Repeat vital signs are unchanged**
Orders ECG before 4 minutes	**Report:** 'ECG shows no change'
At 4 minutes	**Cue SP to change presentation**
Orders repeat **ECG**	**Pause** briefly, provide designated ECG
Orders **cardiac monitor**	**Apply** three cardiac dots and **report**: 'Sinus rhythm and pulse **80**'
Orders **oxygen**	**Apply** nasal prongs
Requests O$_2$ **saturation level**	**Apply** nasal prongs **report** specified O$_2$
Orders IV	**Set up** IV as requested
Orders blood **lab tests**	**Simulate** then **report**: 'Done, it's about 10–15 minutes for results'
Orders pain medication	**Cue** SP to the appropriate response for the medication and route
Ask for beta blocker	**Ask:** 'How do you want it to be given doctor?'
Orders **chest X-ray**	**Report:** 'I will order stat.'
Any other orders	**Report:** 'I will order' or 'I will set up stat.'
Note	

Some guidelines have been removed.

Station 1 Resources required

Makeup	Pallor and clamminess, perspiration on forehead and nostril area
Clothing	Shorts and socks, hospital gown
Furniture	Examination table/stretcher, pillows, sheets, two chairs
Medical equipment	IV pole, ER kit, cardiac dots, BP cuff, two stopwatches or clocks, clipboard ECGs – Labelled for nurses Nurse's charts – With columns for tracking candidate actions

Case Study

OSCE for PGY-1 Resident Physicians –
Madigan Army Medical Center

8

OSCE for Postgraduate Year-1 Resident Physicians – Madigan Army Medical Center	
Title	Assessing Intern Core Competencies with an OSCE
Author	Matthew W. Short and Patricia A. Short*
School/institution	Madigan Army Medical Center, Washington, USA
Professional background	Medicine
Course including level	Postgraduate Year 1 (PGY-1)
Short description	PGY-1 residents from 10 medical specialties were evaluated with an OSCE at the beginning and end of internship. The OSCE included eight 12-minute stations that collectively evaluated the six Accreditation Council for Graduate Medical Education (ACGME) core competencies using human patient simulators, standardised patients and clinical scenarios. Residents were scored by standardised patients and faculty using objective and subjective criteria with a maximum score of 100 for each competency. Stations included death notification, abdominal pain, transfusion consent, suture skills, wellness history, chest pain, altered mental status and computer literature search. These stations were chosen by specialty programme directors, created with input from board-certified specialists, and were peer reviewed.
Role of examination	Formative programme evaluation. The OSCE was used to test for interval improvement in resident core competencies. Results were shared with programmes to assess programme performance in teaching the competencies and station topics. Programmes not showing significant improvement in resident scores used the data to implement changes in their programme curriculum.
Venue	Simulation centre with rooms arranged as clinical and emergency exam rooms
Number of students	106 PGY-1 residents
Number of stations, duration of stations and length of exam	8 stations each 12 minutes with a total exam time of 96 minutes
Number of circuits and timing	Four circuits were used. 32 residents, with 8 residents allocated to each circuit from 7.30 a.m. to 5.30 p.m. This was repeated the second day for up to 64 residents. This testing was repeated at the end of the academic year and the study spanned 2 years for a total of 106 residents.

OSCE for Postgraduate Year-1 Resident Physicians – Madigan Army Medical Center—cont'd

Examiners	Board-certified physicians and standardised patients
Patients	Human patient simulators (SimMan) and standardised patients)
Criteria for pass/fail decision	This OSCE was used to evaluate the effectiveness of residency education during the internship year in 10 specialties. Pre- and post-internship scores were compared among specialties to provide feedback to programme directors on whether their programme curricula provided adequate education on the station topics
Feedback provided	The same OSCE was used at the beginning and end of the academic year for the purpose of programme improvement. In order to minimise the 'practice effect' bias, residents were not provided with feedback after testing, nor were they told that the end of year OSCE would include the same stations.
Experience gained with exam	6 years
Publications describing exam	Lee et al. (2008); Short et al. (2009); Stevens (2010); Opar et al. (2010); O'Brien et al. (2010); Fargo et al. (2011)

*The views expressed are those of the authors and do not reflect the official policy of the Department of the Army, the Department of Defense or the U.S. Government.

List of stations

No.	Station	Patient representation	Competencies assessed	
			Faculty physician	*Standardised patient*
1	Death notification	Standardised patient	ICS	ICS
2	Abdominal pain	Standardised patient	PC, MK, ICS, Pro, SBP	ICS, Pro
3	Suture skills	Pigs' feet	PC, SBP	–
4	Transfusion consent	Standardised patient	PC, MK, ICS, Pro	ICS, Pro
5	Wellness history	Standardised patient	PC, ICS, Pro, SBP	ICS, Pro
6	Altered mental status	Human patient simulator (SimMan)	PC, MK, ICS, Pro, SBP	–
7	Literature search	Computer	PBLI	–
8	Chest pain	Human patient simulator (SimMan)	PC, MK, SBP	–

ICS, interpersonal and communication skills; MK, medical knowledge; PBLI, practice-based learning and improvement; PC, patient care; Pro, professionalism; SBP, systems-based practice. Empty cell means there was no standardised patient at that OSCE station, so there was no standardised patient assessment of competencies.

Station 1 Death notification

Station title: Death notification

Station type: Standardised 'patient' (family member)

Station scenario: The examinee is asked to notify a family member of a patient's death while rotating in the Intensive Care Unit (ICU).

Competencies tested: Interpersonal and communication skills

Station objectives:

• Provide a realistic experience of giving bad news to a family member in a low-risk environment.

• Provide a means for self-evaluation and reflection on interpersonal and communication skills in a simulated high-stakes situation.

Station organisation: Standardised family member is pacing in the doorway to the room. Examinee is briefed on scenario outside of the room. Evaluator watches video recording in real time.

Station 1 Instructions to resident

You are the PGY-1 resident on call in a multidisciplinary Intensive Care Unit (ICU). It seems all parts of the hospital are busy – the ICU, the wards, and the Emergency Department (ED). You and your resident (ENT PGY-2) are called to come down to evaluate a stroke patient who is being 'coded' by the emergency medicine (EM) staff and who will presumably need admission to the ICU. You and your resident join in the resuscitation trying to stabilise the patient enough to transport her up to the ICU.

The patient is a 79-year-old woman who was taking aspirin and warfarin as an outpatient. Upon arrival to the ED she was comatose and found to have a large volume intracranial haemorrhage with significant herniation. Neurosurgery has reviewed her studies from home, discussed the case with the EM staff and does not feel that an emergent surgical intervention would increase this patient's chance for meaningful survival. She became bradycardic and ultimately developed asystole soon after arrival at the ED. You and the EM staff coded her for approximately 15 minutes but were never able to re-establish a rhythm.

Minutes after the code is called the patient's daughter arrives in the ED. The EM staff have moved on to other patients and your resident has to head back to the ICU to take care of an unstable patient. They ask you to let the patient's daughter know that her mother is dead.

The daughter is currently waiting in a private room. The patient's body is behind the curtain. At this time you do not need to inquire about an autopsy or organ donation.

Station 1   Examiner's checklist

Death notification faculty and SP evaluation form	Name:					
Interpersonal and communication skills	Did not perform	Needs improvement	Below average	Average	Above average	Excellent
Marking schedule	0	1	2	3	4	5

Communication skills

1. Greets family member respectfully

2. Introduces self and title

3. Offers family member a seat

4. Maintains calm and concerned affect

5. Maintained appropriate eye contact

6. Used appropriate physical contact

7. Used appropriate pace, volume and tone of speech

8. Appeared comfortable with silence

9. Uses appropriate body language (face family, sit close)

10. Avoids medical jargon and vague descriptions

Continued

11. Expresses sympathy and shows compassion

12. Allowed the bereaved to express emotion

13. Gives family time to talk and ask questions

14. Offers family member a tissue

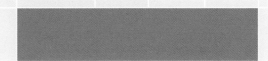

Content issues

15. Describes status of patient on arrival to ED to present

16. Asks family what they understand of the events

17. Able to explain sequence of events in layman's terms

18. Used appropriate language to tell family patient was dead

19. Answers all questions in a straightforward manner

Station 1 Examiner's checklist—cont'd

Follow-up

20. Asks the family if they wish to view body

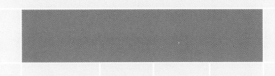

21. Tells family what they will see when viewing the body

22. Tells family okay to touch/hold body

23. Asks if they want to be alone with the body

24. Prepares the body for family viewing

25. Offers support services (chaplain, social worker, counsellor)

Comments:

Note

Items 1, 2, 3, 14, 15, 20, 22, 23 and 25 were considered binomial.

Station 1 Instructions to standardised patient

You have been called to the Emergency Department and are waiting in a private room for news of your elderly mother who has been brought to hospital in a serious condition. You are pacing the room as the resident arrives. The resident tells you that your mother has died. You are crying profusely and are emotional and inconsolable. Please say that you don't understand when the resident tries to explain what happened to your mother.

Station 1 Resources needed

Room with video capability and closable door, two chairs, one box of tissue. Realism can be enhanced in two ways: (1) this would occur in a place where it is noisy and hectic in the hallway outside the room, and (2) there should be a manikin or other simulated dead patient on a gurney behind a curtain in the room that the examinee will enter with the simulated family member.

9

Case Study

Dundee Undergraduate BSc in Nursing Programme – First-year OSCE

Dundee Undergraduate BSc in Nursing Programme – First-Year OSCE	
Title	Dundee Undergraduate BSc in Nursing Programme – First-Year OSCE
Authors	Arlene Brown and Iain Burns
School/institution	School of Nursing and Midwifery, University of Dundee, UK
Professional background	Nursing
Course including level	**Module name:** Skills and Practice 1 First-year undergraduate nursing students
Short description	An OSCE designed to assess essential foundation skills, techniques and practices associated with nursing. Each station consists of a skill that has been taught and practised during clinical skills sessions, and students have then had the opportunity to practise during their clinical placements. Students are assessed at each OSCE station using a validated checklist for the particular skill being examined.
Role of examination	This is a summative assessment. Students are required to pass this examination before proceeding to the next year of the programme.
Venue	Clinical Skills Centre
Number of students	Approximately 350 students within two campuses (250 in one campus and 100 in the other).
Number of stations, duration of stations and length of exam	8 stations each 5 minutes with a total exam time of 40 minutes. 5 minutes between circuits.
Number of circuits and timing	Identical OSCEs are run on both campuses in the same week. On the Dundee campus 250 students are examined over 3.5 days and 100 students on the Fife Campus over 2 days. Generally one circuit is used but sometimes two depending on numbers and time available in the Clinical Skills Unit. Eight students to each circuit, for example, from 9.00 a.m. to 9.40 a.m. with a 5 minute break. The remaining students are examined on the same circuits every 45 minutes. Breaks are built into each day.

Dundee Undergraduate BSc in Nursing Programme – First-Year OSCE—cont'd

Examiners	Members of academic teaching staff
Patients	Simulated patients, simulators
Criteria for pass/fail decision	Each station has a pre-determined pass mark of 80% determined following internal and external validation of the stations. Stations are assessed using a web-based programme which facilitates effective marking feedback and analysis of results.
Feedback provided	Each checklist has a section for student feedback which the examiner will complete during the OSCE. The student's Learning Team Facilitator (personal tutor) will receive a copy of this to allow feedback to be given post-OSCE. Students are given personal feedback and are provided with their scoring sheet complete with the examiner's comments via an email generated by a web-based programme.
Experience gained with exam	22 years

List of stations

Station	Learning outcomes assessed	Patient representation	Examiner
1	Medicine administration	Simulated patient	Observed and scored by examiner
2	Completion of temperature, pulse and respiration	Simulated patient	Observed and scored by examiner
3	Cardiopulmonary resuscitation	Resuscitation manikin	Observed and scored by examiner
4	Hand decontamination	–	Observed and scored by examiner
5	Urinalysis	Simulated urine and written results	Observed and scored by examiner
6	Completion of a fluid balance chart	Written information and completion of fluid balance chart	Observed and scored by examiner
7	Completion of medicine administration calculations	Written information	Observed and scored by examiner
8	Measurement of blood pressure	Simulated arm	Observed and scored by examiner

Station 1 Medicine administration
Instructions to student

Administer John (or Jane) Watt's medication for 08.00.

The examiner, as the Registered Nurse, will check all details with you.

You will have cleansed your hands prior to commencing this station.

Note, please use hand rub at the end of this procedure before progressing to the next station.

Station 1 Simulated patient script – male/female

Thank you for agreeing to participate in the nursing OSCE.

- You are a co-operative and friendly patient.
- Your name is John/Jane Watt and you were admitted to hospital to be treated for a chest infection and anaemia.
- You have been feeling much better since your treatment commenced.
- The medicines you are taking are fighting the infection and correcting the iron deficiency.
- It is 8.00 a.m. and the nurse will be coming to give you your amoxicillin capsule ('Tic Tac' sweets) followed by a drink.
- If the student asks you to, identify yourself by stating your full name and date of birth (see details below). Your patient identity bracelet also contains this information.
- If the student asks whether you are sensitive/allergic to any medicines or other substances you will answer 'no'.
- The student may want to confirm that you have swallowed the medicine by asking to look in your mouth.
- Please refrain from initiating any conversation with students during the procedure.
- You should not speak to the student about their OSCE performance after they have completed the Medicine Administration Station.

Name: John Watt/Jane Watt

Doctor: Dr Rose

Date of birth: 26 February 1939

Hospital: VHK, Ward 35

Please tick appropriate box to confirm whether each of the criteria has been achieved or not.

Criteria	Yes	No
1. Introduces self and explains procedure to patient, gaining consent and co-operation.		
2. Checks and *demonstrates* that the medication prescription is legal (i.e. the prescriber's and pharmacist's signatures and prescription date).		
3. Asks the patient to confirm their name and date of birth *and* checks this corresponds with the identity band details *and* the prescription.		
4. Checks documented allergies on the prescription *and* confirms this with patient.		
5. Confirms 08.00 medication *only* has not been administered by checking the recording sheet *and* asking the patient.		
6. Checks 08.00 medication and dose *only* corresponds with prescription.		
7. Checks expiry date on container for 08.00 drug *only* has not passed.		
8. Uses non-touch technique to dispense the medication into the medicine receptacle.		
9. Ensures patient swallows medication with a drink and then correctly disposes of used equipment.		
10. Correctly records the administration of the medication on the recording sheet (i.e. writes their initials in the 08.00 box and the date at the top of the column in the date box).		

Notes

NMC Standards for Medicines Management (2008).

See script for simulated patients – male and female. Inform simulated patient that 'Tic Tac'/'Smint' medicines can be held under tongue or in cheek pocket and then disposed at end of OSCE station into appropriate waste disposal container but students *must* demonstrate that swallowing of medicine has been checked.

Marker's No.:_____   **Grade:**_____

Feedback for student:

CASE STUDIES

Station 1   List of resources

Simulated patient

Examiner

Medicine administration trolley

Simulated medicine

Completed drug prescription and administration record

Case Study

OSCE in Undergraduate Dentistry

10

OSCE in Undergraduate Dentistry

Title	OSCE in Undergraduate Dentistry
Author	Anthony Damien Walmsley
School/institution	School of Dentistry, University of Birmingham, UK
Professional background	Dentistry
Level	Undergraduate
Short description	A list of stations typically used in an OSCE is given, with one described in more detail. The OSCE is generally used with other forms of assessment such as written essays, structured oral assessments, clinical portfolios and clinical assessments.
Role of examination	May be used as a formative or summative examination
Venue	Typically in a dental teaching clinic
Number of students	Up to 80 per year
Number and duration of stations and length of exam	Approximately 16 stations, usually 8 minutes allowing 7 minutes for assessment and 1 minute to clean and prepare the station for the next student.
Number of circuits and timing	One or two circuits
Examiners	Teaching and support staff including instructor technicians, dental nurses and Dental Core trainees (house officers)
Patients	Standardised patients, patient models and simulation
Publications relating to exam	Schoonheim-Klein et al. (2005)

List of stations

A typical dental OSCE will have a mixture of stations including practical dentistry, communications and knowledge-based stations. The stations included will be dependent on the student level of experience in the course. A clinical student will have had exposure to a range of clinical practice specialties and the following annotated list provides an example of stations.

Continued

283

List of stations—cont'd

No.	Speciality	Procedure	Type of patient representation	Assesses
1	Periodontology	Root planning of teeth	Simulation	Clinical skill, knowledge
2	Periodontology	Measuring bone depth from a radiograph	Simulation	Diagnostic skill
3	Prosthodontics	Designing a partial denture	Simulation	Knowledge, communication to laboratory technician
4	Oral surgery	Suturing of a simulated wound	Simulation	Manual dexterity, ability to close a wound
5	Paediatrics	Interpreting eruption dates from a radiograph	Standardised patient	Knowledge, diagnostic skill
6	Conservative (operative) dentistry	Rubber dam procedure for endodontics	Simulation	Clinical skill
7	Clinical practice	Listening to dental charting through headphones and marking them on a clinical chart	Simulation	Interpretation of data, knowledge
8	Orthodontics	Designing an appliance	Simulation	Knowledge communication to laboratory technician
9	Behavioural science (communication)	Discussing removal of old amalgam fillings for new white coloured ones	Standardised patient	Communication
10	Infection control	Washing of hands	Simulation	Clinical skill
11	Biomaterials	Light curing a tooth coloured restoration	Simulation	Clinical skill knowledge
12	Prosthodontics	Setting up of anterior teeth on a denture	Simulation	Clinical skill
13	Radiology	Interpreting radiograph	Simulation	Diagnostic skill
14	Medical emergencies	Resuscitation	Simulation	Clinical skill
15	Conservative (operative) dentistry	Assessment of crown procedures	Patient models	Diagnostic skill
16	Oral surgery	Extraction of a tooth on a manikin	Simulation	Clinical skill

Notes

Stations 1, 2, 5, 6, 11, 13 and 16 use a phantom head in a dental chair. Stations 3, 8 and 12 use models/casts of the mouth. Stations 5 and 9 use actors.

Station 3 Prosthetics – Denture design

Instructions for the student

You are provided with a model of a partially dentate upper arch which has been prepared for provision of a removable partial denture to replace:

<u>5 | 56</u>

The upper arch is opposed by a complete lower denture.

Complete a laboratory design *in full* (*sketch the design* and *write instructions*) on the laboratory card provided for the construction of an upper **cobalt-chrome framework denture.**

Incorporating the following features:

- Four rests (corresponding to the positions of rest seats indicated on the cast)
- One cast cobalt-chrome clasp:
  - UL4: Gingivally approaching
- One wrought stainless steel clasp:
  - UR6: Occlusally approaching terminating in the disto-buccal undercut
- Ring major connector and appropriate minor connectors

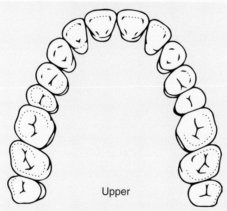

Upper

Marking schedule

Drawn instruction:

Saddles	Two saddles correctly identified on diagram. (One mark per pair)	2	1	0
Support	Two pairs of rests correctly drawn in correct positions. (One mark per pair)	2	1	0
Retention	One mark for each pair of correctly drawn clasps	2	1	0
Reciprocation	One mark for each pair of effectively reciprocated clasps (Note, reciprocation can be from connector)	2	1	0
Major connector:	Ring connector correctly drawn		1	0
Minor connectors:	All components are connected		1	0

Continued

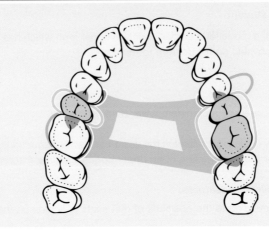

Case Study

Diploma in Veterinary Nursing

11

Diploma in Veterinary Nursing

Title	Veterinary Nursing (DipVN)
Author	Martin Barrow and Denise Burke (collaborator)
School/institution	Central Qualifications (CQ), Examination Board and Awarding Organisation, UK
Professional background	Veterinary Medicine and Surgery
Course including level	Diploma in Veterinary Nursing Level 3 qualification
Short description	A practical examination of essential clinical/practical skills conducted at the end of 2 or 3 years of vocational training. The practical examinations are conducted by CQ appointed external examiners and are run at CQ approved centres throughout the year. One of the challenges is the assessment of small numbers of students at any one time with a limited number of examiners.
Role of examination	Summative. This assessment must be passed in order for the student to achieve the full Diploma in Veterinary Nursing qualification.
Venue	Large rooms at the teaching centre specially prepared for the purpose and used during the weekend.
Number of students	11 students
Number of stations, duration of stations and length of exam	12 stations arranged as three sets of four stations. Each station was 10 minutes. A total exam time of 150 minutes. There were supervised breaks between each set of four stations.
Number of circuits and timing	Three circuits were used. Four students allocated to each circuit from 10.30 a.m. to 1.00 p.m.; the following group of four students were examined on the same circuit from 2.00 p.m. to 4.30 p.m. The final group were examined the following day from 10.30 a.m. to 1.00 p.m.
Examiners	CQ trained and appointed 'external' examiners, and not known to the students. A senior examiner oversaw each examination.
Patients	Simulated patients (models) and task scenarios, e.g. laboratory techniques, wound dressing and X-rays.

Continued

Diploma in Veterinary Nursing—cont'd

Criteria for pass/fail decision	A panel of raters was used to determine the pass mark (Angoff method). Partially completed items were recorded and considered for borderline scores
Feedback provided	Students were given feedback via their centres at the time results were issued. In the instance of a fail they were advised whether the fail was due to critical components not performed or a percentage score below the pass mark.
Experience gained with exam	2 years
Costs or resources required	Venue provided static equipment, e.g. anaesthesia and X-ray machine. Consumables and task equipment supplied by CQ
Publications describing exam	N/A

List of stations
OSCE for veterinary nurses: List of 12 tasks over four stations

Station	Learning outcomes assessed	Patient representation	Examiner
1a	AT003 – Select equipment and calculate the settings for anaesthesia	–	Observed by examiner and scored later
2a	GN003 – Apply bandage using dressing, splint and bandage to immobilise limb	Simulated patient	Observed by examiner and scored later
3a	GN004 – Calculate dosage and administer injection	Model dog	Observed by examiner and scored later
4a	GN007 – Calculate and dispense medication	–	Observed by examiner and scored later
1b	GN009 – Administer fluid via IV cannula and record on hospitalisation record	Model cat	Observed by examiner and scored later
2b	LT003 – Interpretation of urine sample	–	Observed by examiner and scored later
3b	LT005 – Obtain blood sample	Simulation	Observed by examiner and scored later
4b	LT006 – Set up microscope and identify items on slide	–	Observed by examiner and scored later
1c	R004 – Position patient for X-ray	Simulated patient	Observed by examiner and scored later
2c	R005 – Position patient for X-ray	Simulated patient	Observed by examiner and scored later
3c	SN004 – Sterilise and pack instruments	–	Observed by examiner and scored later
4c	SN005 – Prepare instruments	–	Observed by examiner and scored later

Notes

The model dog and model cat used in Stations 3a and 1b are low-tech models. Stations 2a, 1c and 2c use more sophisticated models.

Station 3b does not use a model and covered all procedures up to but excluding the venepuncture.

Station 2a   Apply dressing with splint and bandage to immobilise limb
Task scenario for candidate

Your patient has been admitted to the hospital following a road traffic accident.

Radiography reveals a simple transverse fracture of the right radius and ulna. There is also a minor wound on the lateral aspect of the limb, as indicated by the simulated wound on the model. This has been cleaned and sutured. Surgery to repair the fracture is to be performed the following day.

The veterinary surgeon has requested that you apply a dressing to the wound, together with a splint and bandage as a first aid measure to immobilise the limb until then.

Note, the patient is still anaesthetised following radiography and is being monitored.

Station 2a   Examiner's guidance notes

Task set-up instructions

- Adhere wound to lateral aspect of the right forelimb, just above the carpus with double sided tape. Ensure wound does not get dislodged between candidates
- Place patient in right lateral recumbency between candidates
- An assistant will be required for this task to hold the limb for the candidate
- Place patient on one table and set up equipment on a separate table

Station 2a   Scoring sheet

Step	Task	Guidance for scoring	Partial completion	Tick/ cross
1.	Select wound dressing			
2.	Select small amount of padding for digits	Cotton wool or strips of padding bandage acceptable		

Continued

CASE STUDIES

Step	Task	Guidance for scoring	Partial completion	Tick/ cross
3.	Select padding bandage			
4.	Select conforming bandage			
5.	Select protective layer			
6.	Select scissors	Scissors can be selected at any time. Candidates may use their own scissors, this is also acceptable.		
7.	Select appropriate size of splint.	The longer of the splints should be selected. The other is too short.		
8.	Select and prepare (unwrap) materials and equipment prior to starting.	Scissors can be selected at any time. Candidates may use their own scissors, this is also acceptable.		
9.	Place patient in correct lateral recumbency, affected limb uppermost.	Patient to be placed in left lateral recumbency.		
10.	Ask assistant to support the affected limb to facilitate bandaging.			
11.	Wear gloves	If the candidate fails to put on gloves prior to starting the bandage but remembers halfway through placing the bandage and wishes to start again, the examiner may encourage the candidate to continue with the bandage as starting again may mean the bandage will be incomplete at the end of the 6 minutes. This step is not awarded unless the candidate wears gloves for steps 12–15.		
12.	Apply wound dressing with correct side facing wound.	Shiny side facing wound		
13.	Apply dressing aseptically without touching the side facing the wound.	It is acceptable to secure the primary dressing with a piece of tape. The candidate may only touch the side of the dressing not in contact with the wound.		

Step	Task	Guidance for scoring	Partial completion	Tick/ cross
14.	Apply padding between digits (as far as possible).	It can be difficult to place padding between digits on the model. As long as the candidate demonstrates they are attempting to do this the examiner may ask them to move onto the next step.		
15.	Apply padding layer to the limb, ensuring wound dressing not moved.			
16.	Apply padding to include the foot.	The whole foot must be covered in padding layer.		
17.	Apply padding to include the elbow.			
18.	Apply splint to the caudal aspect of the limb.	Candidates may wish to tape this in place although this is not necessary. Candidates may place another layer of padding over the splint, this is acceptable. It is acceptable to place the cupped end of the splint either at the elbow or the paw.		
19.	Splint includes the elbow.	Splint to fit over elbow.		
20.	Splint includes the carpus.	Carpus must be fully included in splint. If the candidate has selected the correct size of splint and placed it correctly this will be achieved.		
21.	Apply conforming layer to the limb.			
22.	Apply conforming layer to include the foot and the elbow.	Splint to be included in conforming layer to hold in place.		
23.	Apply protective layer to limb.			
24.	Apply outer protective layer to include the foot and the elbow.	Splint to be included in protective layer.		
25.	Bandage applied from distal to proximal limb.	Once the foot is covered, the bandage should travel distal to proximal. (1) At the top it should be snipped off and not travel back down the leg or (2) it may travel down the leg but the entire leg must be recovered and tension must be the same throughout the bandage.		

CASE STUDIES

SECTION D

Step	Task	Guidance for scoring	Partial completion	Tick/ cross
26.	Bandage material applied in correct order ensuring each rotation covers $\frac{1}{2}-\frac{2}{3}$ of previous rotation.	Correct order – dressing, padding, splint, conforming and protective. Candidate may place another layer of padding over the splint, this is acceptable.		
		There should be no gaps between each rotation of bandage layer, an overlap of $\frac{1}{2}-\frac{2}{3}$ should apply. Third layer should stop level with first and second layers.		
27.	Bandage is of suitable tension – not too tight or too loose.	Candidate to demonstrate they are checking tension by placing fingers inside bandage, and not just say they are doing so.		
28.	Check bandage is neatly and professionally presented.	Small amount of padding showing at top of bandage is acceptable, otherwise no other padding or conforming bandage to be showing. The splint should not be showing.		
29.	Limb handled gently throughout.			
30.	Correct limb bandaged.	Right forelimb		
31.	Bandage of correct tension (examiner to check).	Correct tension: There should be room to easily insert two fingers side by side into the top of the bandage. The bandage should be gently pulled to ensure it does not slip off easily. Tension should be even throughout the bandage.		

If at any point during the 6 minutes of the task the candidate realises they have bandaged the wrong limb they will be allowed the remaining time to rectify this. If the candidate runs out of time the examiner may only mark the steps the candidate has performed when bandaging the correct limb.

Notes

1. The examiner scores by putting a tick, cross or 'P' (partial completion) in the box next to each step. (Not all steps have a 'partial completion' option.)

2. A panel of raters previously assigns a value to each step (1–10 scale, where 1 = trivial and 10 = critical). After the OSCE the candidate's score is ascertained by entering the results into a spreadsheet.

Station 2A Equipment list

Equipment	Quantity/ candidate	Notes	Supplier
Model dog	1	Place wound on patient as indicated by scenario	Central Qualifications (CQ)
Melolin non-adhesive dressing (5 cm × 5 cm)	3		CQ
Cotton wool roll	1	Spare to be available	CQ
Synthetic padding roll 5 cm	3		CQ
Synthetic padding roll 7.5 cm	3		CQ
Conforming bandage 5 cm	3		CQ
Conforming bandage 7 cm	3		CQ
Protective bandage 5 cm	3		CQ
Protective bandage 7.5 cm	3		CQ
Scissors	1		CQ
Gloves (non-powdered, non-latex)	1 box of each	Small, medium and large	CQ
Wound – sutured	1	To be adhered to patient	CQ
Splint – correct length for patient	1		CQ
Splint – too short for patient	1		CQ
Double-sided tape	0	To adhere wound to patient	CQ
Zinc oxide tape 2.5 cm	1	Spare to be available	CQ
Elastoplast 2.5 cm	1	Spare to be available	CQ
Normal waste bin	1		Centre

Spare materials to be kept from the task area.

Case Study

12

Summative OSCE for a Clinical
Pharmacy Course, Malaysia

Summative OSCE for a Clinical Pharmacy Course, Malaysia

Title	Summative OSCE for a Clinical Pharmacy Course, Malaysia
Author	Ahmed Awaisu[1], Siti Halimah Bux Rahman Bux[2] and Mohamad Haniki Nik Mohamed[2]
School/institution	Faculty of Pharmacy, International Islamic University, Malaysia
Authors' current affiliations	[1]College of Pharmacy, Qatar University, Doha, Qatar; [2]Faculty of Pharmacy, International Islamic University Malaysia, Kuantan, Malaysia
Professional background	Pharmacy
Course including level	Clinical Pharmacy III course Fourth-professional (final) year undergraduate pharmacy students
Short description	An OSCE was designed to assess clinical competence of final-year pharmacy students with a focus on patient education and communication, clinical pharmacokinetics skills, identification and resolution of drug-related problems, and critical appraisal of drug literature and drug information provision. Students were required to perform specific functions to complete tasks or address certain problems in each station. For example, pharmacy students were required to counsel/educate patients on the use of an insulin delivery device or asthma inhaler device; identify and resolve drug-related problems in a patient with multiple comorbidities using an evidence-based approach; and provide information requested by a physician on a newly approved/marketed medication.
Role of examination	Summative. The OSCE contributed 25% to the course assessment at the end of the second semester.
Venue	Typically, two parallel circuits at departmental offices (Pharmacy Practice Department) and/or clinical skills laboratory rooms and corridors
Number of students	Variable: 42 and 52 students during 2005/2006 and 2007/2008 academic years, respectively

Number of stations, duration of stations and length of exam	During 2007/2008: 13 stations each 15 minutes with a total exam time of 195 minutes and total changeover time of about 30 minutes (length of exam = 3 hours and 45 minutes)
Number of circuits and timing	Two circuits or tracks (i.e. two identical but separate sets of stations) were run simultaneously in parallel for two groups of 13 students each, and repeated in the afternoon. The estimated total time required per circuit/track was 3 hours and 45 mins: • 9.15 a.m.–1.00 p.m. (two morning tracks/circuits) • 2.15 p.m.–6.00 p.m. (two afternoon tracks/circuits)
Examiners	Academic faculty members and hospital-based preceptors
Patients	Standardised or simulated patients and actors
Criteria for pass/fail decision	No standard setting for pass/fail criteria. The OSCE contributed 25% to the course assessments
Feedback provided	Randomly selected stations and students were videotaped with prior consent for the purpose of teaching and learning in subsequent years. Students were provided with feedback on the examination as a group, but no individual student feedback was usually provided.
Experience gained with exam	10 years
Publications describing exam	Awaisu et al. (2007); Awaisu et al. (2010); Awaisu and Nik Mohamed (2010)

Case Study 12 – List of stations

Station	Competency	Learning outcomes assessed	Patient/actor and case description
1	DRPs identification and resolution	To assess a patient's drug related needs in order to identify DRPs and provide evidence-based recommendations for a pharmacist's care plan to resolve and/or prevent the problems.	SP: A 45-year-old male with a history of hypertension and epilepsy; receiving medications on an outpatient basis. He presented with untreated anaemia, PUD, hypokalaemia, non-adherence to drugs and signs/symptoms of phenytoin toxicity. Props needed: Medical records/charts
2	Rest station	–	–

Continued

3	Management of acetaminophen toxicity	To identify the risk of liver damage due to acetaminophen toxicity; use measured serum drug concentration and a nomogram to predict severity of hepatotoxicity; and recommend whether or not to give a specific antidote [N-acetylcysteine].	SD: A physician actor seeks the pharmacist's opinion on the management of the case below: 'A 30-year-old male who presented to the ED after intentional acetaminophen overdose. Decontamination was done upon patient's arrival at the ED. Serum acetaminophen concentration was obtained.' Props needed: TDM report form
4	Preparation station	To give the examinee an opportunity to review pertinent patient's medical records related to Station 5.	Props needed for use by the pharmacist: Medical records/charts
5	DRPs identification and resolution	To assess a patient's drug related needs in order to identify and prioritise DRPs, provide evidence-based recommendations to resolve and/or prevent the identified problems and determine how to monitor the therapeutic regimens.	SP: A 43-year-old male diagnosed with PTB and started on DOTS 3 months prior. Currently complaining of increase in cough intensity along with blood-stained sputum, fever and night sweat for the past 1 week. Liver enzymes are elevated, red cell indices are low and his DM is uncontrolled. Props needed: Medical records/charts including labs
6	Rest station	–	–
7	Education/counselling on the use of insulin delivery devices	To assess the student's competence in educating/counselling a patient with diabetes on the use of NovoMix® 30 FlexPen® (preparation before injection, injection techniques, injection sites and care of insulin).	SP: A 50-year-old female with type 2 DM for 8 years. On a follow-up visit, FBS was 12 mmol/L, HbA$_{1c}$ was 10%, and renal function has recently declined (Clcr = 38 mL/min). The physician decided to discontinue her OHA and prescribed NovoMix® 30 FlexPen® 6 units to be injected two times daily. Props needed: Insulin pen (NovoMix® 30 FlexPen®), sponge.

8	Clinical pharmacokinetics: Dosage regimen design	To interpret TDM results; estimate the patient's pharmacokinetic parameters; and provide individualised maintenance dosing regimen recommendations.	A 60-year-old patient diagnosed with CHF was started on 0.5 mg digoxin PO as a LD. A cardiologist requests TDM analysis 24 hours after the LD. (Result: digoxin level = 0.7 mcg/L). He asks for a recommendation on the maintenance dose. Props needed: TDM report form
9	Rest station	–	–
10	Preparation station	To undertake a quick appraisal of drug literature	Props needed: Two articles regarding a new medication for smoking cessation (varenicline) were provided. After 15 minutes, the candidate enters the next station (Station 11) where a physician will make a drug information inquiry. Props needed: The same articles above will be made available in Station 11.
11	Critical appraisal of the literature and drug information enquiry	To receive a drug information enquiry and formulate a response in a timely manner through evaluation of relevant literature.	SD: A physician makes an enquiry, via the telephone, about a new drug for smoking cessation. Opening statement: 'I am Dr May. I have heard of varenicline, the new drug for smoking cessation. I am thinking of using it for one of my patients. Could you urgently tell me the safety, efficacy and suitability of the drug for the patient?'
12	Clinical pharmacokinetics: Dosage regimen design	To interpret serum drug concentration measurements; design an individualised dosing regimen for a patient receiving phenytoin; and provide appropriate dosing regimen recommendations.	SP: A 42-year-old man with a history of GTC seizures and hepatic cirrhosis has been taking oral phenytoin sodium 100 mg PO tds for 2 weeks. He presents with the symptoms of nystagmus, ataxia, slurred speech and bradycardia. The physican suspects that the patient is experiencing phenytoin toxicity and requests for TDM of the drug as well as the pharmacist's recommendations.
13	Preparation station	To give the examinee an opportunity to review pertinent patient's medical records related to Station 1.	Props needed for use by the pharmacist: Medical records/charts

Notes

- All active OSCE stations were observed and scored by faculty or hospital-based preceptor examiners, except Station 8 which was scored immediately after the examination.
- Station 13 is the preparation for Station 1. The first candidate starts 15 minutes earlier than the other candidates at Station 13. Similarly, Station 4 and 10 are preparation stations.
- Randomly selected stations and randomly selected students were videotaped. Students were informed of this possibility in advance.

DRPs, Drug-related problems; SP or SD, standardised patient or simulated doctor; PUD, peptic ulcer disease; ED, Emergency Department; DOTS, directly observed therapy short-course; FBS, fasting blood sugar; OHA, oral hypoglycaemic agent(s); LD, loading dose; PO, per oral; TDM, therapeutic drug monitoring; GTC, generalised tonic clonic.

Station 7 Counselling on the use of insulin delivery devices
Instructions to the student

You are meeting a patient who has had **type 2 diabetes mellitus for 8 years.**

- She has been taking. Diamicron® tablets 160 mg bd and metformin tablets 1 gm tds for her diabetes.
- Today, on a follow-up visit to her doctor, her FBS was 12 mmol/L, HbA$_{1C}$ was 10%, and her creatinine levels were rising (Clcr = 38 mL/min).
- Her doctor decided to stop her oral hypoglycaemic agents (OHAs) and prescribed NovoMix® 30 FlexPen® 6 units to be injected two times daily.

Your task is to:

- Briefly explain to the patient why the doctor probably stopped her tablets and switched her to this particular insulin injection.
- Teach the patient on the use of NovoMix® 30 FlexPen® (preparation before injection, injection techniques, injection sites and care of insulin).

Do not inject the insulin pen into the patient's or your skin. The sponge provided is to be used as a site for injection in your demonstration.

DO NOT ask the examiner any questions during the task.

Examiner's name/initials .... Student's no. ....

REMEMBER TO WRITE THE **STUDENT'S ID NUMBER** AT THE TOP RIGHT-HAND CORNER OF THE MARK SHEET.

Please circle the appropriate mark for each criterion

Description of criterion	Performed fully competently	Performed not fully competently	Not performed or incompetent
Initial approach to the patient (introduces him/herself, explains what he/she will be doing)	2	1	0
Explanation of the rationale for use of insulin (refer to the guide for the examiner)	2	1	0
Explanation of technique (preparation of penfill before making an injection)	2	1	0
Explanation of technique (making an injection, rotation of sites)	2	1	0
Clarity of instructions to the patient (inviting feedback, encouraging patient to speak); use of layman terms	2	1	0
Communication techniques (smiles, eye contact, tone of voice and volume)	2	1	0
Counselling on care of insulins: Storage (25°C for up to 4 weeks; do not freeze or expose to excessive heat and sunlight)	2	1	0
Counselling on precautions to take while on insulin (preventing hypoglycaemia)	2	1	0
Closing statement (asking patient if he/she has any more questions, thanking patient for their time)	2	1	0
Overall approach to task	2	1	0
Total (max. 20)			

CASE STUDIES

Station 7   Guidelines for the assessor/examiner
Highly confidential – For examiner's use only

Please read carefully the 'Instructions for the student' and the 'Instructions for the stand-ardised patient'.

Please introduce yourself to the student and give him/her the written instructions.

This station evaluates the student's competence to counsel and educate a patient with diabetes on the use of NovoMix® 30 FlexPen® (insulin analogue).

1. **The student should include these points when explaining to the patient the rationale for switching from OHAs to insulin:**

   – OHAs possibly not effective anymore – shown by persistent hyperglycaemia (FBS and HbA$_{1c}$ high) especially if patient confirms adherence.

   – There is kidney impairment (increased creatinine levels). OHAs metabolised in the kidney – will cause more damage to kidneys so have to stop them or adjust the dose.

   – Insulin will not cause damage to the kidneys. (Explain how insulin works in our body and its benefits in relation to complications.)

2. **Use of NovoMix® 30 FlexPen® (before making an injection):**

   – It is a cloudy solution. Roll FlexPen between palms approximately 10 times, then mix by flicking it up and down, i.e. hold in hand and move elbow up and down until the solution turns white.

   – Novomix is 30% insulin aspart and + 70% protaminated insulin aspart; this gives both postprandial glucose control (30% aspart) as well as basal blood glucose control (70% protaminated aspart).

Complete the mark sheet while observing the interaction between the student and the simulated patient.

Please DO NOT interact with the student or simulated patient during or after comple-tion of the task.

Station 7   Instructions for the standardised patient

Please read carefully the 'Instructions for the student' and 'Guidelines for the assessor/examiner' prior to the start of the examination.

Answer questions based on the following scenario. Do not volunteer any information unless asked.

• You were diagnosed with diabetes about 8 years ago and have already been informed that you are on the maximum dose of your oral diabetic medications.

• You have been compliant with taking your medications and diets as instructed and you never miss a dose.

• At today's follow-up with your doctor, you have been switched from taking the tablets to insulin injections.

- The student pharmacist has to tell you why your doctor has stopped your tablets and has prescribed this particular insulin product for your condition.
- The student is going to teach you how to use your FlexPen to deliver insulin into your body.

You may ask the following questions if you have not yet been informed by the student during the session:

1. How many times can I re-use the needle? (Expected response: Max. three times)

2. My friend is on insulin but she always has shivery feelings and sometimes faints. Will I get the same reactions if I go on insulin now? What should I do? (Student should explain about hypoglycaemia and how to overcome it; why you experience it, especially when exercising; if not injected in relation to meal times; overdosing)

3. How long do I have to wait before eating? (Expected response: For this particular insulin preparation you do not have to wait, just inject and eat!)

4. Where do I keep my insulin pen?

13 Case Study

Postgraduate Year 1 – Patient Safety OSCE

Postgraduate Year 1 – Patient Safety OSCE	
Title	Postgraduate Year 1 – Patient Safety OSCE
Authors	Dianne P. Wagner, Ruth B. Hoppe and Carol J. Parker
School/institution	College of Human Medicine, Michigan State University, Michigan, USA
Professional background	Medicine
Course including level	Orientation to residency Recent graduates just beginning residency
Short description	An OSCE designed to assess patient safety-related skills in new postgraduate year 1 residents. 10 stations were developed using residency director input of skills required for safety/success in early residency.
Role of examination	Formative. New residents are required by their programme directors to participate in this half-day experience. Baseline data on strengths and weaknesses were given to programme directors.
Venue	Simulation centre
Number of participants	150–200 participants/year
Number of stations, duration of stations and length of exam	10 stations of 20 minutes each, exam length 200 minutes.
Number of circuits and timing	Two simultaneous circuits per half-day
Examiners	Standardised patients/standardised family members/ standardised healthcare providers.
Patients	Standardised patients, standardised family members, standardised healthcare providers, simulators and the results of investigations, e.g. ECG and X-ray.
Criteria for pass/fail decision	Not applicable as this is a formative examination
Feedback provided	Participants receive immediate, specific, individual feedback on checklist items from standardised patients/standardised healthcare workers and/or exemplars (for things like admission orders or a progress note) and are provided with access to their videos. Participants create personal learning plans at the end of the experience to take back to their programme directors for discussion and for their own personal study planning.

Experience gained with exam   8 years

Publications describing exam   Wagner et al. (2009); Wagner and Lypson (2009)

List of stations

Station	Learning outcomes assessed	Patient representation	Examiner
1	Obtaining informed consent	Standardised patient	Scored by SP
2	Giving bad news	Standardised patient	Scored by SP
3	Aseptic technique	Simulator Standardised nurse	Scored by standardised nurse
4	History taking in a patient with vaginal bleeding Pelvic exam	Standardised patient Pelvic simulator	Scored by SP
5	Progress note construction	Vaginal bleeding case	Scored by programme directors/exemplar revealed
6	Testicular/breast/prostate examinations	Simulators	Findings entered into computer/correct answers revealed
7	Team skills with patient in respiratory distress	Simulator Standardised nurse	Scored by Standardised nurse
8	Admission order writing	Respiratory distress station scenario	Exemplar revealed
9	Critical vitals/lab/X-ray/ECG findings	Lab results X-rays EKGs	Exemplars/answers revealed
10	Cultural competency	Standardised patient	Scored by SP

Notes

Stations 4 and 5 are linked.

Station 6: After the examinee has entered responses into the computer the correct answers can be revealed by clicking on a different link.

Stations 7 and 8 are linked. The examinee has the full time to interact with the nurse and simulator at Station 7 and to receive feedback on the checklist then moves to Station 8 to complete the admission orders and enter them into the computer. These can be accessed by faculty to grade or to discuss with the examinee at a later date. No grade is generated at the time of the examination.

Station 9: The software grades the responses and generates a score.

CASE STUDIES

Stations 7 and 8 – Linked stations: team skills and patient in respiratory distress/admission order writing

Station 7 Examiner's checklist

1	Trainee introduced themselves and role to the patient	Yes	Yes with reservation	No
2	Trainee had ongoing communication with patient	Yes	Yes with reservation	No
3	Trainee introduced themself and role to nurse/team member	Yes	Yes with reservation	No
4	Trainee appropriately undrapes patient	Yes	Yes with reservation	No
5	Trainee assesses patient by looking at neck veins	Yes	Yes with reservation	No
6	Trainee assesses patient by listening to lungs	Yes	Yes with reservation	No
7	Trainee assesses patient by listening to the heart	Yes	Yes with reservation	No
8	Trainee assesses patient by feeling legs for odema	Yes	Yes with reservation	No
9	Trainee assesses patient by acknowledging monitor information	Yes	Yes with reservation	No
10	Trainee interacts appropriately with team member by asking the nurse to tell them about the patient	Yes	Yes with reservation	No
11	Trainee interacts appropriately with team member by clearly communicating intent and requests	Yes	Yes with reservation	No
12	Trainee establishes presence of crash cart	Yes	Yes with reservation	No
13	Trainee recognises need to ask for help	Yes	Yes with reservation	No
14	Comments:			

Station 8 Blank for admission order writing

University hospital

Physician's order

In the text box order sheet below please indicate your admission orders for this patient.

Sample admission order

Orders	Date	Time	Orders	Days
Order 1	13 June 2014	11.30 a.m.	Admit to ICU	
Order 2			Diagnosis: third-degree heart block/ respiratory distress	
Order 3			Condition: Critical	
Order 4			Vitals: Every 15 minutes for 1 hour, then 30 minutes for 4 hours, then ask House Officer to further orders	1
Order 5			Activity: Bedrest with bedside commode	1
Order 6			Diet: Cardiac diet	5
Order 7			Tests: CBC/comprehensive panel/ABGs stat/UA/troponin/12-lead EKG/CPK, CXR PA and lateral, portable	
Order 8			IV: D5/25 NS to keep vein open	1
Order 9			Meds: To be determined	
Order 10			Special tests: Echocardiogram ASAP. Social work evaluation	

Telephone orders read back to physician [ ]

81.   Doctor

Authorisation is granted to supply by non-proprietary name as per formulary policy unless checked here [ ]

82. Noted by

Admit, diagnosis, condition, vitals, activity, diet, tests, IVs, meds, special needs or testing is one organisational strategy for admission orders. Admission orders that are complete and take into account planning for the first few days of a patient's hospitalisation, not just the initial few hours, are optimal. Medication reconciliation guidelines are important, and excellent readable penmanship if orders are handwritten cannot be overemphasised.

Click Submit when you have reviewed the sample admission order

CASE STUDIES

14

Case Study

Basic Abdominal Ultrasound Course

Basic Abdominal Ultrasound Course	
Title	Basic Abdominal Ultrasound Course
Author	Matthias Hofer
School/institution	Medical School, University of Duesseldorf, Germany
Professional background	Medicine, diagnostic radiology
Course including level	Introduction to hands-on skills in abdominal ultrasound for third- and fourth-year undergraduate students in a peer-teaching format
Short description	This OSCE assesses the hands-on skill of how to perform an abdominal ultrasound examination. 12 stations were designed to scan a specific abdominal organ or blood vessel region for the exclusion of focal lesions, enlarged lymph nodes, inflammatory diseases and vascular alterations. The students have to show their scanning algorithm, measure certain key values and identify target structures in frozen images within 4 minutes. They get additional questions concerning background knowledge (1 minute) and subsequent feedback (1.5 minutes) with specific suggestions for improvement = total time of 7 minutes at every station. One station focusses on drawing two cross-sectional anatomy images out of 12 standardised image sections.
Role of examination	Both formative mid-course (to steer the students' exercises in the skills lab – since they do not know which 4 out of 12 they are going to be tested on) as well as summative at the end of the course. Students were required to pass the examination before proceeding to the next year of the programme.
Venue	Three small group training rooms in our skills lab
Number of students	Max. capacity of 126 students in six, 1-hour circuits (21 per circuit)
Number of stations, duration of stations and length of exam	4 out of 14 stations, each 7 minutes with a total exam time of 50 minutes per group of 7 trainees. Each student has to perform an ultrasound examination three times, to be a patient three times and to draw two cross-sectional standard sketches from memory one time.

Number of circuits and timing	Three circuits were performed simultaneously in adjacent rooms: 3 rooms × 7 students = 21 students per hour (10 minutes of pauses, preparation and changing time included). Six circuits (3 hours in the morning and 3 hours in the afternoon) add up to a capacity of 126 students.
Two kinds of examiners	Three experienced sonographers (one attending physician per room) plus 12 senior student tutors (four student tutors per room)
No patients necessary	The students rotate between the roles of the sonographer (n = 3) and the patient model (n = 3), and draw two sketches (n = 1). Students are only patients in tasks where they do not perform the role of the sonographer, and do not know in advance which tasks they will have to perform.
Criteria for pass/fail decision	60% of the maximum score to be achieved, based upon detailed checklists
Feedback provided	Students were given personal feedback and live demonstrations on specific steps on how to improve over 1.5 minutes, if reasonable.
Experience gained with exam	20 years
Publications describing exam	Hofer et al. (2011). See reference list for further details.

List of stations

Station	Learning outcomes assessed	Patient	Examiner
1	Systematic scanning of entire right kidney in long and short axis, measurement of organ size and PPI, identification of pyramids and borderline between parenchyma and pelvis.	Cotrainee (student)	Observed and scored by examiner with detailed checklist/guide.
2	Performance of collapse test of IVC under enhanced inspiration, measurement of maximal and minimal vessel diameter of IVC, identification and measurement of caudate lobe in frozen image.	Co-trainee (student)	Observed and scored by examiner with detailed checklist/guide.
3	Systematic scanning of entire left lobe of thyroid gland in long and short axis, volumetry of thyroid gland, performance of Valsalva manoeuvre and identification of CCA and IJV in frozen image.	Co-trainee (student)	Observed and scored by examiner with detailed checklist/guide.

Continued

SECTION D

Station	Learning outcomes assessed	Patient	Examiner
4	Systematic scanning of hepatic hilum and portal vein (PV), measurement of PV luminal diameter with interpretation/ normal values, identification of common bile duct and hepatic artery in frozen image.	Co-trainee (student)	Observed and scored by examiner with detailed checklist/guide.
5	Systematic scanning of entire gall bladder in sagittal and transverse section, measurement of wall thickness with interpretation and normal values, differentiation NPO ↔ postprandial status.	Co-trainee (student)	Observed and scored by examiner with detailed checklist/guide.
6	Systematic scanning of entire left hepatic lobe in sagittal and axial views, measurement of caudate lobe, comparison with normal values, identification of one branch of hepatic artery and vein.	Co-trainee (student)	Observed and scored by examiner with detailed checklist/guide.
7	Systematic scanning of the spleen, measurement of organ size and comparison with normal values/ interpretation, identification of predilection sites for accessory spleens.	Co-trainee (student)	Observed and scored by examiner with detailed checklist/guide.
8	Systematic scanning of retroperitoneal space and entire pancreas in transverse section, measurement of organ size and pancreatic duct, identification of splenic vein in frozen image.	Co-trainee (student)	Observed and scored by examiner with detailed checklist/guide.
9	Systematic scanning of entire urinary bladder in sagittal and transverse section, measurement of wall thickness and volume, with comparison to normal values; identification of prostate gland versus uterus.	Co-trainee (student)	Observed and scored by examiner with detailed checklist/guide.
10	Systematic scanning of sagittal retroperitoneal space, measurement of suprarenal and infrarenal aortic luminal distances, identification of five hypoechoic, egg-shaped differential diagnoses to LN.	Co-trainee (student)	Observed and scored by examiner with detailed checklist/guide.
11	Performance of FAST algorithm for trauma patients, identification of eight predilection sites for free blood or haematoma in four frozen images.	Co-trainee (student)	Observed and scored by examiner with detailed checklist/guide.

Station	Learning outcomes assessed	Patient	Examiner
12	Systematic scanning of right hepatic lobe in sagittal and axial views, measurement of organ size in right MCL.	Co-trainee (student)	Observed and scored by examiner with detailed checklist/guide.
13	Scanning of right hepatic lobe, measurement of luminal diameter of peripheral hepatic veins, interpretation with normal values and comparison in case of acute RVF.	Co-trainee (student)	Observed and scored by examiner with detailed checklist/guide.
14	Systematic scanning of entire left kidney in long and short axis, measurement of organ size, identification of pyramids and borderline between parenchyma and pelvis.	Co-trainee (student)	Observed and scored by examiner with detailed checklist/guide.
15–26	The task is to draw from memory the sectional anatomy outlines of two standardised abdominal image levels, with topographic shapes, sizes and localisations of involved organs and blood vessels in each section ('pattern recognition'), with normal values and vessel diameters to be included.	–	Immediate feedback, but scored later with detailed checklist.

CASE STUDIES

Guidelines for examiners in hands-on ultrasound OSCE assessment

Please keep in mind to fill out top line: Name of examinee and your own name. Thank you!

Please choose an inadequate zoom factor, so that the examinees have to adjust it, thank you.

Introduction: 'Please take some jelly on the transducer.'

'Are you ready?'

Please wait for the signal of the timekeeper.

Start: Please read the task literally to the examinee, but **without** answers in italics, of course!

Opening: 'Please comment on your actions, whilst you are performing the ultrasound examination.'

Schedule with standardised options for help (if necessary) or interventions.

If the examinee does not perform necessary steps in time, please read the hints literally:

After 30–45 s	*Orientation:*	*Positioning:*	*Connection:*	*Zoom factor:*	*Breathing:*
	→	→	→	→	→
	'Do you think, the transducer is set on the skin correctly?'	'Is the position of the transducer correct in this case?'	'Could you improve image quality by changing your handling of the transducer?'	'Is it an adequate zoom factor in your eyes?'	'Can the patient help you in some way?'
After 1.5 min	*Image level in 3D:* (target structure not found yet)	'Which structure are you looking for?'			

If necessary, please visualise target section yourself – point reduction!

Guidelines for examiners in hands-on ultrasound OSCE assessment—cont'd

After 2 min	**Measurement:**	*Immediately after wrong measurement:* 'Are you confident with your measurement/results?'
	Explanation of frozen image(s):	*Missing measurement:* 'How could you complete the examination?' *Missing explanation:* Please read again the missing part of the initial task (reminder).
After 4 min		'Please store the transducer – now, we come to some theoretical questions.'
Additional questions:		*Please read the question literally to the examinee.*

How to deal with pauses?		*Amount of correct answers:* **>50%** **<50%**
		                                                    'Do you know more about it?'
		            Next question *Please wait 10 seconds…*

In case of verbal diarrhoea:		'Excuse me please, let's talk about the next question.'
Remaining time at the end:		'Let's go back to the previous question – do you know more about…?'
After 4.5 min		*Please ask last question.*
Up to 5 min		'Thank you! We have reached the time limit.'
6.5 min		*Please provide supportive/corrective feedback (not only concerning theoretical aspects).* *Please demonstrate as detailed as possible options for improvement of hands-on approaches.*

Notes

The Examiner's guide seeks to standardise remarks by the examiner and also the time when examiners should intervene.

Text in italics represents the expected action by the examinee, and also to remind examiners not to read the text aloud.

Name of student:_____ **Name of examiner:**_____

Station 10 (Retroperitoneal space with aorta.) *Please read out*:

'A patient presents with suspected lymphoma: Please: (1) examine the entire retroperitoneal space to measure or exclude enlarged lymph nodes (LNs) and (2) determine the diameter of the aortic lumen. (3) Please identify five hypoechoic/anechoic egg-shaped structures in a frozen image, which might be mistaken for LNs.' *Systematic scanning of RP space from L para-aortic to R paracaval sections, following the aorta to its bifurcation, AO-Ø, shows 5 dark/black egg-shaped DDs.*

Initial handling of the transducer

Orientation:

- Correct, initial check by disconnecting the cranial part of the transducer, done by him/herself   2
- Initial problems or forgotten, corrected after examiner's reminder (see guideline)   1
- Needs assessor's help to find the adequate orientation   0

Positioning:

- Correct, puts transducer in place right away   2
- Initial problems, but can adjust after examiner's reminder (see guideline)   1
- Needs assessor's help to position the transducer in the appropriate place   0

Connection:

- Connects the transducer adequately to the skin, adjusts pressure if necessary   2
- Initial problems, but can adjust after examiner's reminder (see guideline)   1
- Insufficient pressure, does not succeed in connecting the transducer to the skin without help   0

Adequate zoom factors:

- Adjusts the zoom factor by him/herself immediately if necessary for the present task   2
- Initial problems, but can adjust after examiner's reminder (see guideline)   1
- Does not achieve an adequate zoom factor even after examiner's feedback/2° to time limits   0

Communication with the patient/model

Breathing commands:

- Correct: 'Please take a deep breath – and hold it' **4**
- Incomplete/initial problems (forgotten)/reminder by examiner necessary (see guideline) **2**
- Even after reminder incomplete or forgets several times to ask the patient to inhale **0**

- Immediately asks the patient to breathe again after freezing the image **2**

Scanning performance

Scanning/following the blood vessels:

- RP space completely scanned – even with left paraaortic and right paracaval spaces **8**
- RP space scanned down to the bifurcation *without* scanning the paravascular areas **4**
- Scanning of the RP space only possible with examiner's help (see guideline) **2**
- Even with examiner's support no adequate scanning possible **0**

Measurement:

- Correct: perpendicular to the long axis of the vessel, vessel walls not included **5**
- Wrong endpoints of the diameter/corrective feedback by examiner necessary (see guideline) **2**
- Wrong or missing measurement – even after examiner's feedback/2° to time limits **0**

Explanation of frozen image

- Identifies five hypoechoic/anechoic egg-shaped structures (as DD to LN) correctly: **0–5**
  Oesophagus **(1)**, crura of the diaphragm **(1)**, confluens PV **(1)**, left renal vein **(1)**, duodenum **(1)**

Overall performance (global rating scale)

Outstanding **8** - **7** - **6** - **5** - **4** - **3** - **2** - **1** Poor **0–8**

Continued

CASE STUDIES

SECTION D

Theoretical background

- LNs are nodular structures – how can you differentiate them from tubular structures?
  Please explain two options:
  Continuous scanning (1) => LN: sudden (dis-)appearance (1); rotation of the transducer by 180° around its cable (1); LN: keeps round shape and does not become tubular (1)

  0–4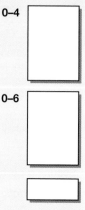

- Please explain with a diagram the increased risk for rupture of a partially thrombosed aneurysm with eccentric lumen in contrast to aneurysm with concentric lumen:
  Diagram of aortic aneurysm with concentric (1) verus eccentric (1) lumina: protective thrombotic ring in case of concentric lumina (2)/correct predilection site for rupture in eccentric cases (2)

  0–6

Station score (max. 50):

Case Study

Dundee Medical School Multiple Mini-Interview (MMI)

15

Dundee Medical School Multiple Mini-Interview

Title	Dundee Medical School Multiple Mini-Interview (MMI)
Authors	Adrian Husbands and Jon Dowell
School/institution	Dundee Medical School, Dundee, UK
Professional background	Medicine
Short description	The Dundee MMIs are designed to measure the following attributes: interpersonal skills and communication (including empathy); logical reasoning and critical thinking; moral and ethical reasoning; motivation and preparation to study medicine; teamwork; and personal integrity is also considered.
Role of examination	To assess candidates applying for undergraduate medicine course
Number of stations, duration of stations and length of exam	Ten 7-minute stations with one assessor at each. Station content is split between five observed interactions with a role player and five traditional face-to-face structured interview stations.
Number of circuits and timing	Two full circuits (10 in each) in the morning and two concurrent sets of circuits (four circuits) in the afternoon.
Examiners	Staff, students and simulated patients
Actors	Standardized students or simulated patient actors
Scoring	Candidates are scored on three domains per station as well as an overall global judgement, all scored on five-point Likert scales. A 'red flag' option is included to allow assessors to express serious concerns about a candidate's suitability.
Experience gained with exam	6 years
Publications describing exam	Ferguson et al. (2002); Albanese et al. (2003); Kreiter et al. (2004); Eva et al. (2004a); Eva et al. (2004b); Reiter et al. (2007); Eva et al. (2009); Siu and Reiter (2009); Dowell et al. (2012); Pau et al. (2013); Husbands and Dowell (2013).

List of stations

Station	Description	Type	Domain 1	Domain 2	Domain 3
1	Counselling interaction with a distressed fellow student	Interactive	Communication	Communication	Critical thinking
2	Candidate plays the role of a peer advisor assessing a student who has admitted wrongdoing	Interactive	Communication	Moral reasoning	Critical thinking
3	Candidate is given a complex card sorting task to accomplish with a helper	Interactive	Teamwork	Teamwork	Communication
4	Candidate and helper complete a puzzle task	Interactive	Teamwork	Teamwork	Communication
5	Candidate interacts with a relative (actor) who has difficulty managing their medications	Interactive	Communication	Communication	Critical thinking
6	Discussion of expectations of career as a doctor	One-to-one	Motivation	Motivation	Critical thinking
7	Discussion of topical issues on the provision of medical care	One-to-one	Moral reasoning	Motivation	Communication
8	Discussion about learning styles	One-to-one	Critical thinking	Motivation	Communication
9	Assessor explores experiences and motivation to apply to study medicine	One-to-one	Communication	Motivation	Critical thinking
10	Discussion about a controversial ethical issue in medicine	One-to-one	Communication	Moral Reasoning	Critical thinking

Notes

Stations 1–5 use a role-player, who may be a student actor.

Stations 1 and 2 are quite intense. Student actors would have attended a training session and been sent scripts in advance. The other interactive stations would have student volunteers learn the station material in the 30 minutes before the MMIs.

Stations 3 and 9 are explained in detail.

In this station, the candidate is asked to sort some cards into spaces. The rules for sorting the cards will be given, and the candidate will be told that you are there to help them with the task, and that they should delegate some of the work to you. The candidate will have the following description and instructions of the task, to which they can refer at any time:

> You have been entered into a competition while volunteering at a centre for young people with learning disabilities. Your task is to read a list of instructions then complete the task using the cards provided within 7 minutes. You also have a helper to whom you should delegate some of the work. If you find a good strategy, the task will go very quickly.

Please read the following instructions before starting:

1. Put cards with prime numbers (a number that is only divisible by one or itself) in space 1. Do not include face cards.

2. Put the cards that are multiples of four in space 2. Do not include face cards.

3. Put all the cards with a heart on them in space 3.

4. Put cards with a red male or a black female in space 4.

5. Complete instruction 3 first and then complete the other instructions with the remaining cards.

Your role

You are playing the part of a helper with a learning disability and you need the candidate to go through the instructions slowly. This is also the first time you are playing with cards (the candidate does not know this) and you are confused and make a number of mistakes as a result.

Take a look at the cards and the rules now. (You don't need to do the sorting; just look through the materials so you understand what the candidate is being asked to do.) Continue reading only after you feel you understand the sorting task.

The most likely thing that a candidate will ask you to do is to take some of the cards and divide them according to the rules. But a candidate might also ask you to take some of the cards and sort them into the space. Whatever the candidate asks you to do, you should do it. However an important part of your role as a 'helper' is actually to not be very helpful at all and to express confusion about parts of the tasks. Details are given below.

Confusion

At the beginning of the interaction you should express confusion if the candidate starts with instruction 3 first (as you think that logically instructions should be completed sequentially, i.e. 1, 2, 3, etc). You should begin by slowly counting on your fingers 1, 2, 3, 4, 5 while pointing out instruction 1. Express confusion **twice**. The candidate should be made to explain (slowly) that they are to begin with instruction 3, not 1. After the candidate explains that they have to begin with instruction 3, not 1 you should say 'Sorry, I understand now' and begin the task.

Continued

The candidate should be made to explain how to identify a heart among the other suits before beginning the instructions, if they attempt to begin without comprehensively doing so. If the candidate does not explain how to identify a heart before beginning the task you should express confusion. You should then express confusion on the differences between a heart and a diamond (as they are both red and have a somewhat similar shape). After the candidate explains the differences you should say 'Sorry, I understand now' and begin the task.

If the candidate enlists your help with instruction 1 (prime numbers) you should express confusion and ask them to explain what prime numbers are. The candidate will likely try to explain that a prime number is a number that is divisible by one or itself. Express confusion **twice**, each time asking the candidate to explain again. The clever candidate will realise that there are four prime number cards: 2, 3, 5 and 7 and ask you to identify those and sort them into spaces.

If the candidate enlists your help with instruction 4 you should express confusion by saying that you do not understand how to tell if a card is 'male' or 'female'. The candidate will likely respond by explaining how to identify each. You should express confusion, saying that the queen looks like a male and the jack like a female. Express confusion **twice**, each time asking the candidate to explain again.

Mistakes

You will make three mistakes while doing the task. These should look like innocent mistakes, but if the candidate discovers them, you will be quite embarrassed and apologetic (use remarks like, 'Oh, I'm really sorry; that was not very helpful at all' or 'I've wasted some of your time; I'm so sorry.'). It is very important that you do BOTH of these behaviours: making the three mistakes and being very apologetic if the candidate notices your mistakes. If the candidate does not notice your mistakes, then carry on with whatever she/he asks you to do. Examples of mistakes are:

1. The candidate asks you to sort all the cards with a heart in space 3. You should sort a few diamonds into the set of hearts.
2. The candidate asks you to place the cards that are multiples of four in space 2. You should place a few other cards in the pile randomly.
3. You place some of the cards in the wrong space.

You should only make three mistakes, otherwise be careful to do exactly as you are asked to do. In general, you should appear very willing to help, but not very rushed.

What if?

We can't anticipate everything that might happen in this station, but one thing seems likely to happen at least once or twice. First, a candidate might decide that the task could be done more easily and faster by themselves (especially after you've made a mistake or two), so they may tell you that they will take over from there. If that happens, you should apologise again and ask, 'Are you sure I can't help in some way? I promise to be more careful.' If they still decline your help, or if they never ask for your help in the first place, make suggestions about the cards they are sorting (e.g. 'I think that goes in space 3...') or read the rules as if you're doing it to help them. Don't be overtly annoying; just stay active in the task, but don't touch the cards if you haven't been asked to help in a specific way.

Station 3 Card sort: Helper training—cont'd

It's very unlikely, but possible, that a candidate could become upset at your (feigned) incompetence. If they do become upset and don't seem to be able to continue, the assessor for the station will ask them if they would like to take a break for a few moments. You should simply go with the flow in this situation and resume your role when the candidate is ready.

When the bell rings to signal that time is up, be sure the assessor has finished scoring the candidate before you reshuffle the cards and set up the station for the next candidate. Please work with the assessor to determine the best way to handle these tasks.

Station 3 Card sort: Assessor training

In this station, we give the candidate a somewhat complex task to accomplish in a short time. The task involves sorting a set of playing cards.

This station is designed to measure **teamwork, critical thinking and communication skills**.

Candidates will have read the following station description:

> You have been entered into a competition while volunteering at a school for young people with learning disabilities. Your task is to read a list of instructions then complete the task using the cards provided within 7 minutes. You also have a helper to whom you should delegate some of the work. If you find a good strategy, the task will go very quickly.

Your role

Please familiarise yourself with the helper's script before assessing this station. You are asked to observe the interaction between the candidate and the actor. You are required to provide FOUR scores: three domain scores and one overall judgment. Descriptors are provided on the score sheet.

Please be aware that each of the three domain scores is independent of the others' i.e. it is entirely possible for a candidate to receive high scores in one category and low scores in another.

Please ensure the candidate can see the sheet with the following instructions:

1. Put cards with prime numbers (a number that is only divisible by one or itself) in space 1. Do not include cards with faces on them.
2. Put the cards that are multiples of four in space 2. Do not include cards with faces on them.
3. Put all the cards with a heart on them in space 3.
4. Put cards with a red male or a black female in space 4.
5. Complete instruction 3 first and then complete the other instructions with the remaining cards.

Continued

Station 3 Card sort: Assessor training—cont'd

What's the best strategy?

A person who approaches this task without thinking strategically will likely take each card in turn, see whether it fits the rules for space 1, and if not, look at the rules for space 2, and so on for spaces 3 and 4. This is a poor strategy because it requires considering the rules for each individual card and while sorting them. A better and faster strategy involves pre-sorting according to these criteria before moving the cards into the spaces. Using appropriate pre-sorting, one can solve the task of sorting the cards in fewer steps.

A helper could be useful in this task by pre-sorting one stack of cards, while the candidate works on the other stack. The helper will have seen the cards before and will have practised sorting them (although the candidate does not know this). The helper will also have been trained to make some deliberate mistakes and express confusion, so as to present inter-personal challenges to the candidate in this station. **Please read the helper instructions to fully understand the station.**

When you have finished scoring, the helper will shuffle the cards thoroughly and place them in a neat stack before the next candidate enters. You can work with the helper to find the fastest way of doing this, so that it does not interfere with your scoring.

Station 3 Card sort: Scoring criteria

Teamwork

Excellent: Very comfortable with leadership role • Exceptional ability to work with helper • Gives clear, logical instructions to the helper • Tactful when helper makes mistakes • Works calmly and effectively under pressure

Poor: Uncomfortable in leadership role • Lacks confidence when giving instructions to helper • Lacks tact when helper makes mistakes • Unable to work well under pressure

Critical thinking

Excellent: Logical approach to problem solving • Most cards are sorted into the correct spaces within the allotted time • Monitors progress of the helper to catch problems early on • Acknowledges the helper's difficulties by changing strategies as needed • Communicates the strategy to the helper

Poor: Problem-solving approach lacks logic • Disjointed, disorganised approach • Few cards sorted in the correct spaces within allotted time • Fails to effectively monitor progress of helper • Ineffective strategy • Fails to effectively communicate strategy to helper

Communication

Excellent: Appropriate tone • Appears engaged, professional and confident • Empathetic • Patient • Treats helper with respect despite mistakes • Adequate command of English

Poor: Inappropriate tone • Displays of anger or frustration toward helper • Limited patience • Lacks confidence • Lacks professionalism • Below average interpersonal skills • Command of English problematic • Manner makes interaction 'hard work'

Station 9 Preparation for medicine: Assessor training

In this station, you will explore the candidate's medical experience and non-medical achievements.

This station is designed to measure **critical thinking, motivation and communication skills.**

Candidates will have read the following station description:

> You will discuss your medical work experience and your non-academic achievements with an assessor. Non-academic experience includes: (1) exceptional talent, (2) competitive achievement and (3) social responsibility. You will be asked to expand on your experiences and elaborate on how they lead you to believe you will be a good physician.

Your role

Medical experience

Ask the candidate to briefly explain specific elements of their medical work experience. You are looking for the following:

- Does the candidate have knowledge about what it will be like to study medicine and to work as a doctor?
- Does it appear that they have taken initiative to gain knowledge and insight about why they are applying to study medicine?
- Do they convey a sense of enthusiasm for learning and for studying medicine in particular?
- You must probe their experiences to confirm they are able to discuss these in detail and that their reported interest is genuine.

After the candidate has described their experiences please ask the following questions:

- **Compare before and after your medical experience. What (if any) new insights about the profession have you learnt?**
- **Based on your experiences, what qualities do you believe are needed for a successful career in medicine and why?**

Non-academic achievement

Ask the candidate to briefly explain specific elements of their non-academic achievements in three categories individually, namely: (1) exceptional talent, (2) competitive achievement and (3) social responsibility. After each element please ask the candidate:

'What lessons have you learnt from these achievements that could be applied to a successful career in medicine?'

If a candidate has no medical experience or lacks specific elements of their non-academic experience, please ask them to draw from other personal experiences.

Continued

Station 9 Preparation for medicine: Assessor training—cont'd

Scoring

As you interact with the candidate, remember that you are not going to score their experiences per se. You are going to score their ability to elaborate on their experiences and how they apply their experiences to a career in medicine.

You are required to provide FOUR scores: three domain scores and one overall judgment. Descriptors for each domain are provided on the score sheet. **Please be aware that each of the three domain scores is independent of the others, i.e. it is entirely possible for a candidate to receive high scores in one category and low scores in another.**

Station 9 Preparation for medicine: Scoring criteria

Critical thinking

Excellent: Demonstrates exceptional ability to apply experiences to a career in medicine
• Aware and able to discuss the need for social responsibility in medicine

Poor: Insensitive to broader complexities/relevance of personal characteristics to a career in medicine • Limited ability to effectively apply experiences to a career in medicine • Application lacks depth and clarity

Motivation

Excellent: Competitive achievements motivated by exceptional drive, desire to excel and succeed • Social responsibility experience motivated by a desire to advance social goals. No indication of demonstrating a 'tick-box' approach to acquiring experiences

Poor: No clear motivation behind achievements • Conveys little genuine motivation in any category • A 'tick-box' approach to acquiring experiences • Appears primarily motivated by challenge of getting in

Communication

Excellent: Excellent interpersonal skills • Appropriate tone • Maintains eye-contact • Appears engaged, professional and confident • Explanations clear, concise and easy to follow • Strong command of English

Poor: Below average interpersonal skills • Limited eye contact • Explanations lack clarity and precision • Lacks confidence • Rambling, incoherent explanations • Manner makes interaction 'hard work' • Command of English problematic

References

Abdelkhalek, N.M., Hussein, A.M., Sulaiman, N., Hamdy, H., 2009. Faculty as simulated patients (FSPs) in assessing medical students' clinical reasoning skills. Educ. Health 22 (3), 323. <http://www.educationforhealth.net/> (accessed 1 November 2014).

Adamo, G., 2003. Simulated and standardized patients in OSCEs: achievement and challenges 1992–2003. Med. Teach. 25 (3), 262–270.

Aeder, L., Altshuler, L., Kachur, E.K., et al., 2007. The 'Culture OSCE' – introducing a formative assessment into a postgraduate program. Educ. Health 20 (1), 11. <http://www.educationforhealth.net/> (accessed 1 November 2014).

Aeder, L., Altshuler, L., Kachur, E., Langenau, E., 2012. *Fostering an Atmosphere of Professionalism in a Residency Program: Learning how to Address the Unprofessional Behavior of Colleagues Through OSCEs*. *MedEdPORTAL Publications* <http://www.mededportal.org/publication/9168> (accessed 30 October 2014).

Ainsworth, M.A., Callaway, M.R., Perkowski, L., 1995. An OSCE assessment of fourth-year students. Acad. Med. 70, 444–445.

Albanese, M., Snow, M., Skochelak, S., Huggett, K., Farrell, P., 2003. Assessing personal qualities in medical school admissions. Acad. Med. 78 (3), 313–321.

Al Rumayyan, A.R., Seefeldt, F.M., Magzoub, M.E., Awad, T., Alalwan, I., 2012. Teaching and assessing clinical competence early in a PBL curriculum. New Egypt. J. Med. 46 (5), 383–388.

Altshuler, L., Kachur, E.K., 2001. A culture OSCE: teaching residents to bridge different worlds. Acad. Med. 76 (5), 514.

Altshuler, L., Sussman, N.M., Kachur, E.K., 2003. Assessing changes in intercultural sensitivity among physician trainees using the Intercultural Development Inventory. Int. J. Intercult. Relat. 27 (4), 387–401.

Artemiou, E., Adams, C.L., Hecker, K.G., Vallevand, A., Violato, C., Coe, J.B., 2014. Standardised clients as assessors in a veterinary communication OSCE: a reliability and validity study. Vet. Rec. August 28. [Epub ahead of print.]

Ault, G., Reznick, R., MacRae, H., et al., 2001. Exporting a technical skills evaluation technology to other sites. Am. J. Surg. 182 (3), 254–256.

Austin, A., O'Byrne, C., Pugsley, J., Munoz, L., 2003. Development and validation processes for an Objective Structured Clinical Examination (OSCE) for entry-to-practice certification in pharmacy: the Canadian experience. Am. J. Pharm. Educ. 67 (3), Article 76.

Awaisu, A., Abd Rahman, N.S., Nik Mohamed, M.H., Rahman Bux, S.H., Mohamed Nazar, N.I., 2010. Malaysian pharmacy students' assessment of an objective structured clinical examination (OSCE). Am. J. Pharm. Educ. 74 (2), Article 34.

Awaisu, A., Nik Mohamed, M.H., Al-Efan, Q.A.M., 2007. Perception of pharmacy students in Malaysia on the use of objective structured clinical examinations to evaluate competence. Am. J. Pharm. Educ. 71 (6), Article 118.

Awaisu, A., Nik Mohamed, M.H., 2010. Advances in pharmaceutical education: an experience with the development and implementation of an objective structured clinical examination (OSCE) in an undergraduate pharmacy program. Pharm. Educ. 10 (1), 32–38.

Azcuenga, J., Valls, M., Martinez-Carretero, J.M., 1998. Cost analysis of three clinical skills assessment (CSA) projects. In: Evolving Assessment: Protecting the Human Dimension: 8th Ottawa Conference, July 12–15, 1998, Philadelphia, Pennsylvania, USA.

Baribeau, D.A., Mukovozov, I., Sabljic, T., Eva, K.W., Delottinville, C.B., 2012. Using an objective structured video exam to identify differential understanding of aspects of communication skills. Med. Teach. 34 (4), e242–e250.

Barrows, H.S., 1993. An overview of the use of standardized patients for teaching and evaluating clinical skills. Acad. Med. 68 (6), 443–453.

Barry, M., Noonan, M., Bradshaw, C., Murphy-Tighe, S., 2012. An exploration of student midwives' experiences of the Objective Structured Clinical Examination assessment process. Nurse Educ. Today 32 (6), 690–694.

Bartfay, W.J., Rombough, R., Howse, E., LeBlanc, R., 2004. The OSCE approach in nursing education: objective structured clinical examinations can be effective vehicles for nursing education and practice by promoting the mastery of clinical skills and decision-making in controlled and safe learning environments. Can. Nurse 100 (3), 18–25.

Bartman, K., Smee, S., Roy, M., 2013. A method for identifying extreme OSCE examiners. Clin. Teach. 10, 27–31.

Barzansky, B., Etzel, S.I., 2011. Medical Schools in the United States, 2010–2011. J. Am. Med. Assoc. 306 (9), 1007–1014.

Battles, J.B., Sprankell, S.J., Carpenter, J.L., Bedford, J.A., Kirk, L.M., 1992. Developing a support system for teaching and assessing clinical competence. J. Biocommun. 19 (4), 19–25.

Benbow, E.W., Harrison, I., Dornan, T.L., O'Neill, P.A., 1998. Pathology and the OSCE: insights from a pilot study. J. Pathol. 184 (1), 110–114.

Bennett, R.E., 2013. Gordon Commission on the Future of Assessment in Education. To Assess, to Teach, to Learn: A Vision for the Future of Assessment (Technical Report). <http://www.gordoncommission.org/rsc/pdfs/gordon_commission_technical_report.pdf> (accessed 08 October 2014).

Bennett, V., Furmedge, D., 2013. The hidden value of a mock OSCE. Clin. Teach. 10 (6), 407–408.

Berg, K., Majdan, J.F., Berg, D., Veloski, J., Hojat, M., 2011. Medical students' self-reported empathy and simulated patients' assessments of student empathy: an analysis by gender and ethnicity. Acad. Med. 86 (8), 984–988.

Berkenstadt, H., Ziv, A., Gafni, N., Sidi, A., 2006. Incorporating simulation-based objective structured clinical examination into the Israeli National Board Examination in Anesthesiology. Anesth. Analg. 102, 853–858.

Bhatnagar, K.R., Saoji, V.A., Banerjee, A.A., 2011. Objective structured clinical examination for undergraduates: is it a feasible approach to standardized assessment in India? Indian J. Ophthalmol. 59 (3), 211–214.

Biran, L., 1991. Self-assessment and learning through GOSCE (group objective structured clinical examination). Med. Educ. 25 (6), 475–479.

Black, N.M.I., Harden, R.M., 1986. Providing feedback to students on clinical skills by using the Objective Structured Clinical Examination. Med. Educ. 20 (1), 48–52.

Black, N.M.I., Urquhart, A., Harden, R.M., 1986. Educational effectiveness of feedback in the objective structured clinical examination. In: International Conference Proceedings: Newer Developments in Assessing Clinical Competence. Ottawa, Canada. Heal Publications, Montreal, Quebec, pp. 157–160.

Bloch, R., Norman, G., 2012. Generalizability theory for the perplexed: a practical introduction and guide: AMEE Guide No. 68. Med. Teach. 34 (11), 960–992.

Bokken, L., Rethans, J.J., van Heurn, L., Duvivier, R., Scherpbier, A., van der

Vleuten, C., 2009. Students' views on the use of real patients and simulated patients in undergraduate medical education. Acad. Med. 84 (7), 958–963.

Boud, D., Associates, 2010. Assessment 2020: Seven Propositions for Assessment Reform in Higher Education. Australian Learning and Teaching Council, Sydney. <http://www.assessmentfutures.com> (accessed 13 October 2014).

Bouhuijs, P.A.J., van der Vleuten, C.P.M., van Luyk, S.J., 1987. The OSCE as a part of a systematic skills training approach. Med. Teach. 9 (2), 183–191.

Boulet, J., 2009. Improving the flexibility and efficiency of testing. Med. Educ. 44 (1), 18–19.

Boulet, J.R., De Champlain, A.F., McKinley, D.W., 2003. Setting defensible performance standards on OSCEs and standardized patient examinations. Med. Teach. 25 (3), 245–249.

Boulet, J.R., Smee, S.M., Dillon, G.R., Gimpel, J.R., 2009. The use of standardized patient assessments for certification and licensure decisions. Simul. Healthc. 4, 35–42.

Boursicot, K.A., Roberts, T., Pell, G., 2007. Using borderline methods to compare passing standards for OSCEs at graduation across three medical schools. Med. Educ. 41, 1024–1031.

Boursicot, K.A.M., Roberts, T.E., Burdick, W.P., 2014. Structured assessments of clinical competence. In: Swanwick, T. (Ed.), Understanding Medical Education Evidence, Theory and Practice, second ed. John Wiley & Sons, Chichester, UK.

Bradley, P., Humphris, G., 1999. Assessing the ability of medical students to apply evidence in practice: the potential of the OSCE. Med. Educ. 33 (11), 815–817.

Brauer, R.B., Kammerloher, A., Stering, K., Womes, G., Ring, J., Friess, H., 2013. Objective structured clinical examination (OSCE) on completion of surgical block practical training – twelve months experience with a hands-on examination. Zentralbl. Chir. 138 (2), 144–150.

Brown, C., Ross, S., Cleland, J., Walsh, K., 2015. Money makes the (medical assessment) world go round: The cost of components of a summative final year Objective Structured Clinical Examination (OSCE). Med. Teach. 37 (4). In press.

Brookhart, S.M., 2008. How to Give Effective Feedback to Your Students. ASCD, Alexandria, Virginia, USA.

Burgess, A., Clark, T., Chapman, R., Mellis, C., 2013. Senior medical students as peer examiners in an OSCE. Med. Teach. 35 (1), 58–62.

Butler, D.L., Winne, P.H., 1995. Feedback and self-regulated learning: a theoretical synthesis. Rev. Educ. Res. 65 (3), 245–281.

Byrne, A., Tweed, N., Halligan, C., 2014. A pilot study of the mental workload of objective structured clinical examination examiners. Med. Educ. 48, 262–267.

Carpenter, J.L., 1995. Cost analysis of objective structured clinical examinations. Acad. Med. 70 (9), 828–833.

Casey, P.M., Goepfert, A.R., Espey, E.L., et al., 2009. To the point: reviews in medical education – the Objective Structured Clinical Examination. Am. J. Obstet. Gynecol. 200 (1), 25–34.

Castel, O.C., Ezra, V., Alperin, M., et al., 2011. Can outcome-based continuing medical education improve performance of immigrant physicians? J. Contin. Educ. Health Prof. 31 (1), 34–42.

Chambers, K.A., Boulet, J.R., Gary, N.E., 2000. The management of patient encounter time in a high-stakes assessment using standardized patients. Med. Educ. 34, 813–817.

Chan, C.-Y., 2011. Is OSCE valid for evaluation of the six ACGME general competencies? J. Chin. Med. Assoc. 74, 193–194.

Chan, J., Humphrey-Murto, S., Pugh, D.M., Su, C., Wood, T., 2014. The objective structured clinical examination: can physician-examiners participate from a distance? Med. Educ. 48 (4), 441–450.

Chander, B., Kule, R., Baiocco, P., et al., 2009. Teaching the competencies: using objective structured clinical encounters for gastroenterology fellows. Clin. Gastroenterol. Hepatol. 7 (5), 509–514.

Charvat, J., McGuire, C., Parsons, V., 1968. A Review of the Nature and Uses of

Examinations in Medical Education. World Health Organisation, Geneva.

Cohen, R., Rothman, A.I, Poldre, P., Ross, J., 1991b. Validity and generalizability of global ratings in an objective structured clinical examination. Acad. Med. 66 (9), 545–548.

Cohen, R., Singer, P.A., Rothman, A.I., Robb, A., 1991a. Assessing competency to address ethical issues in medicine. Acad. Med. 66 (1), 14–15.

College of Massage Therapists of Ontario, 2014. *Examination candidate handbook 2014.* <http://www.cmto.com/cmto-wordpress/assets/CandidateHandbook2014-July10.pdf> (accessed 30 October 2014).

College of Optometrists, 2010. *What is an OSCE?* <http://www.college-optometrists.org/en/qualifying-as-an-optometrist/pre-registration-scheme/sfr-final-assessment/what-is-an-osce.cfm> (accessed 30 September 2014).

Collins, J.P., Harden, R.M., 1998. AMEE Medical Education Guide No. 13: real patients, simulated patients and simulators in clinical examinations. Med. Teach. 20 (6), 508–521.

Colliver, J.A., Barrows, H.S., Vu, N.V., Verhulst, S.J., Mast, T.A., Travis, T.A., 1991. Test security in examinations that use standardized-patient cases at one medical school. Acad. Med. 66 (5), 279–282.

Cook, D., 2014. Personal Communication. AMEE, Milan.

Cook, D.A., Triola, M.M., 2009. Virtual patients: a critical literature review and proposed next steps. Med. Educ. 43 (4), 303–311.

Cookson, J., Crossley, J., Fagan, G., McKendree, J., Mohsen, A., 2011. A final clinical examination using a sequential design to improve cost-effectiveness. Med. Educ. 45, 741–747.

Courteille, O., Bergin, R., Stockeld, D., Ponzer, S., Fors, U., 2008. The use of a virtual patient case in an OSCE-based exam – a pilot study. Med. Teach. 30, e66–e76.

Crisp, G., 2012. Integrative assessment: reframing assessment practice for current

and future learning. Assess. Eval. High. Educ. 37 (1), 33–43.

Cronbach, L.J., Shavelson, R.J., 2004. Measurement of error of examination results must be analysed. Educ. Psychol. Meas. 64 (3), 391–418.

Cullen, L., Fraser, D., Symonds, I., 2003. Strategies for interprofessional education: the Interprofessional Team Objective Structured Clinical Examination for midwifery and medical students. Nurse Educ. Today 23, 427–433.

Cuschieri, A., Gleeson, F.A., Harden, R.M., Wood, R.A.B., 1979. A new approach to a final examination in surgery. Ann. R. Coll. Surg. Engl. 61 (5), 400–405.

Cushing, A., Abbott, S., Lothian, D., Hall, A., Westwood, O.M.R., 2011. Peer feedback as an aid to learning – what do we want? Feedback. When do we want it? Now! Med. Teach. 33, e105–e112.

Cusimano, M.D., Cohen, R., Tucker, W., Murnaghan, J., Kodama, R., Reznick, R., 1994. A comparative analysis of the costs of administration of an OSCE. Acad. Med. 69 (7), 571–576.

Damassa, D.A., Sitko, T.D., 2010. *Simulation Technologies in Higher Education: Uses, Trends, and Implications* (Research Bulletin 3, 2010). EDUCAUSE Center for Applied Research, Boulder, CO. <http://www.educause.edu/ecar> (accessed 18 October 2014).

DaRosa, D.A., Kaiser, S., 2001. Measurement considerations in planning and evaluating an OSCE. In: McCoy, J.A., Merrick, H.W. (Eds.), The Objective Structured Clinical Examination, second ed. Association for Surgical Education, Springfield, IL, USA.

Daud-Gallotti, R.M., Morinaga, C.V., Arlindo-Rodrigues, M., Velasco, I.T., Martins, M.A., Tiberio, I.C., 2011. A new method for the assessment of patient safety competencies during a medical school clerkship using an objective structured clinical examination. Clinics (Sao Paulo) 66 (7), 1209–1215.

Dauphinée, W.D., Blackmore, D.E., Smee, S.M., Rothman, A.I., Reznick, R.K., 1997. Using the judgments of physician examiners in setting the standards for a national multi-center high stakes OSCE. Adv. Health Sci. Educ. Theory Pract. 8, 201–221.

Davis, M.H., 2003. OSCE: the Dundee experience. Med. Teach. 25 (3), 255–261.

Davis, M.H., Harden, R.M., 2003. Competency-based assessment: making it a reality. Med. Teach. 25 (6), 565–568.

Davis, M.H., Ponnamperuma, G.G., McAleer, S., Dale, V.H., 2006. The Objective Structured Clinical Examination (OSCE) as a determinant of veterinary clinical skills. J. Vet. Med. Educ. 33 (4), 578–587.

De Champlain, A.F., 2010. A primer on classical test theory and item response theory for assessments in medical education. Med. Educ. 44 (1), 109–117.

Donnon, T., Lee, M., Cairncross, S., 2011. Using item analysis to assess objectively the quality of the Calgary-Cambridge OSCE Checklist. Can. Med. Educ. J. 2 (1), e16–e22.

Dowell, J., Lynch, B., Till, H., Kumwenda, B., Husbands, A., 2012. The multiple mini-interview in the UK context: 3 years of experience at Dundee. Med. Teach. 34 (4), 297–304.

Dueck, M., 2014. Grading Smarter Not Harder: Assessment Strategies That Motivate Kids and Help Them Learn. ASCD, Alexandria, Virginia, USA.

Duerson, M.C., Romrell, L.J., Stevens, C.B., 2000. Impacting faculty teaching and student performance: nine years' experience with the objective structured clinical examination. Teach. Learn. Med. 12 (4), 176–182.

Durning, S.J., Artino, A., Boulet, J., et al., 2012. The feasibility, reliability and validity of a post-encounter form for evaluating clinical reasoning. Med. Teach. 34, 30–37.

Duvivier, R., van Geel, K., van Dalen, J., Scherpbier, A.J.J.A., van der Vleuten, C.P.M., 2012. Learning physical examination skills outside timetabled training sessions: what happens and why? Adv. Health Sci. Educ. 17 (3), 339–355.

Earl, L., Katz, S., 2006. Rethinking classroom assessment with purpose in mind: assessment *for* learning, assessment *as* learning, assessment *of* learning. Manitoba Education, Citizenship and Youth, Manitoba, Canada. <http://www.edu.gov.mb.ca/k12/assess/wncp/full_doc.pdf> (accessed 3 November 2014).

Earl, L.M., 2005. Thinking About Purpose in Classroom Assessment: Assessment for, as and of Learning. ACSA, Canberra.

Eberhard, L., Hassel, A., Bäumer, A., et al., 2011. Analysis of quality and feasibility of an objective structured clinical examination (OSCE) in preclinical dental education. Eur. J. Dent. Educ. 15 (3), 172–178.

Edgcumbe, D.P., Silverman, J., Benson, J., 2012. An examination of the validity of EPSCALE using factor analysis. Patient Educ. Couns. 87 (1), 120–124.

Elliot, D.L., Fields, S.A., Keenen, T.L., Jaffe, A.C., Toffler, W.L., 1994. Use of a group objective structured clinical examination with first-year medical students. Acad. Med. 69 (12), 990–992.

Epstein, R., 2007. Assessment in medical education. NEJM 356 (4), 387–396.

Erfanian, F., Khadivzadeh, T., 2011. Evaluation of midwifery students' competency in providing intrauterine device services using objective structured clinical examination. Iran. J. Nurs. Midwifery Res. 16 (3), 191–196.

Eva, K., Reiter, H., Rosenfeld, J., Norman, G., 2004b. The ability of the multiple mini-interview to predict preclerkship performance in medical school. Acad. Med. 79 (10), S40–S42.

Eva, K., Reiter, H., Trinh, K., Wasi, P., Rosenfeld, J., Norman, G., 2009. Predictive validity of the multiple mini-interview for selecting medical trainees. Med. Educ. 43 (8), 767–775.

Eva, K.W., Rosenfeld, J., Reiter, H.I., Norman, G.R., 2004a. An admissions OSCE: the multiple mini-interview. Med. Educ. 38, 314–326.

Evidence-based Medicine Working Group, 1992. Evidence-based medicine: a new approach to teaching the practice of medicine. J. Am. Med. Assoc. 268, 2420–2425.

Falcone, J.L., Schenarts, K.D., Ferson, P.F., Day, H.D., 2011. Using elements from an acute abdominal pain Objective Structured Clinical Examination (OSCE) leads to more standardized grading in the surgical clerkship for third-year medical students. J. Surg. Educ. 68 (5), 408–413.

Fargo, M.V., Edwards, J.A., Roth, B.J., Short, M.W., 2011. Using a simulated surgical skills station to assess laceration management by surgical and non-surgical residents. J. Grad. Med. Educ. 3 (3), 326–331.

Feather, A., Kopelman, P.G., 1997. A practical approach to running an Objective Structured Clinical Examination (OSCE) for medical undergraduates. Educ. Health 10 (3), 333–350.

Fenton, G.W., O'Gorman, E.C., 1984. Assessment of clinical psychiatric skills in final-year medical students: the use of videotape. Med. Educ. 18 (5), 355–359.

Ferguson, E., James, D., Madeley, L., 2002. Factors associated with success in medical school: systematic review of the literature. Br. Med. J. 324 (7343), 952–957.

Fidment, S., 2012. The Objective Structured Clinical Exam (OSCE): a qualitative study exploring the healthcare student's experience. Stud. Engage. Exp. J. 1 (1), <http://dx.doi.org/10.7190/seej.v1i1.37> (accessed 3 November 2014).

Freeman, A., van der Vleuten, C., Nouns, Z., Ricketts, C., 2010. Progress testing internationally. Med. Teach. 32, 451–455.

Frenk, J., Chen, L., Bhutta, Z.A., et al., 2010. Health professionals for a new century: transforming education to strengthen health systems in an interdependent world. Lancet 375 (9756), 1923–1958.

Friedman Ben-David, M., 1999. AMEE Guide No. 14: outcome-based education, part 3: assessment in outcome-based education. Med. Teach. 21 (1), 23–25.

Friedman Ben-David, M., 2000a. The role of assessment in expanding professional horizons. Med. Teach. 22 (5), 472–477.

Friedman Ben-David, M., 2000b. Standard setting in student assessment. Med. Teach. 22 (2), 120–130.

Friedman Ben David, M., Davis, M.H., Harden, R.M., Howie, P.W., Ker, J., Pippard, M.J., 2001a. AMEE Medical Education Guide No. 24: portfolios as a method of student assessment. Med. Teach. 23 (6), 535–551.

Friedman Ben-David, M., Hunter, I., Harden, R.M., 2001b. Introduction of a progress test as a tool for defining core undergraduate curriculum. XV Congreso de la Sociedad Nacional de Educacion Medica. Educ. Med. 4 (3), 97–99.

Frohna, J.G., Gruppen, L.D., Fliegel, J.E., Mangrulkar, R.S., 2006. Development of an evaluation of medical student competence in evidence-based medicine using a computer-based OSCE station. Teach. Learn. Med. 18 (3), 267–272.

Fromme, H.B., 2013. OSTE – One Minute Preceptor Skill/Abdominal Pain Case. MedEdPORTAL Publications <https://www.mededportal.org/icollaborative/resource/886> (accessed 16 October 2014).

Frye, A.W., Richards, B.F., Philp, E.B., Philp, J.R., 1989. Is it worth it? A look at the costs and benefits of an OSCE for second-year medical students. Med. Teach. 11 (3/4), 291–293.

Furman, G.E., 2008. The role of standardized patient and trainer training in quality assurance for a high-stakes clinical skills examination. Kaohsiung J. Med. Sci. 24, 651–655.

Garstang, S., Altshuler, E.L., Jain, S., Delisa, J.A., 2012. Designing the objective structured clinical examination to cover all major areas of physical medicine and rehabilitation over three years. Am. J. Phys. Med. Rehabil. 91 (6), 519–527.

General Medical Council, 2007. Professional and Linguistic Assessment Board (PLAB). <http://www.gmc-uk.org/doctors/plab.asp> (accessed 25 September 2014).

General Medical Council, 2008. Gateways guidance: appendix. <http://www.gmc-uk.org/education/undergraduate/appendix.asp> (accessed 01 October 2014).

General Medical Council, 2009. Tomorrow's Doctors: Outcomes and standards for undergraduate medical education. <http://www.gmc-uk.org/Tomorrow_s_Doctors_1214.pdf_48905759.pdf> (accessed 4 April 2015).

General Medical Council, 2011. Assessment in undergraduate medical education. Supplementary advice to Tomorrows' Doctors 2009. <http://www.gmc-uk.org/Assessment_in_undergraduate_web.pdf_38514111.pdf> (accessed 11 November 2014).

General Medical Council, 2014. Video about tests of competence. <http://www.gmc-uk.

org/concerns/doctors_under_investigation/7128.asp> (accessed 2 November 2014).

Gilson, G.J., George, K.E., Qualls, C.M., Sarto, G.E., Obenshain, S.S., Boulet, J., 1998. Assessing clinical competence of medical students in women's health care: use of the Objective Structured Clinical Examination. Obstet. Gynecol. 92 (6), 1038–1043.

Gleeson, F., 1997. AMEE Medical Education Guide No. 9. Assessment of clinical competence using the Objective Structured Long Examination Record (OSLER). Med. Teach. 19 (1), 7–14.

Godden, D., Baddeley, A., 1975. Context dependent memory in two natural environments. Brit. J. Psychol. 66 (3), 325–331.

Gordon Commission on the Future of Assessment in Education, 2013. *To assess, to teach, to learn: a vision for the future of assessment* (Technical Report). <http://www.gordoncommission.org/rsc/pdfs/gordon_commission_technical_report.pdf> (accessed 8 October 2014).

Gordon, M., Uppal, E., Holt, K., Lythgoe, J., Mitchell, A., Hollins-Martin, C., 2012. Application of the Team Objective Structured Clinical Encounter (TOSCE) for continuing professional development amongst postgraduate health professionals. J. Interprof. Care 27, 191–193.

Gormley, G., 2011. Summative OSCEs in undergraduate medical education. Ulster Med. J. 80 (3), 127–132.

Gormley, G., Menary, A., Layard, B., Hart, N., McCourt, C., 2013. Temporary tattoos: a novel OSCE assessment tool. Clin. Teach. 10, 251–257.

Gormley, G., Sterling, M., Menary, A., McKeown, G., 2012a. Keeping it real! Enhancing realism in standardised patient OSCE stations. Clin. Teach. 9, 382–386.

Gormley, G.J., Johnston, J., Thomson, C., McGlade, K., 2012b. Awarding global grades in OSCEs: evaluation of a novel eLearning resource for OSCE examiners. Med. Teach. 34 (7), 587–589.

Govaerts, M.J.B., van der Vleuten, C.P.M., Schuwirth, L.W.T., 2002. Optimising the reproducibility of a performance-based assessment test in midwifery education. Adv. Health Sci. Educ. 7 (2), 113–145.

Graham, J., 1971. Systematic evaluation of clinical competence. J. Med. Educ. 46 (7), 625–627.

Graham, R., Zubiaurre Bitzer, L.A., Anderson, O.R., 2013. Reliability and predictive validity of a comprehensive preclinical OSCE in dental education. J. Dent. Educ. 77 (2), 161–167.

Grand'Maison, P., Blouin, D., Briere, D., 1985. Utilization of the Objective Structured Clinical Examination (OSCE) in gynecology/obstetrics. Proc. Annu. Conf. Res. Med. Educ. 24, 65–71.

Grand'Maison, P., Brailovsky, C.A., Lescop, J., 1996. Content validity of the Quebec licensing examination (OSCE). Assessed by practising physicians. Can. Fam. Physician 42, 254–259.

Griesser, M.J., Beran, M.C., Flanigan, D.C., Quackenbush, M., Van Hoff, C., Bishop, J.Y., 2012. Implementation of an Objective Structured Clinical Exam (OSCE) into orthopedic surgery residency training. J. Surg. Educ. 69 (2), 180–189.

Griffith Med Revue, 2012. *OSCE rap – losin' marks.* <http://www.youtube.com/watch?v=7YzkTdUhvpI> (accessed 1 November 2014).

Gupta, P., Dewan, P., Singh, T., 2010. Objective Structured Clinical Examination (OSCE) revisited. Indian Pediatr. 47 (11), 911–920.

Hall, P., Marshall, D., Weaver, L., Boyle, A., Taniguchi, A., 2011. A method to enhance student teams in palliative care: piloting the McMaster-Ottawa Team Observed Structured Clinical Encounter. J. Palliat. Med. 14 (6), 744–750.

Hambleton, R.K., 1995. Setting standard on performance assessments: promising new methods and technical issues. Paper presented at the meeting of American Psychological Association, New York, August 1995.

Han, M.H., Park, S.G., 2011. Analysis of trends in self-assessment of performance of clinical skills in nursing students after OSCE. J. Korean Acad. Fundam. Nurs. 18 (2), 210–216.

Harden, R.M., 1988. What is an OSCE? Med. Teach. 10 (1), 19–22.

Harden, R.M., 1992. The OSCE: a 15-year retrospective. In: Hart, I.R., Harden, R.M., Des Marchais, J.D. (Eds.), Current Developments in Assessing Clinical Competence. Canadian-Health, Montreal, pp. 41–53.

Harden, R.M., 2007. Learning outcomes as a tool to assess progression. Med. Teach. 29 (7), 678–682.

Harden, R.M., 2013. Outcome-based education. In: Dent, J.A., Harden, R.M. (Eds.), A Practical Guide for Medical Teachers, fourth ed. Churchill Livingstone Elsevier.

Harden, R.M., Cairncross, R., 1980. Assessment of practical skills: the Objective Structured Practical Examination (OSPE). Stud. High. Educ. 5 (2), 187–196.

Harden, R.M., Crosby, J., 2000. The good teacher is more than a lecturer – the twelve roles of the teacher: AMEE Guide No. 20. Med. Teach. 22 (4), 334–347.

Harden, R.M., Crosby, J., Davis, M.H., Howie, P., Struthers, A., 2000. Task-based learning: the answer to integration and problem-based learning in the clinical years. Med. Educ. 34 (5), 391–397.

Harden, R.M., Crosby, J.R., Davis, M.H., 1999a. An introduction to outcome-based education. Med. Teach. 21 (2), 7–14.

Harden, R.M., Crosby, J.R., Davis, M.H., Friedman, M., 1999b. From competency to meta-competency: a model for the specification of learning outcomes. Med. Teach. 21 (6), 546–552.

Harden, R.M., Gleeson, F.A., 1979. ASME Medical Education Booklet No. 8, Assessment of medical competence using an Objective Structured Clinical Examination (OSCE). Med. Educ. 13 (1), 39–54.

Harden, R.M., Laidlaw, J., 2012. Essential Skills for a Medical Teacher: An Introduction to Teaching and Learning in Medicine. Churchill Livingstone, Edinburgh.

Harden, R.M., Stevenson, M., Downie, W.W., Wilson, G.M., 1975. Assessment of clinical competence using an Objective Structured Clinical Examination. Br. Med. J. 1 (5955), 447–451.

Harden, V., Harden, R.M., Haig, A., McManus, N., Lilley, P., 2003. The Objective Structured Clinical Examination (OSCE): Annotated Bibliography and Structured Contents Analysis. Dundee, UK: Association for Medical Education in Europe.

Harrison, C.J., Könings, K.D., Molyneux, A., Schuwirth, L.W.T., Wass, V., van der Vleuten, C.P.M., 2013. Web-based feedback after summative assessment: how do students engage? Med. Educ. 47, 734–744.

Harrison, C.J., Molyneux, A., Blackwell, S., Wass, V.J., 2014. How we give personalised audio feedback after summative OSCEs. Med. Teach. 37 (4), 323–326.

Harvey, P., Radomski, N., 2011. Performance pressure: simulated patients and high-stakes examinations in a regional clinical school. Aust. J. Rural Health 19 (6), 284–289.

Hassell, A.B., 2002. Assessment of specialist registrars in rheumatology: experience of an Objective Structured Clinical Examination (OSCE). Rheumatology (Oxford) 41 (11), 1323–1328.

Hatala, R., Marr, S., Cuncic, C., Bacchus, C.M., 2011. Modification of an OSCE format to enhance patient continuity in a high-stakes assessment of clinical performance. BMC Med. Educ. 11 (23), <http://www.biomedcentral.com/1472-6920/11/23> (accessed 17 October 2014).

Hatala, R., Scalese, R.J., Cole, G., Bacchus, M., Kassen, B., Issenberg, S.B., 2009. Development and validation of a cardiac findings checklist for use with simulator-based assessments of cardiac physical examination competence. Simul. Healthc. 4 (1), 17–21. Spring.

Hattie, J., Timperley, H., 2007. The power of feedback. Rev. Educ. Res. 77 (1), 81–112.

Hay, M., Garvey, L., Navaratnam, P., 2012. Assessing undergraduate medical students' capacity to integrate patient information: a novel OSCE. Ottawa Conference on the Assessment of Competence in Medicine and the Healthcare Professions, Kuala Lumpur, Malaysia. <http://media.wix.com/ugd/bd1cfc_c54c42a6e92b626fbcb65c15e4ad90f4.pdf> (page 4 (accessed 4 April 2015)).

Heard, J.K., Allen, R.M., Cason, G.J., Cantrell, M., Tank, P.W., 1998. Practical issues in developing a program for the objective assessment of clinical skills. Med. Teach. 20 (1), 15–21.

Hecker, K., Read, E.K., Vallevand, A., et al., 2010. Assessment of first-year veterinary students' clinical skills using Objective Structured Clinical Examinations. J. Vet. Med. Educ. 37 (4), 395–402.

Heinke, W., Rotzoll, D., Hempel, G., et al., 2013. Students benefit from developing their own emergency medicine OSCE stations: a comparative study using the matched-pair method. BMC Med. Educ. 13, 138–146.

Higher Education Academy, 2012. *A marked improvement: transforming assessment in higher education*. <https://www.heacademy.ac.uk/node/3950> (accessed 14 October 2014).

Hirsh, D., Gaufberg, E., Ogur, B., et al., 2012. Educational outcomes of the Harvard Medical School – Cambridge Integrated Clerkship: a way forward for medical education. Acad. Med. 87 (5), 643–650.

Hodder, R.V., Rivington, R.N., Calcutt, L.E., Hart, I.R., 1989. The effectiveness of immediate feedback during the Objective Structured Clinical Examination. Med. Educ. 23, 184–188.

Hodges, B., 2003. OSCE! Variations on a theme by Harden. Med. Educ. 37 (12), 1134–1140.

Hodges, B., 2009. The Objective Structured Clinical Examination: A Socio-History. Lambert Academic Publishing, Berlin.

Hodges, B., Lofchy, J., 1997. Evaluating psychiatric clinical clerks with a mini-objective structured clinical examination. Acad. Psychiatry 21 (4), 219–225.

Hodges, B., Regehr, G., Hanson, M., McNaughton, N., 1997. An Objective Structured Clinical Examination for evaluating psychiatric clinical clerks. Acad. Med. 72 (8), 715–721.

Hodges, B., Regehr, G., Hanson, M., McNaughton, N., 1998. Validation of an Objective Structured Clinical Examination in psychiatry. Acad. Med. 73 (8), 910–912.

Hodges, B., Regehr, G., McNaughton, N., Tiberius, R., Hanson, M., 1999. OSCE checklists do not capture increasing levels of expertise. Acad. Med. 74 (10), 1129–1134.

Hodges, B.D., Ginsburg, S., Cruess, R., et al., 2011. Assessment of professionalism: recommendations from the Ottawa 2010 Conference. Med. Teach. 33 (5), 354–363.

Hodges, B.D., Hollenberg, E., McNaughton, N., Hanson, M.D., Regehr, G., 2014. The Psychiatry OSCE: a 20-year retrospective. Acad. Psychiatry 38 (1), 26–34.

Hofer, M., Kamper, L., Sadlo, M., Sievers, K., Heussen, N., 2011. Evaluation of an OSCE assessment tool for abdominal ultrasound courses. Eur. J. Ultrasound 32, 184–190.

Holmboe, E.S., 2004. Faculty and the observation of trainees' clinical skills: problems and opportunities. Acad. Med. 79 (1), 16–22.

Holmboe, E.S., Sherbino, J., Long, D.M., Swing, S.R., Frank, J.R., 2010. The role of assessment in competency-based medical education. Med. Teach. 32 (8), 676–682.

Homer, M., Pell, G., 2009. The impact of the inclusion of simulated patient ratings on the reliability of OSCE assessments under the borderline regression method. Med. Teach. 31 (5), 420–425.

Hope, D., Cameron, H., 2015. Examiners are most lenient at the start of a two-day OSCE. Med. Teach. 37 (1), 81–85. (Early Online.)

Hosny, S., Ghaly, M.S., 2014. Teaching evidence-based medicine using a problem-oriented approach. Med. Teach. 36, S62–S68.

Huang, C.C., Chan, C.Y., Wu, C.L., et al., 2010. Assessment of clinical competence of medical students using the Objective Structured Clinical Examination: first 2 years' experience in Taipei Veterans General Hospital. J. Chin. Med. Assoc. 73 (11), 589–595.

Hubbard, J.P., 1978. Measuring Medical Education: The Tests and the Experience of the National Board of Medical Examiners, second ed. Lea & Febiger, Philadelphia.

Hubbard, J.P., Levit, E.J., Schumacher, C.F., Schnabel, T.G. Jr., 1965. An objective evaluation of clinical competence – new technics used by the national board of medical examiners. NEJM 272 (25), 1321–1328.

Humphrey-Murto, S., Touchie, C., Smee, S., 2013. Objective Structured Clinical Examinations. In: Walsh, K. (Ed.), Oxford

Textbook of Medical Education. Oxford University Press, Oxford (Chapter 45).

Hunkeler, S., Zimmermann, P., 2014. *eOSCE – Robust Real Time Electronic Marking for Clinical Examinations*. <https://www.youtube.com/watch?v=7eqeMgNU1HE> (accessed 11 November 2014).

Husbands, A., Dowell, J., 2013. Predictive validity of the Dundee multiple mini-interview. Med. Educ. 47 (7), 717–725.

ICRE (International Conference on Residency Education), 2011. *ICRE blog: Improving resident feedback skills: real-time vs. remote observation*. <http://icreblog.royalcollege.ca/2011/11/15/improving-resident-feedback-skills-real-time-vs-remote-observation/> (accessed 30 September 2014).

Institute of Medicine, 2000. To Err is Human: Building a Safer Health System. National Academy Press, Washington, DC.

Iramaneerat, C., Yudkowsky, R., Myford, C.M., Downing, S.M., 2008. Quality control of an OSCE using generalizability theory and many-faceted Rasch measurement. Adv. Health Sci. Educ. 13 (4), 479–493.

Iwata, K., Furmedge, D.S., Sturrock, A., Gill, D., 2014. Do peer-tutors perform better in examinations? An analysis of medical school final examination results. Med. Educ. 48 (7), 698–704.

Jahan, F., Sadaf, S., Bhanji, S., Naeem, N., Qureshi, R., 2011. Clinical skills assessment: comparison of student and examiner assessment in an Objective Structured Clinical Examination. Educ. Health 24 (2), 421.

Jefferies, A., Simmons, B., Tabak, D., et al., 2007. Using an Objective Structured Clinical Examination (OSCE) to assess multiple physician competencies in postgraduate training. Med. Teach. 29 (2–3), 183–191.

Joint Committee on Surgical Training, 2014. <http://www.jcst.org/blog/the-evolving-intercollegiate-mrcs-exam> (accessed 4 November 2014).

Joint Committee on Surgical Training, 2014. The evolving Intercollegiate MRCS exam. <http://www.jcst.org/blog/the-evolving-intercollegiate-mrcs-exam> (accessed 30 October 2014).

Jolly, B., 1981. Videotaped case histories in the final MB (psychiatry) examination at St Bartholomew's Hospital Medical College. J. Audiov. Media Med. 4 (4), 123–126.

Joorabchi, B., 1991. Objective Structured Clinical Examination in a pediatric residency program. Am. J. Dis. Child. 145 (7), 757–762.

Kachur, E.K., Altshuler, L., 2004. Cultural competence is everyone's responsibility! Med. Teach. 26 (2), 101–105.

Kachur, E.K., Green, S., Dennis, C., 1990. Written comments on Objective Structured Clinical Examination rating forms: an exploratory study. Teach. Learn. Med. 2 (4), 225–231.

Kachur, E.K., Zabar, S., Hanley, K., Kalet, A., Bruno, J.H., Gillespie, C.C., 2013. Organizing OSCEs (and other SP exercises) in ten steps. In: Zabar, S., Kachur, E.K., Kalet, A., Hanley, K. (Eds.), Objective Structured Clinical Examinations – 10 Steps to Planning and Implementing OSCEs and Other Standardized Patient Exercises. Springer, New York.

Karabilgin, O.S., Vatansever, K., Caliskan, S.A., Durak, H.I., 2012. Assessing medical student competency in communication in the pre-clinical phase: objective structured video exam and SP exam. Patient Educ. Couns. 87 (3), 293–299.

Kaufman, D.M., Mann, K.V., Muijtjens, A.M.M., van der Vleuten, C.P.M., 2000. A comparison of standard-setting procedures for an OSCE in undergraduate medical education. Acad. Med. 75 (3), 267–271.

Kelly, M., Murphy, A., 2004. An evaluation of the cost of designing, delivering and assessing an undergraduate communication skills module. Med. Teach. 26 (7), 610–614.

Kenkel, P., Holcomb, R., Fitzwater, B., 2004. Feasibility assessment templates for producers and cooperatives. In: 2004 Triennial Conference: Change in Rural America – Social and Management Challenges, KY, USA. <http://www.agrisk.umn.edu/TriennialConference/TriennialPubs/16_8AM/C_KENKEL.pdf> (accessed 3 November 2014).

Kennedy, C., 2013. Update on Feedback: Useful Resources on MedEdWorld. AMEE, Dundee, UK.

Khan, K.Z., Gaunt, K., Ramachandran, S., Pushkar, P., 2013. The Objective

Structured Clinical Examination (OSCE): AMEE Guide No. 81. Part II: organisation & administration. Med. Teach. 35 (9), e1447–e1463.

Khan, Z.H., 2011. Perceptions of appropriate appearance in the OSCE. A mixed study analysing viewpoints of students and examiners. Med. Teach. 33, 170.

Kim, K.S., 2010. Introduction and administration of the clinical skill test of the licensing examination, Republic of Korea (2009). J. Educ. Eval. Health Prof. 7, 4.

Kirton, S.B., Kravitz, L., 2011. Objective Structured Clinical Examinations (OSCEs) compared with traditional assessment methods. Am. J. Pharm. Educ. 75 (6), 111.

Kneebone, R., Nestel, D., Wetzel, C., et al., 2006. The human face of simulation: patient-focused simulation training. Acad. Med. 81 (10), 919–924.

Kobrossi, T., Schut, B., 1987. The use of the Objective Structured Clinic Examination (O.S.C.E.) at the Canadian Memorial Chiropractic College Outpatient Clinic. J. Can. Chiropr. Assoc. 31 (1), 21–25.

Konopasek, L., Kelly, K.V., Bylund, C.L., Wenderoth, S., Storey-Johnson, C., 2014. The Group Objective Structured Clinical Experience: building communication skills in the clinical reasoning context. Patient Educ. Couns. 96, 79–85.

Kramer, W.M., Muijtjens, A., Jansen, K., Dusman, H., Tan, L., van der Vleuten, C., 2003. Comparison of a rational and an empirical standard setting procedure for an OSCE. Med. Educ. 37 (2), 132–139.

Kreiter, C.D., Yin, P., Solow, C., Brennan, R., 2004. Investigating the reliability of the medical school admissions interview. Adv. Health Sci. Educ. 9 (2), 147–159.

Kropmans, T.J.B., O'Donovan, B.G.G., Cunningham, D., et al., 2012. An online management information system of Objective Structured Clinical Examinations. Comput. Inf. Sci. 5 (1), e38–e48.

Lambert, L., Pattison, D.J., de Looy, A.E., 2010. Dietetic students' performance of activities in an Objective Structured Clinical Examination. J. Hum. Nutr. Diet. 23 (3), 224–229.

Langley, R.G.B., Tyler, S.A., Ornstein, A.E., Sutherland, A.E., Mosher, L.M., 2009. Temporary tattoos to simulate skin disease: report and validation of a novel teaching tool. Acad. Med. 84 (7), 950–953.

Larkin, G.L., 1999. Evaluating professionalism in emergency medicine: clinical ethical competence. Acad. Emerg. Med. 6 (4), 302–311.

Lavelle, S.M., Harden, R.M., 1986. The OSCE type examination in an objective methods course for clinical studies. In: International Conference Proceedings: Newer Developments in Assessing Clinical Competence. Ottawa, Canada. Heal Publications, Montreal, Quebec.

Lawson, D., 2006. Applying generalizability theory to high-stakes objective structured clinical examinations in a naturalistic environment. J. Manipulative Physiol. Ther. 29 (6), 463–467.

Lazarus, J., Harden, R.M., 1985. The innovative process in medical education. Med. Teach. 7 (3/4), 333–342.

Lee, J.D., Erickson, J.C., Short, M.W., Roth, B.J., 2008. Education research: evaluating acute altered mental status: are incoming interns prepared? Neurology 71 (18), e50–e53.

Lemay, J.-F., Lockyer, J.M., Collin, V.T., Brownell, A.K., 2007. Assessment of non-cognitive traits through the admissions multiple mini-interview. Med. Educ. 41 (6), 573–579.

Lerner, S., Magrane, D., Friedman, E., 2009. Teaching teamwork in medical education. Mt Sinai J. Med. 76 (4), 318–329.

Liew, S.-C., Dutta, S., Sidhu, J.K., et al., 2014. Assessors for communication skills: SPs or healthcare professionals? Med. Teach. 36 (7), 626–631.

Lin, C.-W., Tsai, T.-C., Sun, C.-K., Chen, D.-F., Liu, K.-M., 2013. Power of the policy: how the announcement of high-stakes clinical examination altered OSCE implementation at institutional level. BMC Med. Educ. 13 (8), <http://www.biomedcentral.com/1472-6920/13/8> (accessed 17 October 2014).

Lu, W.-H., Mylona, E., Lane, S., Wertheim, W.A., Baldelli, P., Williams, P.C., 2014. Faculty development on professionalism and medical ethics: the design, development and implementation of Objective

Structured Teaching Exercises (OSTEs). Med. Teach. 36 (10), 876–882.

Macluskey, M., Durham, J., Balmer, C., et al., 2011. Dental student suturing skills: a multicentre trial of a checklist-based assessment. Eur. J. Dent. Educ. 15 (4), 244–249.

Malik, S.L., Manchanda, S.K., Deepak, K.K., Sunderam, K.R., 1988. The attitudes of medical students to the Objective Structured Practical Examination. Med. Educ. 22 (1), 40–46.

Manring, J., Beitman, B.D., Dewan, M.J., 2003. Evaluating competence in psychotherapy. Acad. Psychiatry 27 (3), 136–144.

Manser, T., 2009. Teamwork and patient safety in dynamic domains of healthcare: a review of the literature. Acta Anaesthesiol. Scand. 53 (2), 143–151.

Mark, M.M., Greene, J.C., Shaw, I.F., 2006. Introduction. In: Shaw, I.F., Greene, J.C., Mark, M.M. (Eds.), Handbook of Evaluation Policies, Programs and Practices. Sage Publications, London, Thousand Oaks, New Delhi.

Marshall, D., Hall, P., Taniguchi, A., 2008. Team OSCEs: evaluation methodology or education encounter? Med. Educ. 42, 1129–1130.

Marshall, G., Harris, P., 2000. A study of the role of an Objective Structured Clinical Examination (OSCE) in assessing clinical competence in third year student radiographers. Radiography 6, 117–122.

Martin, I.G., Jolly, B., 2002. Predictive validity and estimated cut score of an Objective Structured Clinical Examination (OSCE) used as an assessment of clinical skills at the end of the first clinical year. Med. Educ. 36, 418–425.

Martin, J.A., Regehr, G., Reznick, R., et al., 1997. Objective Structured Assessment of Technical Skill (OSATS) for surgical residents. Br. J. Surg. 84, 273–278.

Mavis, B., Turner, J., Lovell, K., Wagner, D., 2006. Faculty, students, and actors as standardized patients: expanding opportunities for performance assessment. Teach. Learn. Med. 18 (2), 130–136.

Mavis, B.E., Henry, R.C., Ogle, K.S., Hoppe, R.B., 1996. The emperor's new clothes: the OSCE reassessed. Acad. Med. 71 (5), 447–453.

May, S.A., Head, S.D., 2010. Assessment of technical skills: best practices. J. Vet. Med. Educ. 37 (3), 258–265.

Mazor, K.M., Zanetti, M.L., Alper, E.J., et al., 2007. Assessing professionalism in the context of an Objective Structured Clinical Examination: an in-depth study of the rating process. Med. Educ. 41, 331–340.

McCourt, C., Johnston, J.L., Cooper, S., Gormley, G.J., 2012. The level playing field: the impact of assessment practice on professional development. Med. Educ. 46 (8), 766–776.

McDaniel, M.A., Agarwal, P.K., Huelser, B.J., McDermott, K.B., Roediger, H.L., 2011. Test-enhanced learning in a middle school science classroom: the effects of quiz frequency and ability of a medical school admission process to predict clinical performance and patients' satisfaction. Acad. Med. 75, 743–747.

McFaul, P.B., Howie, P.W., 1993. The assessment of clinical competence in obstetrics and gynaecology in two medical schools by an Objective Structured Clinical Examination. Br. J. Obstet. Gynaecol. 100, 842–846.

McGaghie, W.C. (Ed.), 2013. International Best Practices for Evaluation in the Health Professions. Radcliffe Publishing Ltd.

McKinley, D.W., Norcini, J.J., 2014. How to set standards on performance-based examinations: AMEE Guide No. 85. Med. Teach. 36 (2), 97–110.

McManus, I.C., Thompson, M., Mollon, J., 2006. Assessment of examiner leniency and stringency ('hawk-dove effect') in the MRCP(UK) clinical examination (PACES) using multi-faced Rasch modelling. BMC Med. Educ. 6, 42. <http://www.biomedcentral.com/1472-6920/6/42> (accessed 3 November 2014).

McNaughton, N., Tiberius, R., Hodges, B., 1999. Effects of portraying psychologically and emotionally complex standardized patient roles. Teach. Learn. Med. 11 (3), 135–141.

McWilliam, P., Botwinski, C., 2010. Developing a successful nursing Objective Structured Clinical Examination. J. Nurs. Educ. 49 (1), 36–41.

Meats, E., Heneghan, C., Crilly, M., Glasziou, P., 2009. Evidence-based medicine teaching in UK medical schools. Med. Teach. 31, 332–337.

Medical Council of Canada, 2011. Evidence for the Validity of a Clinical Skill Assessment. Wood, T.J., Roy, M., McConnell, M., Breithaupt, K. (Eds.), <http://mcc.ca/wp-content/uploads/Technical-Reports-Wood-2011.pdf> (accessed 13 October 2014).

Medical Council of Canada, 2013. Guidelines for the Development of Objective Structured Clinical Examination (OSCE) Cases. <http://mcc.ca/wp-content/uploads/osce-booklet-2014.pdf> (accessed 10 November 2014).

Meechan, R., Jones, H., Valler-Jones, T., 2011. Do medicines OSCEs improve drug administration ability? Br. J. Nurs. 20 (13), 817–822.

Merrick, H.W., McCoy, J.A. (Eds.), 2001. The Objective Structured Clinical Examination: Present and Future, second ed. Association for Surgical Education, Springfield, USA.

Miller, G.E., 1990. The assessment of clinical skills/competence/performance. Acad. Med. 65 (9), S63–S67.

Miller, J., 2010. Competency-based training: Objective Structured Clinical Exercises (OSCE) in marriage and family therapy. J. Marital Fam. Ther. 36 (3), 320–332.

Miller, S.D.W., Butler, M.W., Meagher, F., Costello, R.W., McElvaney, N.G., 2007. Team Objective Structured Bedside Assessment (TOSBA): a novel and feasible way of providing formative teaching and assessment. Med. Teach. 29, 156–159.

Mislevy, R.J., 2004. Can there be reliability without 'reliability'? J. Educ. Behav. Stat. 29 (2), 241–244.

Mitchell, M., Henderson, A., Groves, M., Dalton, M., Nulty, D., 2009. The Objective Structured Clinical Examination (OSCE): optimising its value in the undergraduate nursing curriculum. Nurse Educ. Today 29 (4), 398–404.

Mitchell, M.L., Jeffrey, C.A., Henderson, A., et al., 2014. Using an Objective Structured Clinical Examination for Bachelor of Midwifery students' preparation for practice. Women Birth 27 (2), 108–113.

Moineau, G., Power, B., Pion, A.-M.J., Wood, T.J., Humphrey-Murto, S., 2011. Comparison of student examiner to faculty examiner scoring and feedback in an OSCE. Med. Educ. 45, 183–191.

Moretti, F., Fletcher, I., Mazzi, M.A., et al., 2012. GULiVER–travelling into the heart of good doctor–patient communication from a patient perspective: study protocol of an international multicentre study. Eur. J. Public Health 22 (4), 464–469.

Morison, S., Stewart, M., 2005. Developing interprofessional assessment. Learn. Health Soc. Care 4, 192–202.

Morrison, E.H., Lewis, E.M., Gabbert, C.C., Boker, J.R., Kumar, B., Harthill, M., 2003. Evaluating a 'service elective' in clinical teaching for medical students. Med. Teach. 25, 662–663.

Mucklow, J., Bollington, L., Maxwell, S., 2012. Assessing prescribing competence. Br. J. Clin. Pharmacol. 74 (4), 632–639.

Murray Davis, B., Solomon, P., Marshall, D., et al., 2013. A Team Observed Structured Clinical Encounter (TOSCE) for pre-licensure learners in maternity care: a short report on the Development of an Assessment Tool for Collaboration. J. Res. Interprof. Pract. Educ. 1. <www.jripe.org> (accessed 25 October 2014); March.

National Board of Chiropractic Examiners (NBCE), 2014. <http://www.nbce.org/examinations/part4/> (accessed 1 November 2014).

Nayer, M., 1993. An overview of the Objective Structured Clinical Examination. Physiother. Can. 45 (3), 171–178.

Nestel, D., Cecchini, M., Calandrini, M., et al., 2008. Real patient involvement in role development: evaluating patient focused resources for clinical procedural skills. Med. Teach. 30, 534–536.

Nevo, D., 2006. Evaluation in education. In: Shaw, I.F., Greene, J.C., Mark, M.M. (Eds.), Handbook of Evaluation Policies,

Programs and Practices. Sage Publications, London.

Newble, D., 2004. Techniques for measuring clinical competence: Objective Structured Clinical Examinations. Med. Educ. 38, 199–203.

Newble, D., Dauphinee, D., Macdonald, M., et al., 1994. Guidelines for assessing clinical competence. Teach. Learn. Med. 6 (3), 213–220.

Newble, D., Jaeger, K., 1983. The effect of assessment and examinations on the learning of medical students. Med. Educ. 17 (3), 165–171.

Newble, D.I., 1988. Eight years' experience with a structured clinical examination. Med. Educ. 22 (3), 200–204.

Newble, D.I., Swanson, D.B., 1988. Psychometric characteristics of the Objective Structured Clinical Examination. Med. Educ. 22 (4), 325–334.

Newlin-Canzone, E.T., Scerbo, M.W., Gliva-McConvey, G., Wallace, A.M., 2013. The cognitive demands of standardized patients: understanding limitations in attention and working memory with the decoding of nonverbal behaviour during improvisations. Simul. Healthc. 8 (4), 207–214.

Nieman, L.Z., Cheng, L., 2011. Chronic illness needs educated doctors: an innovative primary care training program for chronic illness education. Med. Teach. 33 (6), 340–348.

Norcini, J., Anderson, B., Bollela, V., et al., 2011. Criteria for good assessment: consensus statement and recommendations from the Ottawa 2010 Conference. Med. Teach. 33, 206–214.

Norcini, J.J., 1994. Principles for setting standards on certifying and licensing examinations. In: The Sixth Ottawa Conference on Medical Education. University of Toronto Bookstore, Toronto, Canada.

Norcini, J.J., 2003. Setting standards on educational tests. Med. Educ. 37 (5), 464–469.

Norcini, J.J., Blank, L.L., Duffy, F.D., Fortna, G.S., 2003. The mini-CEX: a method for assessing clinical skills. Ann. Intern. Med. 138 (6), 476–481.

Norman, G., 2002. Research in medical education: three decades of progress. Br. Med. J. 29 (324), 1560–1562.

Norman, G., Neville, A., Blake, J.M., Mueller, B., 2010. Assessment steers learning down the right road: impact of progress testing on licensing examination performance. Med. Teach. 32 (6), 496–499.

Novack, D.H., Cohen, D., Peitzman, S.J., Beadenkopf, S., Gracely, E., Morris, J., 2002. A pilot test of WebOSCE: a system for assessing trainees' clinical skills via teleconference. Med. Teach. 24 (5), 483–487.

O'Brien, K.L., Champeaux, A.L., Sundell, Z.E., Short, M.W., Roth, B.J., 2010. Transfusion medicine knowledge in postgraduate year 1 residents. Transfusion 50 (8), 1649–1653.

Ogden, G.R., Green, M., Ker, J.S., 2000. Student examiners: the use of interprofessional peer examiners in an Objective Structured Clinical Examination: can dental students act as examiners? Br. Dent. J. 189 (3), 160–164.

Oliven, A., Nave, R., Gilad, D., Barch, A., 2011. Implementation of a web-based interactive virtual patient case simulation as a training and assessment tool for medical students. Stud. Health Technol. Inform. 169, 233–237.

Opar, S.P., Short, M.W., Jorgensen, J.E., Blankenship, R.B., Roth, B.J., 2010. Acute coronary syndrome and cardiac arrest: using simulation to assess resident performance and program outcomes. J. Grad. Med. Educ. 2 (3), 404–409.

O'Sullivan, H., van Mook, W., Fewtrell, R., Wass, V., 2012. Integrating professionalism into the curriculum: AMEE Guide No. 61. Med. Teach. 34 (2), e64–e77.

Ottolini, M., Wohlberg, R., Lewis, K., Greenberg, L., 2011. Using observed structured teaching exercises (OSTE) to enhance hospitalist teaching during family centered rounds. Br. J. Hosp. Med. 6 (7), 423–427.

Oxford Brookes University, 2014. Assessment futures – a website to inform development in assessment, In: Assessment standards manifesto. <http://www.brookes.ac.uk/aske/Manifesto/Example%2018%20Assessment%20Futures.pdf> (accessed 13 October 2014).

Palese, A., Bulfone, G., Venturato, E., et al., 2012. The cost of the Objective Structured Clinical Examination on an Italian nursing bachelor's degree course. Nurse Educ. Today 32 (4), 422–426.

Pandya, J.S., Bhagwat, S.M., Kini, S.L., 2010. Evaluation of clinical skills for first-year surgical residents using orientation programme and objective structured clinical evaluation as a tool of assessment. J. Postgrad. Med. 56 (4), 297–300.

Papadakis, M.A., Hodgson, C.S., Teherani, A., Kohatsu, N.D., 2004. Unprofessional behavior in medical school is associated with subsequent disciplinary action by a State Medical Board. Acad. Med. 79 (3), 244–249.

Patricio, M., Juliao, M., Fareleira, F., Vaz Carneiro, A., 2013. Is the OSCE a feasible tool to assess competencies in undergraduate medical education? Med. Teach. 35, 503–514.

Patricio, M., Juliao, M., Fareleira, F., Young, M., Norman, G., Carneiro, A.V., 2015. Is the OSCE a reliable and valid tool to assess clinical competence in undergraduate medical education? Med. Teach. In press.

Patton, M.Q., 1997. Utilization-Focused Evaluation: The New Century Text. Sage, Thousand Oaks, CA.

Pau, A., Jeevaratnam, K., Chen, Y.S., Fall, A.A., Khoo, C., Nadarajah, V.D., 2013. The multiple mini-interview (MMI) for student selection in health professions training – a systematic review. Med. Teach. 35 (12), 1027–1041.

Payne, N.J., Bradley, E.B., Heald, E.B., et al., 2008. Sharpening the eye of the OSCE with critical action analysis. Acad. Med. 83 (10), 900–905.

Peckham, M., 1998. Future health scenarios and public policy. In: Marinker, M., Peckham, M. (Eds.), Clinical Futures. BMJ Books, London.

Peden, N.R., Cairncross, R.G., Harden, R.M., Crooks, J., 1985. Assessment of clinical competence in therapeutics: the use of the Objective Structured Clinical Examination. Med. Teach. 7 (2), 217–223.

Peeraer, G., De Winter, B.Y., Muijtjens, A.M.M., Remmen, R., Bossaert, L., Scherpbier, A.J.J.A., 2009. Evaluating the effectiveness of curriculum change. Is there a difference between graduating student outcomes from two different curricula? Med. Teach. 31 (3), e64–e68.

Pell, G., Fuller, R., Homer, M., Roberts, T., 2010. How to measure the quality of the OSCE: a review of metrics. AMEE Guide 49. Med. Teach. 32 (10), 802–811.

Pell, G., Fuller, R., Homer, M., Roberts, T., 2012. Is short-term remediation after OSCE failure sustained? A retrospective analysis of the longitudinal attainment of underperforming students in OSCE assessments. Med. Teach. 34 (2), 146–150.

Pell, G., Fuller, R., Homer, M., Roberts, T., 2013. Advancing the Objective Structured Clinical Examination: sequential testing in theory and practice. Med. Educ. 47 (6), 569–577.

Petrusa, E.R., 2002. Clinical performance assessments. In: Norman, G.R., van der Vleuten, C.P.M., Newble, D.I. (Eds.), International Handbook of Research in Medical Education. Kluwer Academic Publishers, Dordrecht, pp. 673–709.

Petrusa, E.R., Blackwell, T.A., Ainsworth, M.A., 1990. Reliability and validity of an Objective Structured Clinical Examination for assessing the clinical performance of residents. Arch. Intern. Med. 150 (3), 573–577.

Phillips, D., Zuckerman, J.D., Strauss, E.J., Egol, K.A., 2013. Objective Structured Clinical Examinations: a guide to development and implementation in orthopaedic residency. J. Am. Acad. Orthop. Surg. 21 (10), 592–600.

Pierre, R.B., Wierenga, A., Barton, M., Branday, J.M., Christie, C.D.C., 2004. Student evaluation of an OSCE in paediatrics at the University of the West Indies, Jamaica. BMC Med. Educ. 4, 22. <http://www.biomedcentral.com/1472-6920/4/22> (accessed 11 November 2014).

Poenaru, D., Morales, D., Richards, A., O'Connor, H.M., 1997. Running an Objective Structured Clinical Examination on a shoestring budget. Am. J. Surg. 173 (6), 538–541.

Police Training Council for England and Wales, 1987. Evaluating for Assessment. National Police Training, Harrogate, UK.

Popham, W.J., 2009. Unraveling reliability. Assoc. Superv. Curriculum Dev. February, 77–78.

Posner, G.D., Hamstra, S.J., 2013. Too much small talk? Medical students' pelvic examination skills falter with pleasant patients. Med. Educ. 47, 1209–1214.

Preece, P., Mulholland, H., Wood, R.A.B., Davis, M., Harden, R.M., Cuschieri, A., 1992. Fifteen years of the OSCE in a final examination in surgery. In: Ottawa Conference Proceedings: Approaches to the Assessment of Clinical Competence Part 1. Centre for Medical Education, Dundee, UK.

Preusche, I., Schmidts, M., Wagner-Menghin, M., 2012. Twelve tips for designing and implementing a structured rater training in OSCEs. Med. Teach. 34 (5), 368–372.

Probert, C.S., Cahill, D.J., McCann, G.L., Ben-Shlomo, Y., 2003. Traditional finals and OSCEs in predicting consultant and self-reported clinical skills of PRHOs: a pilot study. Med. Educ. 37 (7), 597–602.

Pugh, D., Touchie, C., Wood, T., Humphrey-Murto, S., 2014. Progress testing: is there a role for the OSCE? Med. Educ. 48 (6), 623–631.

Ramani, S., Krackov, S.K., 2012. Twelve tips for giving feedback effectively in the clinical environment. Med. Teach. 34 (10), 787–791.

Ratzmann, A., Wiesmann, U., Kordaß, B., 2012. Integration of an Objective Structured Clinical Examination (OSCE) into the dental preliminary exams. GMS Z. Med. Ausbild. 29 (1), 1–14.

Rau, T., Fegert, J., Liebhardt, H., 2011. How high are the personnel costs for an OSCE? A financial report on management aspects. Ger. J. Med. Educ. 28 (1), 1–8.

Reader, T.W., Flin, R., Mearns, K., Cuthbertson, B.H., 2009. Developing a team performance framework for the intensive care unit. Crit. Care Med. 37 (5), 1787–1793.

Regehr, G., Freeman, R., Robb, A., Missiha, N., Heissey, R., 1999. OSCE performance evaluation made by standardized patients: comparing checklists and global ratings scores. Acad. Med. 74 (Suppl. 10), S135–S137.

Regehr, G., MacRae, H., Reznick, R.K., Szalay, D., 1998. Comparing the psychometric properties of checklists and global rating scales for assessing performance on an OSCE-format examination. Acad. Med. 73 (9), 993–997.

Reiter, H., Eva, K., Rosenfeld, J., Norman, G., 2007. Multiple mini-interviews predict clerkship and licensing examination performance. Med. Educ. 41 (4), 378–384.

Renaud, G., Jalali, A., 2011. Helping Dyslexic Medical Students Pass Their OSCE Exams. eLearn Magazine <http://elearnmag.acm.org/featured.cfm?aid=2030254> (accessed 1 October 2014).

Rethans, J.-J., Corter, S., Bokken, L., Morrison, L., 2007. Unannounced standardised patients in real practice: a systematic literature review. Med. Educ. 41 (6), 537–549.

Reznick, R.K., Blackmore, D., Cohen, R., et al., 1993a. An objective structured clinical examination for the licentiate of the Medical Council of Canada: from research to reality. Acad. Med. 68 (Suppl. 10), S4–S6.

Reznick, R.K., Blackmore, D.E., Dauphinée, W.D., Rothman, A.I., Smee, S.M., 1996. Large-scale high-stakes testing with an OSCE: report from the Medical Council of Canada. Acad. Med. S71, 19–21.

Reznick, R.K., Blackmore, D.E., Dauphinee, W.D., Smee, S.M., Rothman, A.I., 1997. An OSCE for licensure: the Canadian experience. In: Scherpbier, A.J.J.A., van der Vleuten, C.P.M., Rethans, J.J., van der Steeg, A.F.W. (Eds.), Advances in Medical Education. Springer, pp. 458–461.

Reznick, R.K., Smee, S., Baumber, J.S., et al., 1993b. Guidelines for estimating the real cost of an Objective Structured Clinical Examination. Acad. Med. 68 (7), 513–517.

Reznick, R.K., Smee, S.M., Rothman, A.I., et al., 1992. An objective structured clinical examination for the licentiate: report of the pilot project of the Medical Council of Canada. Acad. Med. 48, 487–494.

Ricciotti, H., 2013. *Implementing an Objective Structured Teaching Exercise (OSTE) in an OBGYN Residency Program*.

MedEdPORTAL Publications <https://www.mededportal.org/publication/9425> (accessed 15 October 2014).

Roediger, H.L., Agarwal, P.K., McDaniel, M.A., McDermott, K.B., 2011. Test-enhanced learning in the classroom: long-term improvements from quizzing. J. Exp. Psychol. Appl. 17, 382–395.

Roseby, R., Marks, M.K., Conn, J., Sawyer, S.M., 2003. Improving medical student performance in adolescent anti-smoking health promotion. Med. Educ. 37 (8), 704–708.

Rothman, A.I., Blackmore, D.E., Dauphinee, W.D., Reznick, R.K., 1996. The use of global ratings in OSCE station scores. In: Scherpbier, A.J.J.A., van der Vleuten, C.P.M., Rethans, J.J., van der Steeg, A.F.W. (Eds.), Advances in Medical Education. Springer, Netherlands.

Rothman, A.I., Blackmore, D.E., Dauphinée, W.D., Reznick, R.K., 1997. Tests of sequential testing in two years' results of Part 2 of the Medical Council of Canada Qualifying Examination. Acad. Med. S72, 22–24.

Royal College of Physicians of the United Kingdom, 2014. Practical Assessment of Clinical Examination Skills (PACES). <http://www.mrcpuk.org/mrcpuk-examinations/paces> (accessed 30 September 2014).

Rudland, J., Wilkinson, T., Smith-Han, K., Thomson-Fawcett, M., 2008. 'You can do it late at night or in the morning. You can do it at home, I did it with my flatmate.' The educational impact of an OSCE. Med. Teach. 30, 2006–2011.

Ruesseler, M., Weinlich, M., Müller, M.P., Byhahn, C., Marzi, I., Walcher, F., 2010. Simulation training improves ability to manage medical emergencies. Emerg. Med. J. 27 (10), 734–738.

Rushforth, H.E., 2007. Objective Structured Clinical Examination (OSCE): review of literature and implications for nursing education. Nurse Educ. Today 27 (5), 481–490.

Rymer, A.T., 2001. The new MRCOG Objective Structured Clinical Examination – the examiners' evaluation. J. Obstet. Gynaecol. 21, 103–106.

Sakurai, H., Kanada, Y., Sugiura, Y., et al., 2013. standardization of clinical skill evaluation in physical/occupational therapist education – effects of introduction of an education system using OSCE. J. Phys. Ther. Sci. 25 (9), 1071–1077.

Salvatori, P., Brown, B., 1995. Objective Structured Clinical Examination (OSCE). In: Evaluation Methods: A Resource Handbook. McMaster University Program for Educational Development, Program for Faculty Development, and Educating Future Physicians of Ontario (EFPO) Project. Program for Educational Development, Hamilton, ON, Canada. (Chapter 5.2)

Sandars, J., Cleary, T.J., 2011. Self-regulation theory: applications to medical education: AMEE Guide No. 58. Med. Teach. 33 (11), 875–886.

Sandilands, D., Gotzmann, A., Roy, M., Zumbo, B.D., De Champlain, A., 2014. Weighting checklist items and station components on a large-scale OSCE: is it worth the effort? Med. Teach. 36 (7), 585–590.

Schneider, J., 2014. Closing the gap … between university and schoolhouse. Phi Delta Kappan 96 (1), 30–35.

Schoonheim-Klein, M., Walmsley, A.D., Habets, L., van der Velden, U., Manogue, M., 2005. An implementation strategy for introducing an OSCE into a dental school. Eur. J. Dent. Educ. 9, 143–149.

Schoonheim-Klein, M.E., Habets, L.L., Aartman, I.H., van der Vleuten, C.P., van der Velden, U., 2006. Implementing an Objective Structured Clinical Examination (OSCE) in dental education: effects on students' learning strategies. Eur. J. Dent. Educ. 10 (4), 226–235.

Schultz, J.H., Nikendei, C., Weyrich, P., Möltner, A., Fischer, M.R., Jünger, J., 2008. Quality assurance of assessments using the example of the OSCE examination format: experiences of the Medical School of Heidelberg University. Ger. J. Evid. Qual. Healthc. 102 (10), 668–672.

Schuwirth, L.W.T., van der Vleuten, C.P.M., 2011. General overview of the theories used in assessment: AMEE Guide No. 57. Med. Teach. 33 (10), 783–797.

Schwartzman, E., Hsu, D.I., Law, A.V., Chung, E.P., 2011. Assessment of patient communication skills during OSCE: examining effectiveness of a training program in minimizing inter-grader variability. Patient Educ. Couns. 83 (3), 472–477.

Scott, D., Cook, S., DuBeau, C., Podrazik, P., 2013. *A Four Station OSTE (Objective Structured Teaching Exercise) in Geriatric Medicine.* MedEdPORTAL Publications <https://www.mededportal.org/publication/9754> (accessed 15 October 2014).

Scriven, M., 1991. Evaluation Thesaurus, fourth ed. Sage, Thousand Oaks, CA.

Selim, A.A., Ramadan, F.H., El-Gueneidy, M.M., Gaafer, M.M., 2012. Using Objective Structured Clinical Examination (OSCE) in undergraduate psychiatric nursing education: is it reliable and valid? Nurse Educ. Today 32 (3), 283–288.

Shanahan, E.M., Murray, A.M., Lillington, T., Farmer, E.A., 2000. The teaching of occupational and environmental medicine to medical students in Australia and New Zealand. Occup. Med. 50 (4), 246–250.

Shih, R., Silverman, M., Mayer, C., 2013. A 5-year study of emergency medicine Intern-Objective Structured Clinical Examination (OSCE) performance does not correlate with emergency medicine faculty evaluation of resident performance. Ann. Emerg. Med. 62 (5), S181.

Short, M.W., Jorgensen, J.E., Edwards, J.A., Blankenship, R.B., Roth, B.J., 2009. Assessing intern core competencies with an Objective Structured Clinical Examination. J. Grad. Med. Educ. 1 (1), 30–36.

Shumway, J.M., Harden, R.M., 2003. AMEE Guide No. 25: the assessment of learning outcomes for the competent and reflective physician. Med. Teach. 25 (6), 569–584.

Shute, V.J., 2008. Focus on formative feedback. Rev. Educ. Res. 78 (1), 153–189.

Siddiqui, T., Ahmed, A., 2013. Reliability of OSTE in the Health Professions Education Exit Examination of College Physicians and Surgeons, Pakistan: a psychometric analysis. J. Coll. Physicians Surg. Pak. 23 (10), 62–66.

Silva, C.C., Lunardi, A.C., Mendes, F.A., Souza, F.F., Carvalho, C.R., 2011. Objective structured clinical evaluation as an assessment method for undergraduate chest physical therapy students: a cross-sectional study. Rev. Bras. Fisioter. 15 (6), 481–486.

Simmons, B., Egan-Lee, E., Wagner, S.J., Esdaile, M., Baker, L., Reeves, S., 2011. Assessment of interprofessional learning: the design of an Interprofessional Objective Structured Clinical Examination (iOSCE) approach. J. Interprof. Care 25, 73–74.

Simpson, J.G., Furnace, J., Crosby, J., et al., 2002. The Scottish doctor – learning outcomes for the medical undergraduate in Scotland: a foundation for competent and reflective practitioners. Med. Teach. 24 (2), 136–143.

Singer, P.A., Robb, A., Cohen, R., Norman, G., Turnbull, J., 1996. Performance-based assessment of clinical ethics using an Objective Structured Clinical Examination. Acad. Med. 17 (5), 495–498.

Singh, R., Singh, A., Fish, R., McLean, D., Anderson, D.R., Singh, G., 2009. A patient safety Objective Structured Clinical Examination. J. Patient Saf. 5 (2), 55–60.

Singleton, A., Smith, F., Harris, T., Ross-Harper, R., Hilton, S., 1999. An evaluation of the Team Objective Structured Clinical Examination (TOSCE). Med. Educ. 33, 34–41.

Siu, E., Reiter, H., 2009. Overview: what's worked and what hasn't as a guide towards predictive admissions tool development. Adv. Health Sci. Educ. 14 (5), 759–775.

Sloan, D.A., Donnelly, M.H., Schwartz, R.W., Strodel, W.E., 1995. The Objective Structured Clinical Examination: the new gold standard for evaluating postgraduate clinical performance. Ann. Surg. 222, 735–742.

Sloan, P.A., Plymale, M.A., Johnson, M., Vanderveer, B., LaFountain, P., Sloan, D.A., 2001. Cancer pain management skills among medical students: the development of a cancer pain objective structured clinical examination. J. Pain Symptom Manage. 21 (4), 298–306.

Smee, S.M., Blackmore, D.E., 2001. Setting standards for an Objective Structured Clinical Examination: the borderline group method gains ground on Angoff. Med. Educ. 35 (11), 1009–1010.

Smee, S.M., Blackmore, D.E., Rothman, A.I., Reznick, R.K., Dauphinée, W.D., 2000. Pioneering a sequenced OSCE for the Medical Council of Canada: an administrative overview. In: Melnick, D.E. (Ed.), Proceedings of Eighth International Ottawa Conference – Evolving Assessment: Protecting the Human Dimension. National Board of Medical Examiners, Philadelphia, pp. 234–240.

Smee, S.M., Dauphinée, W.D., Blackmore, D.E., Rothman, A.I., Reznick, R., Des Marchais, J., 2003. A sequenced OSCE for licensure: administrative issues, results and myths. Adv. Health Sci. Educ. Theory Pract. 8, 223–236.

Smith, M.A., Burton, W.B., Mackay, M., 2009. Development, impact, and measurement of enhanced physical diagnosis skills. Adv. Health Sci. Educ. 14 (4), 547–556.

Sola Pola, M., Martínez Castela, D., Molins, I., Mesalles, A., Pulpón Segura, A.M., 2011. Testing Objective Structured Clinical Evaluation (OSCE) for nursing students experience developed during the years 1995–2009. Rev. Lat. Am. Enfermagem 34 (7–8), 32–39.

Solomon, P., Marshall, D., Boyle, A., et al., 2011. Establishing face and content validity of the McMaster-Ottawa Team Observed Structured Clinical Encounter (TOSCE). J. Interprof. Care 25, 302–304.

Stern, D.T. (Ed.), 2006. Measuring Medical Professionalism. Oxford University Press, UK.

Stevens, N. (Ed.), 2010. The Objective Structured Clinical Examination for the Resident Physician: An Instructional Manual for Program Directors. CreateSpace, Scotts Valley, CA, USA.

Stojan, J.N., Schiller, J.H., Mullan, P., et al., 2014. Medical school handoff education improves postgraduate trainee performance and confidence. Med. Teach. 36, 1–8. (Early Online.)

Stokes, J., 1974. The Clinical Examination – Assessment of Clinical Skills: Medical Education Booklet 2. Association for the Study of Medical Education, Dundee, UK.

Stroud, L., Herold, J., Tomlinson, G., Cavalcanti, R.B., 2011. Who you know or what you know? Effect of examiner familiarity with residents on OSCE scores. Acad. Med. 86 (10 Suppl.), S8–S11.

Sturpe, D.A., 2010. Objective Structured Clinical Examinations in doctor of pharmacy programs in the United States. Am. J. Pharm. Educ. 74 (8), 148.

Sudan, R., Clark, P., Henry, B., 2014. Cost and logistics for implementing the American College of Surgeons Objective Structured Clinical Examination. Am. J. Surg. <http://www.americanjournalofsurgery.com/article/S0002-9610(14)00529-7/abstract> (accessed 14 November 2014).

Swanson, D.B., Clauser, B.E., Case, S.M., 1999. Clinical skills assessment with standardized patients in high-stakes tests: a framework for thinking about score precision, equating, and security. Adv. Health Sci. Educ. 4 (1), 67–106.

Swing, S.R., 2007. The ACGME outcome project: retrospective and prospective. Med. Teach. 29 (7), 648–654.

Symonds, I., Cullen, L., Fraser, D., 2003. Evaluation of a formative Interprofessional Team Objective Structured Clinical Examination (ITOSCE): a method of shared learning in maternity education. Med. Teach. 25, 38–41.

Szerlip, H., Anderson, D.S., Garris, J.B., Stanton, M., 1998. Development and implementation of a pelvic examination station for a high-stakes OSCE. In: Evolving Assessment: Protecting the Human Dimension: 8th Ottawa Conference, July 12–15, 1998, Philadelphia, Pennsylvania, USA.

Tamblyn, R.M., Klass, D.J., Schnabl, G.K., Kopelow, M.L., 1991. The accuracy of standardized patient presentation. Med. Educ. 25 (2), 100–109.

Tavakol, M., Dennick, R., 2011. Post-examination analysis of objective tests: AMEE Guide 54. Med. Teach. 33 (6), 447–458.

Tavakol, M., Dennick, R., 2012. Post-examination interpretation of objective test data: monitoring and improving the quality of high-stakes examinations: AMEE Guide No. 66. Med. Teach. 34 (3), e161–e175.

Tavares, W., Eva, K.W., 2013. Exploring the impact of mental workload on rater-based assessments. Adv. Health Sci. Educ. 18, 291–303.

Taylor, C.A., Green, K.E., 2013. OSCE feedback: a randomized trial of effectiveness, cost-effectiveness and student satisfaction. Creat. Educ. 4 (6A), 9–14.

Townsend, A.H., McIlvenny, S., Miller, C.J., Dunn, E.V., 2001. The use of an Objective Structured Clinical Examination (OSCE) for formative and summative assessment in a general practice clinical attachment and its relationship to final medical school examination performance. Med. Educ. 25, 841–846.

Treadwell, I., 2006. The usability of personal digital assistants (PDAs) for assessment of practical performance. Med. Educ. 40 (9), 855–861.

Troncon, L.E., 2004. Clinical skills assessment: limitations to the introduction of an 'OSCE' (Objective Structured Clinical Examination) in a traditional Brazilian medical school. Sao Paulo Med. J. 122 (1), 12–17.

Trowbridge, R.L., Snydman, L.K., Skolfield, J., Hafler, J., Bing-You, R.G., 2011. A systematic review of the use and effectiveness of the Objective Structured Teaching Encounter. Med. Teach. 33 (11), 893–903.

Tuckman, B.W., 1975. Measuring Educational Outcomes: Fundamentals of Testing. Harcourt Brace Jovanovich, Inc, Chicago, USA.

Tudiver, F., Rose, D., Bank, B., Pfortmiller, D., 2009. Reliability and validity testing of an evidence-based medicine OSCE station. Innov. Fam. Med. Educ. 41 (2), 89–91.

Turner, J.L., Dankoski, M.E., 2008. Objective structured clinical exams: a critical review. Fam. Med. 40 (8), 574–578.

Turner, R., Nicholson, S., 2011. Reasons selectors give for accepting and rejecting medical applications before interview. Med. Educ. 45 (3), 298–307.

Tweed, M.J., Thompson-Fawcett, M., Wilkinson, T.J., 2013. Decision-making bias in assessment: the effect of aggregating objective information and anecdote. Med. Teach. 35, 832–837.

van de Ridder, J.M., Stokking, K.M., McGaghie, W.C., ten Cate, O.T., 2008. What is feedback in clinical education? Med. Educ. 42 (2), 189–197.

van den Berk, I.A., van de Ridder, J.M., van Schaik, J.P., 2011. Radiology as part of an Objective Structured Clinical Examination on clinical skills. Eur. J. Radiol. 78 (3), 363–367.

van der Vleuten, C.P.M., 1996. The assessment of professional competence: developments, research, and practical implications. Adv. Health Sci. Educ. 1 (1), 41–67.

van der Vleuten, C.P., Schuwirth, L.W., 2005. Assessing professional competence: from methods to programmes. Med. Educ. 39 (3), 309–317.

van der Vleuten, C.P.M., Schuwirth, L.W.T., Driessen, E.W., et al., 2012. A model for programmatic assessment fit for purpose. Med. Teach. 34, 305–314.

van der Vleuten, C.P.M., Swanson, D.B., 1990. Assessment of clinical skills with standardized patients: state of the art. Teach. Learn. Med. 2, 58–76.

Van Schoor, A.N., Navsa, N., Meiring, J.H., Treadwell, I., Bosman, M.C., Greyling, L.M., 2006. Perspectives on the use of PDAs as assessment tools. Clin. Teach. 3 (3), 170–174.

van Zanten, M., Boulet, J.R., Norcini, J.J., McKinley, D., 2005. Using a standardised patient assessment to measure professional attributes. Med. Educ. 39 (1), 20–29.

Vargas, A.L., Boulet, J.R., Errichetti, A., Van Zanten, M., Lopez, M.J., Reta, A.M., 2007. Developing performance-based medical school assessment programs in resource-limited environments. Med. Teach. 29 (2–3), 192–198.

Vaughan, B., Florentine, P., 2013. The OSCE in a pre-registration osteopathy program: introduction and psychometric properties. Int. J. Osteopath. Med. 16 (4), 198–206.

Verma, A., Bhatt, H., Booton, P., Kneebone, R., 2011. The Ventriloscope® as an innovative tool for assessing clinical examination skills: appraisal of a novel method of simulating auscultatory findings. Med. Teach. 33 (7), e388–e396.

Vu, N.V., Marcy, M.M., Colliver, J.A., Verhulst, S.J., Travis, T.A., Barrows, H.S., 1992. Standardized (simulated) patients' accuracy in recording clinical performance check-list items. Med. Educ. 26 (2), 99–104.

Wagner, D., Lypson, M., 2009. Centralized Assessment in Graduate Medical Education: cents and sensibilities. J. Grad. Med. Educ. 1 (1), 21–27.

Wagner, D.P., Hoppe, R.B., Parker Lee, C., 2009. The patient safety OSCE for PGY-1 residents: a centralized response to the challenge of culture change. Teach. Learn. Med. 21 (1), 8–14.

Wallace, J., Rao, R., Haslam, R., 2002. Simulated patients and Objective Structured Clinical Examinations: review of their use in medical education. Adv. Psychiatr. Treat. 8, 342–350.

Wallace, P., 2007. Coaching Standardized Patients for Use in the Assessment of Clinical Competence, first ed. Springer Publishing Company, New York.

Wallenstein, J., Heron, S., Santen, S., Shayne, P., Ander, D., 2010. A core competency–based Objective Structured Clinical Examination (OSCE) can predict future resident performance. Soc. Acad. Emerg. Med. 17 (Suppl. 2), S67–S71.

Walsh, M., Bailey, P.H., Koren, I., 2009. Objective structured clinical evaluation of clinical competence: an integrative review. J. Adv. Nurs. 65 (8), 1584–1595.

Walters, K., Osborn, D., Raven, P., 2005. The development, validity and reliability of a multimodality Objective Structured Clinical Examination in psychiatry. Med. Educ. 39, 292–298.

Ward, H., Barratt, J., 2005. Assessment of nurse practitioner advanced clinical practice skills: using the Objective Structured Clinical Examination (OSCE): Helen Ward and Julian Barratt examine how OSCEs can be developed to ensure a robust assessment of clinical competence. Prim. Health Care 15 (10), 37–41.

Wass, V., van der Vleuten, C., Shatzer, J., Jones, R., 2001. Assessment of clinical competence. Lancet 357, 945–949.

Waterston, T., Cater, J.I., Mitchell, R.G., 1980. An objective undergraduate clinical examination in child health. Arch. Dis. Child. 55, 917–922.

Watson, R., Stimpson, A., Topping, A., Porock, D., 2002. Clinical competence assessment in nursing: a systematic review of the literature. J. Adv. Nurs. 39 (5), 421–431.

Webb, E.A., Davis, L., Muir, G., Lissauer, T., Nanduri, V., Newell, S.J., 2012. Improving postgraduate clinical assessment tools: the introduction of video recordings to assess decision making. Med. Teach. 34 (5), 404–410.

Weller, J., Boyd, M., Cumin, D., 2014. Teams, tribes and patient safety: overcoming barriers to effective teamwork in healthcare. Postgrad. Med. J. 90, 149–154.

Wessel, J., Williams, R., Finch, E., Gémus, M., 2003. Reliability and validity of an Objective Structured Clinical Examination for physical therapy students. J. Allied Health 32 (4), 266–269.

Whelan, G.P., Boulet, J.R., McKinley, D.W., et al., 2005. Scoring standardized patient examinations: lessons learned from the development and administration of the ECFMG Clinical Skills Assessment (CSA®). Med. Teach. 27 (3), 200–206.

White, C.B., Ross, P.T., Gruppen, L.D., 2009. Remediating students' failed OSCE performances at one school: the effects of self-assessment, reflection, and feedback. Acad. Med. 84 (5), 651–654.

Widyandana, D., Majoor, G.D., Scherpbier, A.J.J.A., 2011. Effects of partial substitution of pre-clinical skills training by attachments to primary health care centers: an experimental study. Med. Teach. 33 (6), e313–e317.

Wilkinson, T.J., Newble, D.E., Frampton, C.M., 2001. Standard setting in an Objective Structured Clinical Examination: use of global ratings of borderline performance to determine the passing score. Med. Educ. 35 (11), 1043–1049.

Wilkinson, T.J., Newble, D.I., Wilson, P.D., Carter, J.M., Helms, R.M., 2000. Development of a three-centre simultaneous Objective Structured Clinical Examination. Med. Educ. 34 (10), 798–807.

Williams, R., Miler, R., Shah, B., et al., 2011. Observing handoffs and telephone management in GI fellowship training. Am. J. Gastroenterol. 106 (8), 1410–1414.

Wilson, G.M., Lever, R., Harden, R.M., Robertson, J.I.S., MacRitchie, J., 1969. Examination of Clinical Examiners. Lancet 293 (7584), 37–40.

Wood, L., Hassell, A., Whitehouse, A., Bullock, A., Wall, D., 2006. A literature review of multi-source feedback systems within and without health services, leading to 10 tips for their successful design. Med. Teach. 28 (7), e185–e191.

Woodburn, J., Sutcliffe, N., 1996. The reliability, validity and evaluation of the Objective Structured Clinical Examination in podiatry (chiropody). Assess. Eval. High. Educ. 21 (2), 131–156.

Yang, Y.Y., Lee, F.Y., Hsu, H.C., et al., 2010. A core competence-based Objective Structured Clinical Examination (OSCE) in evaluation of clinical performance of postgraduate year-1 (PGY1) residents. J. Chin. Med. Assoc. 74 (5), 198–204.

Yap, K., Bearman, M., Thomas, N., Hay, M., 2012. Clinical psychology students' experiences of a pilot Objective Structured Clinical Examination. Aust. Psychol. 47, 165–173.

Yazbeck-Karam, V., Bahous, S.A., Faour, W., Khairallah, M., Asmar, N., 2014. Influence of standardized patient body habitus on undergraduate student performance in an Objective Structured Clinical Examination. Med. Teach. 36 (3), 240–244.

Young, J.Q., van Merrienboer, J., Durning, S., ten Cate, O., 2014. Cognitive Load Theory: implications for medical education: AMEE Guide No. 86. Med. Teach. 36, 371–384.

Young, W.W., Barthold, J.C., Birenbaum, D., Long, P., Dion, M., Hamilton, L.A., 1995. An objective structured clinical exam in multisite obstetrics and gynecology clerkship. Teach. Learn. Med. 7 (3), 177–181.

Yudkowsky, R., 2009. Performance tests. In: Downing, S.M., Yudkowsky, R. (Eds.), Assessment in Health Professions Education. Routledge, New York and London.

Zartman, R.R., McWhorter, A.G., Seale, N.S., Boone, W.J., 2002. Using OSCE-based evaluation: curricular impact over time. J. Dent. Educ. 66 (12), 1323–1330.

Zink, T., Power, D.V., Finstad, D., Brooks, K.D., 2010. Is there equivalency between students in a longitudinal, rural clerkship and a traditional urban-based program? Fam. Med. 42 (10), 702–706.

Bibliography

The following publications may be of interest to the reader who wishes to explore some aspects of the OSCE in more depth; to consult books, reviews and reports on the theme of the OSCE; to see some examples of OSCE stations; or to look at the OSCE from a broader perspective of assessment methodology. Some useful online videos are also included.

Many books and other resources relating to the OSCE are available, and the list below is just a small sample. A web search will reveal many other relevant publications and videos.

Aspects explored in more depth

How to measure the quality of the OSCE: A review of metrics. AMEE Guide no. 49
Pell, G., Fuller, R., Homer, M. and Roberts, T. (2011). Dundee: Association for Medical Education in Europe (AMEE).
A review of the metrics that are available for measuring quality in assessment and indicating how a rounded picture of OSCE assessment quality may be constructed by using a variety of measures.

Post-examination analysis of objective tests: AMEE Guide no. 54
Tavakol, M. and Dennick, R. (2012). Dundee: Association for Medical Education in Europe (AMEE).
An overview of the practical importance of analysing questions to ensure quality and fairness of the test.

Post-examination interpretation of objective test data: Monitoring and improving the quality of high-stakes examinations: AMEE Guide no. 66
Tavakol, M. and Dennick, R. (2013). Dundee: Association for Medical Education in Europe (AMEE).
Logical and empirical evidence for medical teachers to improve their objective tests by appropriate interpretation of post-examination analysis. A description and explanation of some basic statistical and psychometric concepts are included.

345

Generalisability theory for the perplexed: A practical introduction and guide: AMEE Guide no. 68
Bloch, R. and Norman, G. (2014). Dundee: Association for Medical Education in Europe (AMEE).
Some practical examples and an introduction to the use of a web-based tool to facilitate understanding of this important theory, both as it relates to the OSCE and more generally.

General overview of the theories used in assessment: AMEE Guide no. 57
Schuwirth, L.W.T. and van der Vleuten, C.P.M. (2012). Dundee: Association for Medical Education in Europe (AMEE).
As assessment is modified to suit student learning, it is important to understand the theories that underpin which method of assessment are chosen. This guide provides an insight into the essential theories used.

Standard setting in student assessment: AMEE Guide no. 18
Friedman Ben-David, M. (2000). Dundee: Association for Medical Education in Europe (AMEE).
An introduction to the principles, key concepts and practical considerations of standard-setting approaches.

How to set standards on performance-based examinations: AMEE Guide no. 85
McKinley, D.W. and Norcini, J.J. (2014). Dundee: Association for Medical Education in Europe (AMEE).
A resource to help those responsible for determining passing scores on tests, which explains methods for setting passing scores.

The assessment of learning outcomes: AMEE Guide no. 25
Shumway, J.M. and Harden, R.M. (2003). Dundee: Association for Medical Education in Europe (AMEE).
An overview of assessment approaches relevant to the categories of learning outcomes in the healthcare professions.

The use of real patients, simulated patients and simulators in clinical examinations: AMEE Guide no. 13
Collins, J.P. and Harden, R.M. (1999). Dundee: Association for Medical Education in Europe (AMEE).
The range of patient representations that can be chosen for an OSCE and advice on when they may be more appropriately used.

A systemic framework for the progress test: Strengths, constraints and issues: AMEE Guide no. 71
Wrigley, W., van der Vleuten, C., Freeman, A. and Muijtjens, A. (2013). Dundee: Association for Medical Education in Europe (AMEE).
A generic framework to help identify and explore improvements in the quality and defensibility of progress test data.

Books and reports on the theme of the OSCE

Criteria for good assessment: Consensus statement and recommendations from the Ottawa 2010 Conference
Norcini, J., Anderson, B., Bollela, V., Burch, V., Costa, M.J., Duvivier, R., Galbraith, R., Hays, R., Kent, A., Perrott, V. and Roberts, T. (2011). Medical Teacher 33 (3): 206–214.
A summary of the criteria for good assessment, including validity, reproducibility, equivalence, feasibility, educational effect, catalytic effect and acceptability.

Performance in assessment: Consensus statement and recommendations from the Ottawa Conference
Boursicot, K., Etheridge, L., Setna, Z., Sturrock, A., Ker, J., Smee, S. and Sambandam, E. (2011). Medical Teacher 33 (5): 370–383.
A summary of recommendations for individuals and institutions when designing and implementing OSCEs and workplace-based assessments.

The objective structured clinical examination: A socio-history
Hodges, B. (2009). Saarbrücken: Lambert Academic Publishing.
How discourses of performance, psychometrics and production have led to substantial changes in the way competence is understood, facilitating the worldwide adoption of the OSCE.

Objective structured clinical examinations: 10 steps to planning and implementing OSCEs and other standardized patient exercises
Zabar, S., Kachur, E., Kalet, A. and Hanley, K. (2012). New York: Springer.
Tips for designing OSCE cases and on recruiting, training and using standardised patients for remediation and assessment in clinical settings.

The objective structured clinical examination (OSCE): AMEE Guide no. 81
Khan, K.M., Gaunt, K., Ramachandran, S. and Pushkar, P. (2014). Dundee: Association for Medical Education in Europe (AMEE).
A practical overview of the OSCE, from early theoretical beginnings to developing an assessment programme.

Objective structured clinical examinations
Humphrey-Murto, S., Touchie, C. and Smee, S. (2013). In: Oxford Textbook of Medical Education, Chapter 45. Walsh, K. (Ed.) Oxford: Oxford University Press.
A short review of the OSCE, including the theoretical underpinnings, together with suggestions on how to run an OSCE.

The use of the objective structured clinical examination (OSCE) in dental education
Schoonheim-Klein, M. (2008). Thesis: Academic Centre for Dentistry Amsterdam (ACTA), The Netherlands.
The OSCE as it relates to dentistry.

Objective structured clinical evaluation of clinical competence: An integrative review
Walsh, M., Hill Bailey, P. and Koren, I. (2009). Journal of Advanced Nursing 65 (8): 1584–1595.
A literature review on use of the OSCE to measure clinical competence in nursing.

A best evidence medical education (BEME) review on the feasibility, reliability and validity of the objective structured clinical examination (OSCE) in undergraduate medical studies
Patricio, M. (2012). PhD dissertation. Faculty of Medicine of the University of Lisbon, Portugal. http://hdl.handle.net/10451/7600 (accessed 14 November 2014).
Madalena Patricio's PhD dissertation on the topic of the OSCE.

Performance tests
Yudkowsky, R. (2009). In: Assessment in Health Professions Education, Chapter 9. Downing, S.M. and Yudkowsky, R. (Eds.) London: Routledge.
The purposes, advantages and limitations of performance tests and guidelines for the use of standardised patients.

Structured assessments of clinical competence
Boursicot, K.A.M., Roberts, T.E. and Burdick, W.P. (2014). In: Understanding Medical Education Evidence, Theory and Practice, Chapter 17. Second Ed. Swanwick, T. (Ed.) Chichester, UK: John Wiley & Sons.
A summary of the theoretical principles underlying the development of modern structured assessments of clinical competence and some practical aspects of designing and implementing OSCEs, including standard setting methods.

Clinical performance assessments
Petrusa, E.R. (2002). In: International Handbook of Research in Medical Education, Part Two, Chapter 21, Norman, G.R., van der Vleuten, C.P.M. and Newble, D.I. (Eds.) Dordrecht: Kluwer Academic Publishers.
An in-depth look at research into the OSCE.

Examples of OSCE stations

Core clinical skills for OSCEs in medicine
Dornan, T. and O'Neill, P. (2006). Philadelphia: Churchill Livingstone Elsevier.
Designed for students, the book provides hints on approaching an OSCE and contains 90 OSCE stations.

OSCEs for anaesthetists
Shambrook, A.S., Appadurai, I.R. and Vickers, M.D. (Eds.) (1995). London: Chapman & Hall Medical.
Contains 120 conventional OSCE stations in anaesthesiology. Answers and explanatory notes are provided, together with some key references.

OSCE and clinical skills handbook
Hurley, K.F. (2011) (Second Ed.). Toronto: Elsevier Saunders.
A study aid for medical students preparing for OSCEs.

The easy guide to OSCEs for communication skills
Akunjee, M., Akunjee, N., Siddiqui, S. and Mallick, A. (2010). Milton Keynes: Radcliffe Publishing Ltd.
Designed for students, includes common dilemmas in clinical and examination settings relating to communication skills.

Clinical skills for OSCEs
Burton, N. (2011). Oxfordshire: Scion Publishing Ltd.
Designed for students, with comprehensive coverage of the clinical skills examined in a final year OSCE.

A broader perspective of assessment methodology

International best practices for evaluation in the health professions
McGaghie, W.C. (Ed.) (2013). London: Radcliffe Publishing Ltd.
The book aims to provide a better understanding of assessment principles, concepts, tools and technologies to help medical educators to respond to assessment challenges.

Assessment in health professions education
Downing, S.M. and Yudkowsky, R. (Eds.) (2009). New York: Routledge
The fundamentals of testing and assessment, specifically written for health professions educators.

A practical guide for medical teachers
Dent, J.A. and Harden, R.M. (Eds.) (2014). (Fourth Edn.) London: Churchill Livingstone Elsevier.
Section 6 provides a general perspective on principles of assessment and the tools available. It also looks at giving feedback and evaluating professionalism.

Essential skills for a medical teacher
Harden, R.M. and Laidlaw, J.M. (2012). Edinburgh: Churchill Livingstone Elsevier.
A useful introduction to medical education and the principles of assessment. Five questions are asked relating to assessment: what to assess; how to assess; why assess; who should assess; when and where assessment should occur.

Standard setting, the next generation: Where few psychometricians have gone before
Berk, R.A. (1993). Applied Measurement in Education 9 (3): 215–235.
The pros and cons of the various methods of standard setting.

Videoclips

Measurement and improvement of the OSCE: Recognition and remediation of station level problems (part 1)
Fuller, R. and Pell, G. (2013). http://www.mededworld.org/stream/display.aspx?video=Fuller_Richard_Pell_Godfrey_26_Feb_2013_0900_WEB.mp4 (accessed 14 November 2014).
Common OSCE standard-setting techniques, with special reference to the borderline methods, with a discussion of the use and interpretation of a variety of psychometric indicators using 'real' data from the presenters' own high stakes assessment.

Measurement and improvement of the OSCE: Recognition and remediation of station level problems (part 2)
Fuller, R. and Pell, G. (2013). http://www.mededworld.org/stream/display.aspx?video=Fuller_Richard_Pell_Godfrey_05_March_2013_0900_WEB.mp4 (accessed 14 November 2014).
A range of 'diagnostic' exercises on interpreting station level metrics and remediation of station level problems, ranging across checklist/station design issues and the impact of aberrant assessor behaviour, proposing solutions and carrying out subsequent monitoring.

Standard setting for clinical competence examinations
Boursicot, K. (2012). http://www.mededworld.org/stream/display.aspx?video=Boursicot_Kathy_0900_WEB.mp4 (accessed 14 November 2014).
The principles of standard setting, with worked-through examples of the Angoff method. Standard setting for OSCEs is also covered.

An introduction to generalisability theory and its application to common medical education problems
De Champlain, A.F. (2012). http://www.mededworld.org/Webinars/Webinar-Items/An-introduction-to-generalizability-theory-and-its.aspx (accessed 14 November 2014).
An overview of generalisability theory models and related key concepts and includes several illustrative practical examples.

The ABCs of item response theory
De Champlain, A.D. (2011). http://www.mededworld.org/Webinars/Webinar-Items/The-ABC-s-of-IRT-(Item-Response-Theory).aspx (accessed 14 November 2014).
An introduction to common item response theory (IRT) models, including the Rasch model, as well as two- and three-parameter logistic models, and a discussion of practical applications of IRT in various aspects of medical education and assessment.

Pass-fail decisions – How do we make them fairly?
Harley, D. (2013). http://www.mededworld.org/Webinars/Webinar-Items/Pass-fail-decisions – how-do-we-make-them-fairly.aspx (accessed 14 November 2014).
Problems of and possible solutions for setting a defensible standard. Three common methods of standard setting are addressed using realistic examples.

Professional and linguistic assessments board (PLAB) OSCE examination
http://www.gmc-uk.org/doctors/plab/osce_briefing.asp (accessed 1 November 2014).
The PLAB test is the main route by which International Medical Graduates (IMGs) demonstrate that they have the necessary skills and knowledge to practise medicine in the UK. This helpful video briefs candidates about what to expect during the PLAB Part 2 OSCE examination.

OSCE rap – Losin' marks
Griffith Med Revue (2012). http://www.youtube.com/watch?v=7YzkTdUhvpI (accessed 1 November 2014).
A humorous look at the perceived stresses involved in the OSCE by medical students at Griffith Medical School, Australia, through the medium of rap.

Interview with Ronald Harden
https://vimeo.com/67224904 (accessed 10 March 2015).
Ronald Harden discusses the development of the OSCE.

Index

Page numbers followed by "*f*" indicate figures, "*t*" indicate tables, and "*b*" indicate boxes.